Foundations of Nursing Research

Seventh Edition

Rose Marie Nieswiadomy, PhD, RN
Professor Emerita
Texas Woman's University
College of Nursing

Catherine Bailey PhD, RN, CNE
Associate Professor
Texas Woman's University
College of Nursing

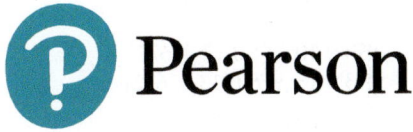

330 Hudson Street, NY, NY 10013

Publisher: Julie Alexander
Portfolio Manager: Pamela Fuller
Editorial Assistant: Erin Sullivan
Managing Content Producer: Melissa Bashe
Content Producer: Michael Giacobbe
Development Editor: Barbara Price
Interior and Cover Designer: Maria Guglielmo-Walsh
Vice President of Sales and Marketing: David Gesell
Vice President, Director of Marketing: Margaret Waples
Senior Product Marketing Manager: Phoenix Harvey
Director, Digital Studio: Amy Peltier
Digital Project Manager: Jeff Henn
Full-Service Project Management: iEnergizer Aptara®, Ltd.
Cover Image: Shutterstock

Copyright © 2018, 2012, 2008 by Pearson Education, Inc. All rights reserved. Manufactured in the United States of America. This publication is protected by Copyright, and permission should be obtained from the publisher prior to any prohibited reproduction, storage in a retrieval system, or transmission in any form or by any means, electronic, mechanical, photocopying, recording, or likewise. For information regarding permissions, request forms and the appropriate contacts within the Pearson Education Global Rights & Permissions Department, please visit www.pearsoned.com/permissions/

Library of Congress Cataloging-in-Publication Data
Names: Nieswiadomy, Rose Marie, author.
Title: Foundations of nursing research / Rose Marie Nieswiadomy, PhD, RN,
 Professor emerita, Texas Woman's University, College of Nursing.
Description: Seventh edition. | Boston : Pearson, [2018] | Includes
 bibliographical references and index.
Identifiers: LCCN 2017001635| ISBN 9780134167213 | ISBN 013416721X
Subjects: LCSH: Nursing—Research—Methodology.
Classification: LCC RT81.5 .N54 2018 | DDC 610.73072—dc23 LC record available at https://lccn.loc.gov/2017001635

2011000025

2   17

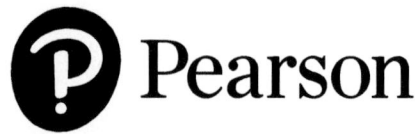

ISBN 10:   0-13-416721-X
ISBN 13: 978-0-13-416721-3

To Dr. Rose Nieswiadomy
May this edition of Foundations of Nursing Research become a tribute to your life's work and may it continue to nurture those who seek to understand and promote research in nursing.

About the Author

Catherine A. Bailey, PhD, RN, CNE

Catherine Bailey is a registered nurse. She graduated from a diploma program in Germantown, Pennsylvania and received her BS, MS, and PhD from Texas Woman's University (TWU) College of Nursing in Denton, Texas. She is an Associate Professor at Texas Woman's University, College of Nursing in Dallas, Texas. Her primary interests are in nursing education, adult healthcare and research in nursing. She has taught undergraduate baccalaureate nursing students in the classroom, the simulation lab, and the clinical setting since 2001. She teaches research to master's level graduate nursing students and she has chaired Professional Projects for Family Nurse Practitioner students. She also works with doctoral students who are seeking the degree of Doctor of Nursing Practice. She has published textbook chapters on the use of high-fidelity simulations for nursing students and case scenarios that are appropriate for simulation experiences. She has presented the findings from her studies in podium and poster presentations at METI HPSN Conferences and Sigma Theta Tau International Conferences as well as other regional and local venues.

Dr. Bailey has chaired the TWU Institutional Review Board for the Texas Woman's University, Dallas Campus. She has worked as a research consultant for the Department of Veterans Affairs, VA North Texas Health Care System, Nursing Service, and participated in the planning of four biennial National Nursing Research conferences in Dallas, Texas. She is a past president of the Board of Directors for Sigma Theta Tau International, Beta Beta Chapter. She is an editorial review board member of the *Journal of Theory Construction and Testing*. She volunteers as a mentor of the Nursing Research and Evidence Based Practice Council at the UT Southwestern Medical Center William P. Clements Jr. University Hospital. Dr. Bailey is also a member of the International Association of Clinical Simulation and Learning, the American Association of the Colleges of Nursing, the American Nurses Association and the Texas Nurses Association.

Contributors

We extend a sincere thanks to our contributors who so willingly gave their time, effort, and expertise for the development and writing of resources that promote understanding of nursing research in the pursuit of nursing excellence.

Renae L. Dougal, MSN, RN, CLNC, CCRP
Clinical Assistant Professor
Idaho State University School of Nursing,
Accelerated Program
Meridian, ID

Stephanie Huckaby, MSN, RN-BC
UT Southwestern Medical Center
William P. Clements, Jr. University Hospital
Dallas, TX

Peggy Mancuso, PhD, RN, CNM, CNE
Professor
Texas Woman's University, College of Nursing
Denton, TX

Verdell Marsh, PhD, RN
Colonel (Retired), Army Nurse Corps
Nurse Consultant
Garland, TX

Dawna Martich, MSN, RN
Nursing Education Consultant
Subject Matter Expert
Pittsburgh, Pennsylvania

Connie G. Maxwell, MLS
Dallas Public Library
Preston Royal Branch Manager
and Texas Woman's University
Assistant Dean of Libraries (Retired)
Denton, TX

Charles E. McConnel, PhD
Professor of Health Care Sciences and Family and Community Medicine
U. T. Southwestern Medical Center in Dallas
Dallas, TX

Michael L. Nieswiadomy, PhD, BA
Professor of Economics
Editor, Journal of Legal Economics
University of North Texas, Dept. of Economics
Denton, TX

Sharon Souter, RN, PhD, CNE
Dean and Professor
University of Mary Hardin-Baylor, College of Nursing,
Belton, TX

Becky Spencer, PhD, RN, IBCLC
Texas Woman's University, College of Nursing
Denton, TX

Jo-Ann Stankus, PhD, RN
Assistant Professor and Coordinator RN BS/MS Program
Texas Woman's University, College of Nursing
Denton, TX

Donna Scott Tilley, PhD, RN, CNE, CA SANE
Assistant Provost for Promotion of Research and Sponsored Programs
Professor, College of Nursing
Denton, TX

Vicki L. Zeigler, PhD, RN
Texas Woman's University, College of Nursing
Denton, TX

Reviewers

Thank You
Our heartfelt thanks go out to our colleagues from schools of nursing across the country who have generously given their time to help us create this exciting new edition of our book. We have reaped the benefit of your collective experience as nurses and teachers, and have made many improvements due to your efforts. Among those who gave us their encouragement and comments are:

Tracy Arnold, DNP, RN
Assistant Professor of Nursing
Gardner-Webb University
Boiling Springs, NC

Judy Frain, PhD, RN
Assistant Professor
Goldfarb School of Nursing at Barnes Jewish College
St. Louis, MO

Cheryl Hewlett, PhD, MBA, MSN, RN, NEA-BC
Director for Professional Practice, Quality, Wound Care and Infection Prevention
Bon Secours Maryview Medical Center
Portsmouth, VA

Kimberly D. Johnson, PhD, RN, CEN
Assistant Professor
University of Cincinnati
Cincinnati, OH

Elise A. Jolade, DNP, FNP-BC, ACNS, APRN, CCRN
Adjunct Assistant Professor
Hunter Bellevue School of Nursing
City University of New York
New York, NY

Jane Leach, PhD, RNC, CNE
Graduate Coordinator Nurse Educator Program
Midwestern State University
Wichita Falls, TX

Carole A. McKenzie, PhD, CNM, RN
Associate Professor
Texas A&M University Commerce
Commerce, TX

Jeanette Peterson, MSN, RN, CHSE, VA-BC
Assistant Professor & Simulation Coordinator
Chaminade University of Honolulu, School of Nursing
Honolulu, HI

Jill Price, PhD, MSN, RN
Dean, RNBSN Online Option
Chamberlain College of Nursing
Downers Grove, IL

Maureen Schoch
Assistant Professor
Wilkes University
Scranton, PA

Kathleen L. Slyh, RN, MSN
Nursing Instructor
Technical Collegef the Lowcountry
Beaufort, SC

Robyn B. Tobias, MSN, APN, NP-C
Lecturer
University of Tennessee at Chattanooga
Chattanooga, TN

Dr. Kathleen M. Williamson, PhD, RN
Associate Professor & Chair
Midwestern State University
Wichita Falls, TX

Preface

Our main purpose in writing the seventh edition of this book is to promote an interest in nursing research. Like Dr. Rose Nieswiadomy, we firmly believe that research is essential to an evidence-based nursing practice and the growth of the nursing profession. The results of nursing research studies improve patient care and demonstrate that nurses are not only caring but also cost-effective providers of healthcare.

Research can be interesting and exciting. We have tried to present the material in this textbook in an inspirational manner that memorializes the voice of our original author, Rose. Nursing students and practicing nurses have reported that they have actually read the past editions of this book, which is not the case for most of their textbooks or other books that they read.

After reading this introductory research book, you will not be expected to have the skills to conduct research independently or to critique research reports with a great deal of confidence. However, our goals will have been achieved if you:

- recognize the importance of research to evidence-based nursing practice.
- are willing to use research findings in your practice.
- have gained knowledge about the research process.
- possess beginning skills necessary to evaluate research findings.
- discuss research study results with your colleagues, family, and friends.
- begin to think about conducting your own research study in the future.

For those of you just beginning your careers in nursing, the future of the profession depends on you. This book is intended primarily for individuals with little research experience, particularly undergraduate nursing students. However, many students in graduate programs have used this text to supplement their other research textbooks in order to gain a better understanding of nursing research. They have commented that this text explains the research simply and clearly. It is our hope that practicing nurses will also use this book as they evaluate study findings for use in practice, and as they begin to conduct their own studies.

Features of the Book

The informal writing style has been maintained in this seventh edition of the text. Readers have made many positive comments about the writing style. Students have said that they often feel as if they are talking with the author. The book continues to be learner-friendly, just like the previous six editions. Please interact with us as you read this text. Get involved! This is the best way to learn about research.

Readers are referred to websites throughout the book for additional information and resources. References from recent nursing research studies are interspersed throughout this book. These research study excerpts are presented to illustrate various aspects of the research process. Most of these studies were conducted in the United States. A number were conducted in other countries.

New terms are highlighted and defined the first time they are discussed. Each chapter in the book concludes with a summary of the content presented in that chapter. While Chapter 2 provides an overview of evidence-based practices (EBPs), the newly organized Chapter 3 introduces the reader to ways in which EBPs can be promoted. Chapter 4 and the ends of Chapters 6 through 17 with the exception of Chapter 11, provide ideas for critiquing the specific parts of the research process found in a research report. Chapter 19 provides numerous examples of nursing research studies with a focus on healthcare economics. This chapter was added because nurses should be aware of the monetary issues involved in healthcare and demonstrate that they are not only caring but cost-effective providers of healthcare. Chapter 20 presents guidelines for critiquing both quantitative and qualitative study reports.

Appendix B presents a critiquing exercise. To become engaged in this strategy, you are asked to obtain a copy of a specific research article then critique this article, using the questions listed.

The Self-Tests at the end of each chapter provide readers an opportunity to see how well they have mastered the chapter content. Answers to all of the questions with their rationales are provided at the back of the book.

For each chapter, resources include:

- Chapter Objectives
- Key Terms
- Chapter Review
- Review Questions
- Research Links
- Critical Thinking Exercises/Challenges

The knowledge you gain from reading this book will help you to provide evidence-based care for your patients/clients. We also hope you will gain a greater appreciation of research and can actually picture yourself conducting a research study in the future.

Acknowledgments

When I agreed to assist Dr. Rose with the work of this seventh edition, I never dreamed that she would be called to her heavenly reward prior to its completion. The value of this book, first published in 1985, is evident by its continued use in the United States and other countries throughout the world with translations into several other languages. Thus, it seemed appropriate that I should commit to continue the legacy of her life's work.

Instructors usually make the decision about textbooks for their courses. I and my co-authors are so grateful to the instructors who have chosen this textbook or recommended it as a reference source for their students.

We cannot give enough praise to all of the students who have given this textbook great reviews. We continue to receive comments about how learner-friendly the book is and how it is one of the few textbooks that they have read from cover to cover. Of course, it helps that this textbook is much smaller than some of their other textbooks!

Master's and doctoral level nursing students have remarked they use this book to supplement their course research textbooks. They believe this text presents the research process clearly and succinctly. When they review content in this book, they achieve a greater recall and understanding of research concepts.

Heartfelt thanks go to practicing nurses who have had the courage to pick up this research textbook. It demonstrates their awareness of the importance of nursing research, particularly in this day of evidence-based nursing practice.

Once again, Connie Maxwell, now employed by the Dallas Public Library, has contributed to the revision of the chapter dedicated to the review of the literature. This chapter is always a challenge because of the continued changes in the ways we access information. As was true with Dr. Rose, I am especially grateful for the services provided by Texas Woman's University librarians, especially Eula Oliphant and Elaine Cox, who never failed to find whatever articles were necessary for the work of this book.

Many people at Pearson Education deserve my gratitude, especially Barbara Price, Development Editor, who provided advice as the various chapters of this edition evolved. I appreciate her patience as she kept me on task with the many details of coordinating my responsibilites with the publishing team and the other contributors for this book. She was always available to answer questions, set up phone conferences, and coordinate the copyeditors' workflow, as I reviewed everyone's work.

Although the task of perpetuating Dr. Rose's work at times seemed daunting, I never felt alone. Instead, I was surrounded by Dr. Rose, through so much support from her family, and many colleagues and friends. Dr. Rose's daughter, Anne, frequently offered to help, and her son, Michael, and his colleague, Charles McConnel, contributed to the information on nursing research as it relates to healthcare economics in Chapter 19. A special word of appreciation is directed to Dr. Rose's colleagues and special friends from Texas Woman's University, College of Nursing (Drs. Mancuso, Marsh, Spencer, Stankus, Scott Tilley, and Zeigler), who eagerly volunteered to contribute to this work in honor of her memory. I am grateful to Stephanie Huckaby, who shared her experiences of implementing an EBP in her hospital as we co-authored Chapter 3. Finally, I wish to thank Renae Dougal, Dawna Martich, and Sharon Souter, who also worked to complement this work.

Lastly, but not least, I wish to recognize my family, who patiently overlooked my piles of printed pages that eventually filled every room of our home. I am grateful to my parents, who prepared me to be the person that I am, and my husband, Barney, and my children, who continued to encourage me as I worked through the many processes of writing this edition.

Catherine Ann Bailey, PhD, RN, CNE

Contents

PART I   Introduction to Nursing Research   1

1 Development of Nursing Research   1

Importance of Research to Nursing   1
   Definitions of Nursing Research   2
   Sources of Nursing Knowledge   2
   Scientific Research   3
   Purposes of Nursing Research   3
   Funding of Nursing Research   4
Goals for Conducting Nursing Research   4
   Promote Evidence-Based Nursing Practice   4
   Ensure Credibility of the Nursing Profession   5
   Provide Accountability for Nursing Practice   5
   Document the Cost-Effectiveness of Nursing Care   5
Quantitative and Qualitative Research   6
Nurses and Research   7
   Roles of Nurses in Research   7
   History of Nursing Research   8
   National Institute of Nursing Research   11
   The Cochrane Collaboration and the Cochrane Nursing Care Field   12
Research Priorities into the Future   12
   National Association of Orthopaedic Nurses   12
   Mental Health Nursing   13
   Oncology Nursing Society   13
   Institute of Emergency Nursing Research   13
   Association of Community Health Nurse Educators   13
   Research in Nursing Education   13
   Future Strategies for Improved Healthcare Quality   14
   Summary   14
   Self-Test   15
   References   16

2 Evidence-Based Nursing Practice   18

Defining Evidence-Based Practice   18
   Why we use evidence-based practice   19
   Research Utilization versus Evidence-Based Practice   20

Evidence-Based Nursing Practice   20
   Benefits of EBP   20
   Asking Clinical Questions   21
   Sources for Evidence for Practice   21
The Cochrane Collaboration   22
   The Cochrane Library   22
   Cochrane Database   22
   Cochrane Centers   23
   Cochrane Nursing Care Field   23
Agency for Healthcare Research and Quality   23
   Evidence-Based Practice Centers   24
   U.S. Preventive Services Task Force   25
   National Guideline Clearinghouse   25
Evidence-Based Nursing Practice Centers   26
   Joanna Briggs Institute   27
   ACE Center for Advancing Clinical Excellence   27
   Sarah Cole Hirsh Institute   27
   Summary   28
   Self-Test   29
   References   30

3 Research Evidence in Nursing Practice   32

The Evolving Nature of Evidence-Based Practice   32
Models to Promote Evidence-Based Practice in Nursing   33
   The Stetler Model   33
   The Iowa Model   33
   Discussion of Iowa Model Concepts   34
Barriers Associated with EBP   36
Facilitators of Evidence-Based Practice   36
Application of the Iowa Model   37
   Summary   38
   Self-Test   39
   References   40

4 Ethical Issues in Nursing Research   42

Development of Ethical Codes and Guidelines   42
   Historical Overview   42
   Unethical Research in the United States   43
   Ethical Research Guidelines   44
Institutional Review Boards   45
   Members of Institutional Review Boards   46
   IRB Review   46

    Elements of Informed Consent   47
        Description of Purpose of Study and Study Procedures   47
        Description of Unforeseeable Risks   48
        Description of Benefits   48
        Disclosure of Appropriate Alternative Procedures   48
        Description of Maintenance of Confidentiality or Anonymity   49
        Plans for Unforeseeable Injuries   49
        Contact Information for Questions Relevant to the Study   49
        Assurance of Freedom to Volunteer for or Withdraw from the Study   50
        Documentation of Informed Consent   50
    Integrity in Research   51
    Research Guidelines for Nurses   52
        Nurse Researcher as a Patient Advocate   52
    Critiquing the Ethical Aspects of a Study   53
        Summary   54
        Self-Test   54
        References   56

5   An Overview of Quantitative and Qualitative Research   58

    Introduction   58
    Comparison of Qualitative and Quantitative Research   58
    Steps in Quantitative Research   59
        Identify the Research Problem   60
        Determine the Purpose of the Study   60
        Formulate the Research Question   61
        Review the Literature   61
        Develop a Theoretical/Conceptual Framework   61
        Identify the Study Assumptions   62
        Acknowledge the Limitations of the Study   62
        Formulate the Hypothesis   62
        Define the Study Variables/Terms   63
        Select the Research Design   63
        Identify the Population   64
        Select the Sample   64
        Conduct a Pilot Study   65
        Collect the Data   65
        Organize the Data for Analysis   65
        Analyze the Data   66
        Interpret the Findings   66
        Communicate the Findings   66
        Utilize the Findings   67
    Qualitative Nursing Research   67
        Types of Qualitative Research   68
        Identify the Problem of the Study   68

State the Purpose   68
Select the Research Design   69
Review the Literature   69
Select the Sample   69
Gain Entry to the Research Site   70
Protect the Rights of Participants   70
Collect the Data   70
Analyze the Data   72
Interpret the Data   72
Communicate the Study Results   72
Utilize the Study Results   73
Combining Qualitative and Quantitative Methods   73
- Summary   74
- Self-Test   74
- References   75

PART II   Preliminary Steps in the Research Process   77

6   Identifying Nursing Research Problems   77

Introduction   77
Sources of Nursing Research Problems   78
- Personal Experiences   78
- Literature Sources   78
- Existing Theories   79
- Previous Research   79

Research Problem Considerations   80
- Ethical Issues   80
- Significance to Nursing   80
- Personal Motivation   81
- Researcher Qualifications   81
- Feasibility of Study   81

Research Question Criteria   83
- Written in Interrogative Sentence Form   83
- Includes the Population   83
- Includes the Variable(s)   83
- Empirically Testable   85

Research Question Format   85
Critiquing Problem Statements, Purpose Statements, and Research Questions   86
- Problem Statement   86
- Purpose Statement   87
- Research Questions   87
- Summary   88
- Self-Test   89
- References   90

7 Review of the Literature 91

Introduction 91
Purposes of the Literature Review 91
Literature Sources 92
    Types of Information Sources 92
    Primary and Secondary Sources 92
    Grey Literature 93
Search Strategies 94
    Develop a Search Strategy 94
    Ask a Librarian 95
    Finding Tools 96
    Selected Databases for Nursing Students 97
Writing the Literature Review 99
    Extracting Information from Literature Sources 99
    Critiquing the Literature Review in a Research Article 100
    Components of a Literature Review 100
    Summary 101
    Self-Test 101
    References 102

8 Theory and Nursing Research 103

Introduction 103
Theory Terminology 104
    Theory 104
    Concept 104
    Construct 105
    Propositional Statements 105
    Empirical Generalization 105
    Hypothesis 105
    Model 105
    Conceptual Models 106
    Paradigm and Metaparadigm 106
Types and Scope of Theories in Nursing Research 106
    Paradigms and Metaparadigms 106
    Nursing Conceptual Models 107
    Orem's Self-Care Model 107
    Rogers's Science of Unitary Human Beings 108
    Roy's Adaptation Model 108
    Neuman's Systems Model 109
    Middle-range and Practice Theories 110
Integrating Theory into Nursing Research 112
    Theories from Nursing 112
    Combining Two Nursing Theories 113

Theories from Other Disciplines   113
  Combining Theories from Nursing and Other Disciplines   114
  Theoretical and Conceptual Frameworks   115
Theoretical Development, Testing, and Critique   115
  Theory Generation and Development   116
  Theory Testing in Nursing Research   116
  Critiquing the Theoretical Framework of a Study   117
  Summary   118
  Self-Test   119
  References   120

9   Hypotheses   124

Introduction   124
Hypotheses Overview   124
  Purposes of Hypotheses   125
  Sources or Rationale for Hypotheses   125
Classifications of Hypotheses   126
  Simple and Complex Hypotheses   126
  Nondirectional and Directional Research Hypotheses   127
  Causal and Associative Research Hypotheses   128
  Null and Research Hypotheses   129
Developing Hypotheses   130
  Hypothesis Format   131
  Hypotheses and Theory Testing   132
  Critiquing Hypotheses   132
  Summary   134
  Self-Test   134
  References   136

PART III   Research Designs   137

10   Quantitative Research Designs   137

Introduction   137
Exploratory, Descriptive, and Explanatory Studies   138
  Research Designs   138
Experimental Research   139
  Validity of Experimental Designs   139
  Threats to Internal Validity   140
  Threats to External Validity   142
  Symbolic Presentation of Research Designs   143
Types of Experimental Designs   143
  True Experimental Designs   143
  Quasi-Experimental Designs   146
  Pre-Experimental Designs   147

Nonexperimental Research 148
    Types of Nonexperimental Designs 148
    Survey Studies 148
    Correlational Studies 149
    Comparative Studies 150
    Methodological Studies 151
    Secondary Analysis Studies 151
    Settings for Research 152
Critiquing Quantitative Research Designs 152
    Summary 153
    Self-Test 155
    References 156

11 Qualitative and Mixed Methods Research Designs 158

Introduction 158
Qualitative Research Designs 159
    Phenomenology 159
    Ethnographic Studies 160
    Grounded Theory 161
    Narrative Inquiry 162
    Case Studies 162
    Action Research Studies 163
Mixed Methods Research 164
Strategies for Mixed Methods Research 164
    Summary 165
    Self-Test 166
    References 167

PART IV Obtaining Study Participants and Collection of Data 169

12 Populations and Samples 169

Introduction 169
Populations 170
Samples and Sampling 170
    Probability Sampling Methods 171
    Nonprobability Sampling Methods 175
    Time Frame for Studying the Sample 177
Sampling Concepts and Factors 179
    Sample Size 179
    Sampling Error and Sampling Bias 181
    Randomization Procedures in Research 182
Critiquing the Sampling Procedure 182
    Summary 183
    Self-Test 184
    References 185

13 Measurement and Data Collection   187

Introduction   187
Measurement   187
    Level of Measurement   188
    Converting Data to a Lower Level of Measurement   189
    Determining the Appropriate Level of Measurement   189
Data-Collection Process   190
    Data-Collection Methods   190
    Data-Collection Instruments   191
Criteria for Selection of a Data-Collection Instrument   192
    Practicality of the Instrument   192
    Reliability of the Instrument   193
    Validity of the Instrument   195
    Relationship between Reliability and Validity   198
Utilizing the Data   199
    Sources of Error in Data Collection   199
    Preparing Data for Analysis   199
    Critiquing Data-Collection Procedures   199
    Summary   200
    Self-Test   201
    References   202

14 Data-Collection Methods   204

Introduction   204
Questionnaires   204
    Overall Appearance of Questionnaire   205
    Language and Reading Level of Questions   205
    Length of Questionnaire and Questions   206
    Wording of Questions   207
    Types of Questions   207
    Placement of Questions   209
    Cover Letter   209
    Completion Instructions   209
    Distribution of Questionnaires   210
    Factors Influencing Response Rates   210
    Advantages of Questionnaires   210
    Disadvantages of Questionnaires   210
Interviews   211
    Types of Interviews   211
    Interview Instruments   212
    Interview Questions   212
    Interviewer Training   212
    Timing and Setting for Interviews   213
    Interviewer Guidelines   213

Influence of Interviewers on Respondents   213
Advantages of Interviews   214
Disadvantages of Interviews   214
Observation Methods   214
   Determining Behaviors to be Observed   214
   Research Observers   214
   Observation Procedures   215
   Relationship between Observer and Subjects   215
   The Role of the Nurse versus the Researcher   216
Attitude Scales   216
   Likert Scale   216
   Semantic Differential Scales   218
Physiological and Psychological Measures   219
   Psychological Tests   219
Other Data-Collection Methods   220
   Q Sort   220
   Delphi Technique   221
   Visual Analogue Scale   221
   Preexisting Data   222
Critiquing Data-Collection Methods   222
   Summary   224
   Self-Test   225
   References   226

PART V   Data Analysis   229

15   Descriptive Statistics   229

Introduction   229
Key Concepts in Statistics   230
   Statistical Symbols   230
   Classifications of Statistics   230
Descriptive Statistics   230
   Measures to Condense Data   231
   Measures of Central Tendency   236
   Measures of Variability   238
Measures of Relationships   240
   Correlation Coefficients   241
   Intraocular Method of Data Analysis   245
   Critiquing Descriptive Statistics in Research Reports   246
   Summary   247
   Self-Test   248
   References   249

16 Inferential Statistics   250

Introduction   250
Purposes of Inferential Statistics   251
    Estimating Population Parameters   251
    Sampling Distribution of the Mean   252
    Confidence Intervals   253
    Testing Hypotheses   255
    The Study Hypothesis   255
    Choosing a Statistical Test   256
    Level of Significance   257
    One-Tailed and Two-Tailed Tests   257
    Calculating the Test Statistic   258
    Comparing Calculated Value and Critical Value   258
    Support for the Study Hypothesis   259
Factors Affecting Choice of Statistical Measures   259
    Parametric and Nonparametric Statistical Tests   259
    Power of a Statistical Test   260
    Type I and Type II Errors   260
Statistical Tests Used in Nursing Research   261
    t Test   261
    Analysis of Variance   262
    Chi-Square   263
    Testing the Significance of Correlation Coefficients   265
    Advanced Statistical Tests   266
    Critiquing Inferential Statistics in Research Reports   268
    Summary   268
    Self-Test   270
    References   271

17 Presentation and Discussion of Study Findings   273

Introduction   273
Presentation of Findings of the Study   274
    Findings of the Study   274
    Ethical Issues in Presenting Research Findings   274
    Narrative Presentation of Findings   274
    Tables   275
    Figures   275
Discussion of Findings and Significance   276
    Discussion of Study Hypotheses   276
    Statistical and Clinical Significance   277
Conclusions, Implications, and Recommendations   278
    Conclusions   278

Implications 279
Recommendations 279
Replication of the Research Study 279
Consideration of Study Limitations in Future Research 280
Extensions of the Research Study 280
Critiquing the Presentation of Study Findings 281
- Summary 282
- Self-Test 283
- References 284

PART VI Research Findings and Nursing Practice 285

18 Communication and Utilization of Nursing Research 285

Introduction 285
Communication of Nursing Research Findings 286
- Preparing a Research Report 286
- Presenting Research Results at Professional Conferences 286
- Presenting a Research Paper 287
- Presenting a Research Poster 288
- Publishing a Journal Article 288
- Choosing Between Refereed and Nonrefereed Journals 290
- Preparing Research Reports for Funding Agencies 292
- Preparing Theses and Dissertations 292

Utilization of Nursing Research Findings 292
- Additional Barriers to Nursing Research Utilization 293
- Inadequate Dissemination of Research Findings 293
- Bridging the Gap between Research and Practice 294
- Summary 296
- Self-Test 297
- References 298

19 Nursing Research and Healthcare Economics 300

Healthcare Economics and Nursing 301
- Understanding Market Forces Affecting Nurses 301
- Determining the Value of Nursing 302
- The Dall Study 302

Nursing Research Cost-Effectiveness Studies 303
- Telephonic Nursing Studies 305
- Need For More Research Studies on Nursing Care 306

Impacts of Governmental Agencies and Related Organizations 307
- Affordable Care Act 307
- Regulatory Agencies 308

Public Health   308
Summary   309
Self-Test   309
References   310

20 Critique of Research Reports   313

Introduction   313
Critiquing Quantitative Research Reports   314
   Researcher Qualifications   315
   Title   315
   Abstract   315
Introduction   315
   Identifying the Problem   315
   Purpose   316
   Review of the Literature   316
   Theoretical/Conceptual Framework   316
   Assumptions   316
   Limitations   317
   Hypothesis(es)   317
   Definition of Terms   317
   Research Design   317
   Setting   318
   Population and Sample   318
   Collection of Data   318
   Data-Collection Instruments   318
   Analysis of Data   319
   Discussion of Findings   319
   Conclusions   319
   Implications   319
   Recommendations   320
   Other Considerations   320
Critiquing Qualitative Research Reports   320
   Researcher Qualifications   321
   Title   321
   Abstract   321
   Introduction   321
     Problem of the Study   321
     Purpose   322
     Research Question   322
     Research Design   322
     Review of the Literature   322
     Selection of Sample   322
     Collection of Data   323

Analysis of Data 323
Interpretation of Data 323
Recommendations 323
Other Considerations 323
Summary 324
Self-Test 324
References 325

Self-Test Answers 327

Appendix A Consent Form 366

Appendix B Critiquing Exercise 368

Glossary 372

Credits 386

Index 388

PART I Introduction to Nursing Research

Chapter 1
Development of Nursing Research

Rose Nieswiadomy, PhD, RN, and Catherine Bailey, PhD, RN

Objectives

On completion of this chapter, you will be prepared to:

1. Identify the importance of research to nursing
2. Describe four goals for conducting nursing research
3. Compare qualitative and quantitative research
4. Describe the various roles of nurses in research
5. Summarize the development of nursing research and future priorities

Importance of Research to Nursing

Many people are still unaware that nurses conduct research. A similar statement has been included in each of the previous editions of this book. What kind of response do you think you would receive if you were to ask 10 friends to describe nursing research? Their answers would probably be quite interesting. My guess is that you would hear about some aspect of medical research, such as which drug might be most effective for some specific health problem. As nurses, we must seek more opportunities to discuss our research and make our research results readily available to the general public.

In 2006 the American Association of Colleges of Nursing recommended that educational guidelines for baccalaureate nurses should assure high quality and safe patient care. The application of research and evidence-based knowledge from nursing and the sciences were identified as the basis for practice. Polit and Beck (2012) reported that the translation of research into practice is full of challenges, but changes in our healthcare system are supporting this effort. Nurses now have an opportunity to show that they make a difference in the lives of the American people. However, in other countries, nurses are also emphasizing the importance of nursing research.

In a conversation about nursing research in the February 2010 issue of *Canadian Nurse*, Smadu, Murphy, and Petrucka remarked that nursing research must become more visible. They stated that researchers have a responsibility to familiarize those in practice with research and ensure that it is meaningful in content and process. Ultimately, nurses must take the lead to communicate their results and encourage the use of research findings in the practice setting.

Right now, you are probably attempting to convince yourself that nursing research is important (or you wouldn't be reading this textbook). You may be trying to meet educational requirements for a baccalaureate degree, or someone has convinced you that you need more knowledge about research.

Sometimes a hard sell is necessary on the first day of an undergraduate nursing research class. The folded arms and facial expressions of students suggest that they are not convinced of the importance of learning about research.

Research knowledge will help you become an excellent nurse. As you read this book, you will be challenged to question every intervention you perform or see performed. Questions to ask include: Am I performing this intervention because someone told me to or maybe even because this is the intervention that has *always* been used? What evidence exists that this is the most effective intervention for the problem?

If an intervention is not based on research evidence, there is no way to determine that the intervention is the optimum one. It is hoped that your instructor or your nurse colleagues, if you are already a nurse, will not have to do a hard sell to convince you that research is of utmost importance to the nursing profession. Your efforts to learn about nursing research will be rewarded in your nursing career in the future.

Definitions of Nursing Research

There is some discrepancy among authors about the definition of nursing research. Polit and Beck (2012) have broadly defined nursing research as "systematic inquiry designed to develop trustworthy evidence about issues of importance to the nursing profession, including nursing practice, education, administration, and informatics" (p. 3). Grove, Burns, and Gray (2013) have more narrowly defined nursing research as "a scientific process that validates and refines existing knowledge and generates new knowledge that directly and indirectly influences the delivery of evidence-based nursing practice" (p. 2). Thus, by their narrow definition, to be called nursing research, study results must directly or indirectly affect clinical nursing practice.

In this book, the term **nursing research** is defined as the systematic, objective process of analyzing phenomena of importance to nursing. Using this definition, nursing research includes all studies concerning nursing practice, nursing education, and nursing administration. Studies concerning nurses themselves are also included in the broad category of nursing research. The term **clinical nursing research** indicates nursing research that involves clients or studies that have the potential to affect the care of clients, such as studies with patients or with so-called normal participants. To learn about nursing research and how to conduct research, it is important to gain an understanding of what scientific research is all about, and why this method of gaining knowledge is valuable to nurses. The scientific method is only one source of nursing knowledge. It is, however, generally considered to be the most reliable source of knowledge.

Sources of Nursing Knowledge

Nurses have relied on several sources of knowledge to guide nursing practice. A great storehouse of knowledge for nurses has been tradition. Tradition involves the handing down of knowledge from one generation to another and leads to actions that occur because "we've always done it that way."

Another source of knowledge for nurses has been found in authority. Experts or authorities in a given field often provide knowledge for other people. In the past, nurses looked to physicians for a great deal of their practice knowledge. It has only been fairly recently that nurses have begun to build a unique body of nursing knowledge.

Nurses have also used trial and error as a means of discovering knowledge. If one approach did not work, another one was used. When a certain approach was found to be effective, the trial-and-error process ceased. Frequently, the reasons behind the failure or success of a certain method were not determined. The goal was "if it works, we'll use it."

Scientific Research

Several features characterize traditional scientific research. The researcher uses systematic, orderly, and objective methods of seeking information. The scientific method is based on **empirical data,** which are data gathered through the sense organs. Information is gained in the form of data or facts that are obtained in an unbiased manner from some aspect of the real world. The researcher tries to exercise as much control as possible over the research situation, to minimize biased results. Various means of exercising such control are discussed throughout this book. The researcher's opinions and personal biases should not influence the findings of a study.

Many similarities exist between scientific research and the problem-solving approach familiar to most nurses. Both processes involve identifying a problem area, establishing a plan, collecting data, and evaluating the data. These two activities, however, have very different purposes. Problem solving attempts to seek a solution to a problem that exists for a person or persons in a given setting. The purpose of scientific research is much broader. Scientific research seeks to obtain knowledge that can be generalized to other people and to other settings. For example, the nursing staff might be concerned about the best approach to use in teaching Mrs. Smith, a blind patient, how to operate an insulin pump. This would be an example of an immediate problem that needs a solution. Scientific research, in contrast, would be concerned with the best approach to use in teaching blind people, in general, how to operate insulin pumps.

Purposes of Nursing Research

Research may be classified as basic or applied according to the general purpose of each study. **Basic research** is concerned with generating new knowledge; **applied research** is concerned with using knowledge to solve immediate problems.

Basic research is conducted to develop, test, and refine theories and generate new knowledge (Kerlinger, 1986; Oman, Krugman, & Fink, 2003; Polit & Beck, 2012). Sometimes it is said that basic research seeks knowledge for knowledge's sake. Whether basic research seeks to generate or develop theories, an immediate application of the results usually does not occur. In fact, years may pass before the social usefulness of the results of the research is determined or acknowledged. Basic research often uses laboratory animals as subjects. The following example of a basic research study was conducted with the use of syringe pumps that are used to deliver medications through intravenous lines. One of the objectives of the study was to assess the effect of different syringe pump settings on the flushed amount.

Applied research is directed toward generating knowledge that can be used in the near future. It is often conducted to seek solutions to existing problems (Grove, Burns, & Gray, 2013; Polit & Beck, 2012). We have found that the majority of nursing studies have been examples of applied research that focus on addressing issues in nursing practice.

The distinction between basic and applied research is really not as clear-cut as it may seem. Sometimes the findings of basic research are applied rather quickly in the clinical setting, whereas applied research findings actually lead to basic studies. The distinction between basic and applied research may have more to do with financial support for the project than with the purpose of the study. In this sense, basic research

> ### Basic Research
>
> Kawakami et al. (2013) conducted a study concerning the effects of flow rate, occlusion alarm settings, syringe sizes, and syringe pump models on bolus amounts. In the presence of different alarm settings, the researchers used either 10 ml or 50 ml plastic syringes that were connected to a 100 cm extension tube then collected the bolus with a syringe at the end of the extension tube. The infusion was started at flow rates of 3 ml or 10 ml per hour and a stopcock was used to release the bolus of fluid from the extension tubing when the occlusion alarm sounded. After releasing the occlusion (with the stopcock) the amount of flushed fluid was higher with high occlusion alarm settings compared with low alarm settings. When a 50 ml syringe was used, the bolus was significantly larger than when a 10 ml syringe was used. The researchers concluded that the use of a smaller-sized syringe, a lower alarm setting, and the use of pumps with protective functions against accidental bolus reductions are associated with decreased inadvertent bolus amounts if the occlusion is inappropriately released. These findings are especially important for nurses caring for patients who must depend on accurately titrated doses of vasoactive drugs for blood pressure control in intensive care units.

may imply that the researcher is provided support to work on a particular project without having to indicate the immediate practical usefulness of the findings.

Funding of Nursing Research

The federal government provides the most money for research in this country. Nurses receive the largest amount of government funding through the National Institute for Nursing Research (NINR). The budget enacted in 2015 for this institute was $140.9 million; and the proposed 2016 budget was more than $144.5 million. More information on this topic can be found on the NINR website.

Other sources of funding for nursing research include private foundations, corporations, and professional organizations, such as Sigma Theta Tau International, Honor Society of Nursing. This organization, in conjunction with its chapters and grant partners (corporations, associations, and foundations), provides more than $200,000 annually for nursing research through grants, scholarships, and monetary awards. This information is located on the Sigma Theta Tau International website. The American Nurses Foundation (ANF) awarded more than $185,000 in research grants for the 2013 cycle. This information is located on the ANF website.

Goals for Conducting Nursing Research

The importance of nursing research cannot be emphasized enough. Some of the goals for conducting research are (a) to promote evidence-based nursing practice, (b) to ensure the credibility of the nursing profession, (c) to provide accountability for nursing practice, and (d) to document the cost-effectiveness of nursing care.

Promote Evidence-Based Nursing Practice

The major reason for conducting nursing research is to foster optimum care for clients. **Evidence-based nursing practice** (EBNP) means that nurses make clinical decisions based on the best research evidence, their clinical expertise, and the healthcare preferences of their patients/clients. Although EBNP may be based on factors other than research findings, such as patient preferences and the expertise of clinicians, the aim of EBNP is to provide the best possible care based on the best available research.

To back up the importance of EBNP, Sigma Theta Tau International, Honor Society of Nursing, and Blackwell Publishing initiated a journal in 2004 titled, *Worldviews on Evidence-Based Nursing*. It is a quarterly peer-reviewed journal.

The nursing profession exists to provide a service to society, and this service should be based on accurate knowledge. Research has been determined to be the most reliable means of obtaining knowledge.

Ensure Credibility of the Nursing Profession

In the past, nursing was frequently thought of as a vocation rather than a profession. In fact, the struggle to gain professional status has been long and difficult. One of the criteria for a profession is the existence of a body of knowledge that is distinct from that of other disciplines. Nursing has traditionally borrowed knowledge from the natural and social sciences, and only recently have nurses concentrated on establishing a unique body of knowledge that would allow nursing to be clearly identified as a distinct profession. Through research, nurses can demonstrate what they do that distinguishes them from other groups in the healthcare field.

Nurses must demonstrate to the general public that nursing makes a difference in the health status of people. In 1999, for the first time, the nursing profession was included in the Gallup Poll that ranked professionals in regard to honesty and ethical standards. Since then, nurses have ranked highest every year (except for 2001, when firefighters scored higher following the terrorist attack on the World Trade Center towers on September 11). Nurses must build on this ranking and the admiration of the general public and continue to show what is unique about their services.

Provide Accountability for Nursing Practice

As nurses have become more independent in making decisions about the care of clients, this independence has brought about a greater need for accountability. There is an old saying that every privilege is accompanied by a corresponding duty. The privilege of being independent practitioners brings with it the duty of being accountable to those who receive our care. Although nurses have generally been glad to achieve some degree of independence from the medical profession, in some ways life was easier when physicians were considered to be responsible for all aspects of healthcare. At that time, if a nurse made an error in providing care, the physician (and sometimes the hospital) was held responsible. The idea of a lawsuit being brought against a nurse was almost unthinkable. In today's culture, the public has higher expectations for nurses to be accountable for more of what they do.

To be accountable for their practice, nurses must have a sound rationale for their actions, based on knowledge that is gained through scientific research. Nurses have the responsibility of keeping their knowledge base current, and one of the best sources of current knowledge is the research literature. The ability to critique research articles and determine findings that are appropriate for practice is a skill that is needed by all nurses.

Document the Cost-Effectiveness of Nursing Care

Because of nursing's humanistic and altruistic traditions, it has been difficult for nurses to consider the cost-effectiveness of nursing care. The goal has been to help people achieve or maintain health, regardless of cost. But the reality of the healthcare picture has forced nurses to think in monetary terms. Some nurses have acquired additional educational preparation in business and finance to help them better understand the financial aspects of healthcare. With the increased cost of healthcare, all disciplines within the healthcare field have been called on to demonstrate their value in a dollar-and-cents fashion.

Consumers are now more aware of the cost of healthcare and are asking for explanations of services they receive. These consumers need to be made aware of the importance of nursing care in maintaining the health of well clients and promoting patient outcomes among those who are ill and recovering.

Nursing services can consume a large percentage of a hospital's budget. With prospective payment systems dictating the amount of reimbursements that hospitals receive, nursing care services are being closely examined. If nursing care can be shown to be cost-effective, hospitals will look to other sources for saving money before considering the curtailment of nursing services. If effective nursing care enables patients to leave hospitals in better condition and in less time than predicted, hospitals will make more profit or lower operating budgets will be needed for nonprofit hospitals. To determine that nursing care is effective, research is needed. Unfortunately, only a small percentage of a hospital's budget is allocated for nursing research.

Many studies in the literature demonstrate the cost-effectiveness of nursing care. In a classic study cited many times, Brooten et al. (1986) examined early hospital discharge and home follow-up care of very-low-birth-weight infants. They found that follow-up care by a nurse specialist is safe and cost-effective. This type of care potentially decreases iatrogenic illness and hospital-acquired infections, enhances parent–infant interaction, and significantly reduces hospital costs for care.

As cost savings have become a serious concern in healthcare, nurses need to have an appreciation for the ways in which the economic market forces have an impact on nursing. Nursing research efforts may contribute positively to the financial well-being and healthcare of members of society.

Quantitative and Qualitative Research

Nurse researchers conduct both quantitative and qualitative categories of studies. **Quantitative research** is concerned with objectivity, tight controls over the research situation, and the ability to generalize findings. Quantitative research studies are typically designed to collect numerical data, which are statistically analyzed to study research questions or hypotheses (LoBiondo-Wood & Haber, 2014). For example, the researcher could be looking for relationships or differences among variables or testing for the effectiveness of interventions. **Qualitative research** is concerned with the subjective meaning of experiences to individuals. Qualitative research usually occurs in a natural setting with a small number of research participants who are willing to share their information about a phenomenon in a narrative format (LoBiondo-Wood & Haber, 2014).

In the past, nurse researchers have primarily conducted quantitative research. Quantitative research has been the traditional scientific approach used by many other disciplines. Some people do not consider qualitative research to be scientific. Others view quantitative research as hard science and qualitative research as soft science. Still others view both research approaches as scientific.

The number of nurse researchers who conduct qualitative research has increased. In 1985 Madeleine Leininger wrote that there were approximately 50 qualitative nurse researchers. Although the exact number of nurses conducting qualitative research more than 25 years later is not known, the numbers have increased dramatically.

The difference between quantitative and qualitative research can be illustrated by considering patients who experience chronic pain. Quantitative research would be concerned with the level of pain that these people were experiencing and how to reduce it, whereas qualitative research would be concerned with what it means to be living with chronic pain. This book focuses more on quantitative research than on qualitative research. However, the book does provide an overview of qualitative research and specific qualitative designs are described.

Nurses and Research

The membership of the American Association of College of Nursing (AACN) approved a research position statement in October 1998, with revisions approved in 1999 and 2006. This statement lists research expectations and outcomes for graduates of baccalaureate programs, master's programs, practice-focused doctoral programs, research-focused doctoral programs, and postdoctoral programs.

Nurses prepared at the baccalaureate level should be able to understand and apply research findings from nursing and other disciplines in their clinical practice. They should be able to work with others to identify potential research problems and collaborate on research teams.

Masters-prepared nurses should be able to evaluate research findings and develop and implement evidence-based practice guidelines. They should identify practice and systems problems that require research, and collaborate with scientists to initiate research.

Graduates of practice-focused doctoral programs are prepared for the highest level of nursing practice expertise and use advanced leadership knowledge and skills to evaluate and translate research into practice. Thus, they are also prepared to collaborate with scientists on new health policy research opportunities that evolve from the translation and evaluation processes.

Graduates of research-focused doctoral programs are prepared to conduct independent research. They are expected to plan and implement an independent program of research and begin to involve others (students, clinicians, and other researchers) in their research interest area.

Finally, postdoctoral study provides a time for graduates of research-focused doctoral programs to fully develop their research skills. They are able to develop their research program with the help of formal mentoring by senior investigators.

Roles of Nurses in Research

Overall, nurses can assume many roles in association with research projects. Some of these roles include the following, and are described in the ensuing sections:

1. Principal investigator
2. Member of a research team
3. Identifier of researchable problems
4. Evaluator of research findings
5. User of research findings
6. Patient/client advocate during studies
7. Subject/participant in studies

Nurses can and should serve as principal investigators in scientific investigations. To be a principal investigator, special research preparation is necessary. It might be possible for a beginning researcher to conduct a small-scale survey study, but preparation beyond the baccalaureate, or even the master's level, is necessary for independent investigator status in most nursing studies.

Nurses can serve as members of a research team. They may act as data collectors or administer the experimental intervention of the study. As nurses increasingly participate in research, it is possible that interest and enthusiasm to conduct their own investigations may grow. In 1982 Rittenmeyer wrote that research would become a higher priority as knowledge of the benefits of research increased. She predicted that by 1990 research would be part of the nurse's normal workload. Unfortunately, the 20th century closed without her prediction coming true. Maybe the 21st century will begin the magic millennium.

Nursing research does seem to be gathering momentum because bedside nurses and healthcare leaders are trying to validate the impact of nursing on patient outcomes and the healthcare system in general.

We can only hope that the trend continues, as evidence-based practice becomes the standard for nursing care.

All nurses, from associate degree to doctoral-level preparation, have the responsibility of trying to identify areas of needed research. Nurses at the bedside are particularly well situated to identify patient-related researchable problems.

Nurses should be involved in the evaluation of research findings. As research consumers, nurses have the obligation to become familiar with research findings and determine the usefulness of these findings in the practice area. Beginning researchers should critique research articles, first with the help of an experienced researcher and eventually on their own. They may gain knowledge in a structured research course (either in their basic nursing education program or in a continuing education course). The evaluation of research is not an easy task. This book will help you to acquire some of the skills needed to critique research articles and reports.

Through the years, nurses have tended to carry out nursing procedures and provide nursing care "the way we've always done it." Change is difficult to bring about, but research findings have no value if they are not put into use. After evaluating research findings, nurses should use relevant findings in their practice. The primary goal of nursing research, as mentioned earlier, is quality nursing care of clients. However, nurses must be judicious in their use of research findings. The results of one small study conducted with a sample of 15 volunteers, for example, would not provide sufficient evidence for a change in nursing practice.

Research utilization and evidence-based nursing practice (EBNP) are related because both processes emphasize research findings. However, **research utilization** focuses on the implementation of findings from specific research studies. The goal of research utilization is to see that the findings of research studies are actually put into action in nursing practice. EBNP is broader and involves searching for the best evidence to use in nursing practice, which includes searching for the best research evidence available.

All nurses have the responsibility to act as advocates when their patients/clients are involved in research. This advocacy involves making sure that the ethical aspects of research are upheld. Nurses should help answer questions and explain about a study to potential participants before the study begins. They also might be available during the study to answer questions or provide support to study participants.

Some of the questions that research participants need to have answered include: Why is the study being conducted? Who is conducting the study? Who is going to be in the study? What kinds of tests and treatments are involved? How long will the study last? (Habel, 2005). Nurses should serve as valuable resources for information about clinical trials, both in healthcare settings and in the community.

Nurses may act as subjects or participants in research. Many nurses are involved in a long-term survey study, the Nurses' Health Study, being conducted by researchers at Harvard Medical School. The study was designed to examine some of the health risks that pose special threats to women. Nurses were chosen as participants, according to Frank Speizer, the principal investigator, because the study called for subjects knowledgeable about health issues in order to obtain more accurate reporting on exposure and diseases than the general population could provide("Massive Nurses' Health Study," 1983, p. 998). The study was begun in 1976 and was originally intended to last for 4 years, but with additional funding the study has continued for over 39 years. In 1989 a new cohort of younger nurses was added to the study in what is called Nurses' Health Study II. Hundreds of publications have resulted from the data obtained in these studies.

History of Nursing Research

Nursing research was slow to develop in the United States, as well as in the rest of the world. Some of this slow growth is related to the development of nursing education. Despite her skill in independent scientific investigation, Florence Nightingale derived the foundation for modern nursing education from the military tradition, which emphasized the concept of authority. The authoritarian system of training deterred the development of inquiring minds (Simmons & Henderson, 1964). Many schools of nursing throughout the world have been influenced by British nursing education and have relied on tradition and authority, as did British schools.

Nursing research was able to develop and expand only as nurses received advanced educational preparation. The growth of nursing research seems to be directly related to the educational levels of nurses. Although the first university-based nursing program in the United States was begun in 1909, the number of such programs increased very slowly. In the early part of the 20th century, nurse leaders were more concerned with increasing the number of nurses and establishing hospital-affiliated nursing schools than with establishing university programs.

Because nurses were not prepared to conduct research, members of other disciplines conducted many of the early nursing studies. Beginning with a 1923 study, titled the Goldmark Report, non-nurses became involved in studying nurses and nursing. Sociologists were particularly interested in the "learning, living, and working" experienced by nurses (Abdellah & Levine, 1965, p. 4). Research conducted by sociologists and behavioral scientists added to their respective bodies of knowledge but did not necessarily expand nursing's body of knowledge (Henderson, 1956).

As nurses received advanced educational preparation and became qualified to conduct research, many of the studies they conducted were in nursing education because before 1950 most nurses received their advanced degrees in education. However, even during the early half of the 20th century, the need for clinical nursing research was evident. In an article in the *American Journal of Nursing* in 1927, Marvin proposed many research questions involving procedures. What was the safest, simplest, quickest method of preparing a hypodermic? How long should the hands be scrubbed, by what method, and with what kind and strength of soap? By the 1950s, interest in nursing care studies began to rise. During the late 1970s, practice-related research expanded rapidly.

Although Florence Nightingale recommended clinical nursing research in the mid-1800s, most nurses did not follow her advice until more than 100 years later. Some of the studies that she recommended, such as those concerning environmental health hazards, are being conducted today. It is only in recent years that Nightingale has come to be appreciated for the extraordinary woman that she was. If nurses had begun sooner to follow their first leader's example, nursing would be much further along in establishing a body of nursing knowledge. However, there is reason for optimism as both the number and quality of nursing studies have increased dramatically.

The historical development of nursing research has many noteworthy events, including:

- 1850s   Florence Nightingale studied nursing care during the Crimean War. She called for research that focused on nursing practice. Nightingale admonished nurses to develop the habit of making and recording observations systematically. She used statistics to clearly illustrate her findings.
- 1902   Lavinia Dock reported a school nurse experiment that was begun by Lillian Wald. Nurses gave free care to school children and visited the homes of sick children.
- 1906   Adelaide Nutting conducted a survey of the educational status of nursing.
- 1909   The first university-based nursing program was established at the University of Minnesota.
- 1923   A well-known study of nursing and nursing education was conducted by the Committee for the Study of Nursing Education and funded by the Rockefeller Foundation. The results, known as the Goldmark Report, recommended advanced educational preparation for teachers, administrators, and public health nurses, and were instrumental in the establishment of early collegiate nursing schools at Yale, Vanderbilt, and Western Reserve (now Case Western Reserve) universities.

1924   The first doctoral program for nurses was established at Teachers College, Columbia University. The EdD degree was offered to nurses preparing to teach at the college level.

1927   Jean Broadhurst and her colleagues researched handwashing procedures. Edith S. Bryan became the first nurse to earn a doctoral degree when she received a PhD in psychology and counseling from Johns Hopkins University.

1928   Ethel Johns and Blanche Pfefferkorn published a study concerning the activities in which nurses were involved. This was the first of many studies that focused on nurses.

1932   Elizabeth Ryan and Virginia B. Miller investigated thermometer-disinfecting techniques.

1936   Sigma Theta Tau, National Honor Society for Nursing, began funding nursing research.

1948   Esther Lucille Brown, a social anthropologist, published her famous study on nursing education, Nursing for the Future, which called for nursing education to take place in university settings. The Brown Report, as the study was called, recommended research in nursing and pointed to the need for nurse educators to be involved in research. Doris Schwartz documented the effectiveness of nursing care for inducing sleep in patients and for decreasing their intake of medications.

1949   The Division of Nursing Resources was organized within the U.S. Public Health Service. Esta H. McNett demonstrated that masks helped to prevent the spread of tuberculosis.

1952   The first issue of Nursing Research was published.

1953   The Institute of Research and Service in Nursing Education was founded at Teachers College, Columbia University. A full-time staff studied nursing and nursing education.

1955   The American Nurses Foundation was established with the goal of promoting high-level wellness and the improvement of patient care. This foundation funds nursing research. The Nursing Research Grants and Fellowship Programs were established by the U.S. Public Health Service.

1957   The first unit directed primarily toward research in nursing practice was established at the Department of Nursing of the Walter Reed Army Institute of Research. The Western Council for Higher Education in Nursing (WCHEN) sponsored a nursing research conference at the University of Colorado.

1962   The federally supported Nurse Scientist Graduate Training Grants Programs were begun.

1963   Lydia Hall published her 5-year study of chronically ill patients who were cared for at the Loeb Center in New York.

1970   The National Commission for the Study of Nursing and Nursing Education, established by the American Nurses Association (ANA) and the National League for Nursing (NLN), published the results of a 3-year study on nursing. The report, titled An Abstract for Action, was called the Lysaught Report, after Jerome Lysaught, director of the project. The report recommended that research be financed in nursing practice and nursing education. A center for nursing research was established at Wayne State University.

1972   The ANA established a Department of Nursing Research.

1974   At its national convention, the ANA delineated nursing practice as the area to which nursing research should be directed in the next decade.

1976   The Commission on Nursing Research of the ANA recommended that research preparation be included in undergraduate, graduate, and continuing education programs.

1977   The Veterans' Administration began employing nurse researchers.

1978   The first issue of Research in Nursing and Health was published.

1979	The first issue of Western Journal of Nursing Research was published.
1980	The ANA Commission on Nursing Research identified research priorities for the 1980s
1982	Eleven volumes were published of the work of the Conduct and Utilization of Research in Nursing (CURN) project.
1983	The first Center for Nursing Research was established. It encompassed the American Nurses Foundation and the American Academy of Nursing.
1986	The National Center for Nursing Research (NCNR) was established within the National Institutes of Health.
1987	Dr. Ada Hinshaw, director of the NCNR, called for nursing organizations to identify their research priorities.
1988	The NCNR convened the first Conference on Research Priorities (CORP #1) to establish research priorities through 1994. The first issues of Applied Nursing Research and Nursing Science Quarterly were published.
1992	The first issue of Clinical Nursing Research was published.
1993	The National Institute of Nursing Research (NINR) was established within the National Institutes of Health (NIH). This organization replaced the NCNR. The second Conference on Research Priorities (CORP #2) was held to establish research priorities for 1995–1999.
1994	The first issue of Qualitative Nursing Research was published.
1997	The International Council of Nurses convened a group of experts to establish worldwide nursing research priorities.
1999	The first issue of Biological Research for Nursing was published.
2001	The budget for NINR reached almost $90 million.
2004	The first issue of Worldviews on Evidence-Based Nursing was published.
2005	The budget for NINR was more than $138 million.
2009	The Cochrane Nursing Care Network (CNCN) was registered as one of the networks within the Cochrane Collaboration, which produces and disseminates systematic reviews.
2010	The name of the CNCN was changed to the Cochrane Nursing Care Field (CNCF).
2011	The American Nurses Association established a Nursing Research Agenda.
2015	The NINR budget was more than $140.8 million.

National Institute of Nursing Research

The National Institute of Nursing Research (NINR) was officially established within the National Institutes of Health (NIH) on June 10, 1993. It replaced the National Center for Nursing Research (NCNR), which had been established in 1986. It is one of the 27 institutes that comprise the National Institute of Health (NIH). With the creation of the NINR, nursing research received a big boost in respectability. Funding for nursing research has increased a great deal. In 1986 the NCNR had a budget of $16 million. In 1995 the NINR received an appropriation of close to $50 million from Congress. By 2014 funding allocations were increased to more than $140 million. More information on this topic may be found on the NINR website.

The NINR mission statement indicates support for clinical and basic research and research training on health and illness across the lifespan. Areas of research emphasis are: promoting health and preventing disease and disability, managing symptoms, and improving palliative and end-of-life care.

The Cochrane Collaboration and the Cochrane Nursing Care Field

The Cochrane Collaboration (CC), established in 1993, is an international nonprofit organization of people with the goal of helping healthcare providers, policy makers, patients, and their advocates and caretakers to make evidence-informed decisions about healthcare. Visit the Cochrane website for more information on this topic.

The CC has more than 25,000 contributors from more than 120 countries. Its goals are achieved through the preparation, updating, and promoting of systematic reviews based on research studies. These reviews are accessible online through the Cochrane Library portal. In the healthcare community, these reviews are generally considered to be the most comprehensive, reliable, and relevant sources of evidence on which to base healthcare decisions. Each review addresses a clearly formulated question, such as "Can antibiotics help in alleviating the symptoms of a sore throat?" Stringent guidelines are used to establish whether there is conclusive evidence about a certain treatment or the accuracy of a diagnostic test. Many of the 5,000 + reviews in the Cochrane Library have relevance to nursing care. The reviews are updated regularly.

The CC established a nursing entity, the Cochrane Nursing Care Network (CNCN), in March 2009. It became one of the 12 fields and networks within the CC. The first inaugural CNCN symposium was held in Singapore in October 2009. More than 135 people from 11 countries attended. The name of the CNCN was officially changed in April 2010 to the Cochrane Nursing Care Field (CNCF). The CNCF is coordinated from Adelaide, Australia.

Some of the objectives of the CNCF are to identify priority topics, to search for studies related to nursing care, to promote the field's perspectives, to raise awareness of the CC among practitioners of nursing, and to disseminate summaries of nursing-care relevant Cochrane Reviews. The CNCF is in the process of developing resources such as nursing care Cochrane Review Summaries, nursing care-relevant podcasts, and online and face-to-face involvement of its members in preparing summaries and other materials. Volunteers are needed to help with all of these projects and are asked to register their interests at the website.

Research Priorities into the Future

Professional nursing organizations and individual nurse leaders are united in identifying the need for research that will help build a scientific knowledge base for nursing practice. In 1980 the ANA Commission on Nursing Research identified priorities for nursing research. These priorities included research concerned with health promotion and preventive health practices for all age groups, healthcare needs of high-risk groups, life satisfaction of individuals and families, and the development of cost-effective healthcare systems.

In November 1987 Dr. Ada Sue Hinshaw, director of the National Center for Nursing Research (NCNR), invited nursing organizations to identify their research priorities. Since then, many nursing organizations have conducted surveys of their membership to determine research priorities.

National Association of Orthopaedic Nurses

The National Association of Orthopaedic Nurses identified a list of priorities in 1990 (Salmond, 1994). They used a Delphi technique to survey experts in the field. Some of the highest ratings were given to preventing confusion in elderly patients following a hip fracture, determining the most effective safety measures to use with patients with acute confusional states, and differentiating pain responses according to diagnoses, ages, and pain management interventions. In 1997 Sedlak, Ross, Arslanian, and Taggart (1998) replicated the 1990 study. Their respondents expressed the need for more research on pain and patient complications, such as deep vein thrombosis (DVT). Sedlak et al. called for an ongoing and wider dissemination of research results.

Mental Health Nursing

In 1999 Pullen, Tuck, and Wallace published a list of priorities in mental health nursing. These priorities were obtained by examining the published literature from 1990 to 1996. Six broad categories were identified: support, holism, mental health nursing practice, quality care outcomes, mental health etiology, and mental health delivery systems. In 2013, the members of 194 countries whose health ministers attended the World Health Organization (WHO) World Health Assembly adopted the Comprehensive Mental Health Action Plan (DeSilva, Samele, Saxena, Patel, & Darzi, 2014). The WHO-supported action plan has four objectives that should be met by all of the involved countries by 2020. In addition to the provision of comprehensive, integrated, and responsive mental healthcare services in community-based settings, the plan also calls for a strengthening of information systems, evidence, and research related to mental health. As there is a shortage of empirical evidence to guide policy makers on the integration of mental health into a general healthcare system, there is a need to study interventions that would provide cost-effective mental health programs that are responsive to the needs of persons with mental health issues.

Oncology Nursing Society

A survey was conducted in 2013 among members of the Oncology Nursing Society (ONS) to determine research priorities for research and evidence-based initiatives (LoBiondo-Wood et al., 2014). Responses were received from 895 members. The top 20 research priorities were identified. These included symptom management, screening and early detection activities, the development of effective interventions for those at risk of cancer, and prevention of central line infections and prevention of medicine errors. Results from this survey were intended to guide the ONS and ONS Foundation with the goal of providing the highest levels of care and quality for patients with cancer and their caregivers.

Institute of Emergency Nursing Research

According to the Emergency Nurses Association (ENA) website, the ENA's research priorities include investigations that address the generation, dissemination, and translation of research related to the organization's strategic framework. These priorities are related to crowding, boarding, psychiatric emergency patient care, and workplace violence. Other Joint Commission National Patient Safety Goals include research related to improving the effective communication among caregivers, the safe use of medications, the recognition and response to changes in the patients' condition, and reducing the risks of infections, falls, and healthcare-associated pressure ulcers.

Association of Community Health Nurse Educators

Priorities for public health nursing were published by the Association of Community Health Nursing Educators (ACHNE) Research Committee in the January 2010 issue of *Public Health Nursing*. They identified the most important priorities as population-focused outcomes, and workforce issues. This research committee called for "multisite studies, clinical trials, community-based participatory research, development and/or analysis of existing large data sets" (p. 94). According the information currently on the ACHNE website, these priorities remain the same.

Research in Nursing Education

Although clinical nursing research is essential for the profession, other types of research are also needed. Tucker-Allen (2003) wrote an editorial in which she called for nurse educators to conduct research on both clinical issues and educational issues. A National League for Nursing (NLN) task group worked for 7 years to compile research in nursing education and to publish a book on their results (Schultz, 2009). Some of the studies reviewed concerned learner developmental stages, aptitude, motivation, and learning styles. The taskforce concluded that more research is needed on effective teaching and that there is a need to build a science of nursing education. Later, the findings of a small sample of responses from schools of nursing affirmed this same concern over a scarcity of research in nursing education (Broome, Ironside, & McNelis, 2012).

Future Strategies for Improved Healthcare Quality

The story associated with evidence-based practice (EBP) in nursing has shown many successes, but much remains to be accomplished (Stevens, 2013). In an editorial statement, Melnyk (2014) advised that there is a need for a collective vision for improved healthcare and better patient outcomes among researchers, clinicians, educators, policy makers, and healthcare systems. The vision needs to focus on the "so what" outcomes that include improved healthcare quality, cost control, and patient outcomes. To accomplish these goals, Stevens (2013) reported that researchers will not only need to generate evidence-based practices, but also focus on the implementation of the EBP and provide research evidence to guide the management decisions associated with the evidence-based quality improvement of care. Stevens believes the nursing profession is central to the interdisciplinary changes necessary to achieve the goals of effective, safe, and efficient care.

Summary

Nursing research is defined as the systematic, objective process of analyzing phenomena of importance to nursing. It includes studies concerning nursing practice, nursing education, nursing administration, and nurses themselves. Clinical nursing research is research that has the potential to affect the care of clients.

Nursing knowledge has come from tradition, authority, trial and error, and scientific research. Scientific research uses empirical data (data gathered through the senses) and is a systematic, orderly, and objective method of seeking information.

Basic research is concerned with generating new knowledge; applied research seeks solutions to immediate problems. Most nursing studies have been applied research. Many studies, however, contain elements of both basic and applied research.

The most important goal for conducting nursing research is the promotion of evidence-based nursing practice. Evidence-based nursing practice (EBNP) means that nurses make clinical decisions based on the best research evidence, their clinical expertise, and the healthcare preferences of their patients/clients. Other goals for research are to ensure credibility of the nursing profession, provide accountability for nursing practice, and document the cost-effectiveness of nursing care.

Quantitative research is concerned with objectivity, tight controls over the research situation, and the ability to generalize findings. Qualitative research is concerned with the subjective meaning of an experience to an individual.

Nurses act as principal investigators, members of research teams, identifiers of researchable problems, evaluators of research findings, users of research findings, patient/client advocates during studies, and subjects/participants in research.

Research utilization focuses on the implementation of findings from specific research studies. Members of other disciplines conducted many of the early nursing studies because nurses were not prepared at the time to conduct research. Some of these studies, such as the Goldmark Report in 1923 and the Brown Report in 1948, contributed important information about nursing and nursing education. As nurses began to receive advanced degrees, these degrees were generally in the field of education. Many of the studies conducted by the first nurse researchers in this country were in the area of nursing education. Florence Nightingale recommended clinical nursing research in the mid-1800s, but this type of research was scarce until the 1970s. Many nursing organizations have identified clinical nursing research priorities for the future. The National Institute of Nursing Research (NINR) was established in 1993. Funding by Congress has increased from $16 million in 1986 to the National Center for Nursing Research, the precursor to the NINR, to more than $140.8 million to NINR in 2015.

The Cochrane Nursing Care Network (CNCN) was registered in March 2009 as one of the fields and networks within the Cochrane Collaboration. The name was changed in April 2010 to the Cochrane Nursing Care Field (CNCF).

Professional nursing organizations and individual nurse leaders are united in identifying the need for research that will help build a scientific knowledge base for nursing practice. Some priorities include research concerned with health promotion and preventive health practices for all age groups, healthcare needs of high-risk groups, life satisfaction of individuals and families, and the development of cost-effective healthcare systems. There is especially a need to implement evidence-based practices that have shown to influence improved healthcare quality, cost control, and patient outcomes.

Self-Test

1. The most reliable means of obtaining nursing knowledge is through
   A. trial and error.
   B. tradition.
   C. scientific research.
   D. authority.
2. Applied research
   A. often leads to basic research.
   B. depends on the existence of healthy participants.
   C. usually occurs in a laboratory.
   D. is not usually based on an immediate practical need.
3. The major reason for conducting nursing research is to
   A. promote evidence-based care for patients/clients.
   B. promote the growth of the nursing profession.
   C. document the cost-effectiveness of nursing care.
   D. ensure accountability for nursing practice.
4. What statement explains how research is establishing the credibility of nursing as a profession?
   A. Nursing has traditionally borrowed knowledge from the natural sciences.
   B. Through research, nursing has been establishing a body of knowledge that is distinct from other professions.
   C. Nurses were included on the Gallup Poll as professionals with an ethical standard.
   D. The nursing profession exists to provide service to society.
5. What type of research provides a statistical analysis of the relationships among variables?
   A. quantitative research studies
   B. qualitative research studies
   C. a tightly controlled study
   D. a cost-effectiveness study
6. Describe the usual setting for research during a qualitative study.
   A. The setting is usually a remote place where the participant responds to a survey.

B. A small numbers of participants usually share their information in a natural setting.
C. Large numbers of participants respond to computer-based surveys from their homes.
D. A proctored and quiet test setting is used to collect information.
7. What is a graduate of a practice-focused doctoral nursing program academically prepared to do? Choose all that apply.
A. Use advanced leadership knowledge.
B. Evaluate research.
C. Translate research into practice.
D. Begin an independent program of research.
E. Carry out research.
8. All nurses should be able to
A. identify researchable problems for nursing research studies.
B. explain the details of a medical research study to potential participants.
C. determine when most study findings are ready for use in nursing practice.
D. confidently critique the majority of published nursing research studies.
9. As nurses first began to receive advanced educational preparation and became qualified to conduct research, many of their studies concerned
A. nursing education.
B. characteristics of nurses.
C. nursing administration.
D. nursing care.
10. Identify which topics are listed as research priorities among the members of the Oncology Nursing Society. Choose all that apply.
A. Quality of life
B. falls
C. Pain
D. domestic violence
E. quality assurance

See answers to Self-Test in the Answer Section at the back of the book.

References

Abdellah, F. G., & Levine, E. (1965). *Better patient care through nursing research.* New York: Macmillan.

American Association of College of Nursing. (2006). *AACN Position statement on nursing research.* http://aacn.nche.edu/Publications/positions/NsgRes

American Association of Colleges of Nursing. (2006). Leading Initiatives. *Hallmarks of Quality and Patient Safety.* http://www.aacn.nche.edu/publications/white-papers/hallmarks-quality-safety

American Nurses Association. (2011). American Nurses Association Research Agenda. http://nursingworld.org/MainMenuCategories/ThePracticeofProfessionalNursing/Improving-Your-Practice/Research-Toolkit/ANA-Research-Agenda/Research-Agenda-.pdf

Association of Community Health Nursing Educators (ACHNE) Research Committee. (2010). Research priorities for public health nursing. *Public Health Nursing, 27,* 94–100. doi:10.1111/j.1525–1446.2009.00831.x

Broome, M. E., Ironside, P. M., & McNelis, A. M. (2012). Research in nursing education: State of the science. *Nursing Education, 51,* 521–524. doi:10.3928/01484834-20120820-10

Brooten, D., Kumar, S., Brown, L. P., Butts, P., Finkler, S. A., Bakewell-Sachs, S., . . . Delivoria-Papadopoulos, M. (1986). A randomized clinical trial of early hospital discharge and home follow-up of very-low-birth-weight infants. *New England Journal of Medicine, 315,* 934–939. http://www.nejm.org/

Canadian Nurse. (2010, February). In conversation about nursing research. *Canadian Nurse.* http://www.canadian-nurse.com/articles/issues/2010/february-2010/in-conversation-about-nursing-research

DeSilva, M., Samele, C., Saxena, S., Patel, V., & Darzi, A. (2014). Policy actions to achieve integrated community-based mental health services. *Health Affairs, 33,* 1595–1602. doi:10.1377/hlthaff.2014.0365

Dougherty, M. D. (2010). Evidence-based practice and nursing research [Editorial]. *Nursing Research, 59*, 1. http://www.nursingworld.org/

Grove, S. K., Burns, N., & Gray, J. (2013). *The practice of nursing research: Appraisal, synthesis, and generation of evidence* (7th ed.). St. Louis, MO: Saunders Elsevier.

Habel, M. (2005, March 14). Can you answer patients' questions about clinical trials? *NurseWeek—South Central Edition*, pp. 23–25. http://news.nurse.com/article/

Henderson, V. (1956). Research in nursing practice—when? *Nursing Research, 4*, 99. http://journals.lww.com/nursingresearchonline/pages/default.aspx

Kawakami, H., Miyashita, T., Yanaizumi, R., Mihara, T., Sato, H., Kariya, T., Mizuno, Y., & Goto, T. (2013). Amount of accidental flush by syringe pump due to inappropriate release of occluded intravenous line. *Technology and Health Care 21*, 581–586. doi:10.3233/THC-130754

Kerlinger, F. (1986). *Foundations of behavioral research* (3rd ed.). New York: Holt, Rinehart & Winston.

LoBiondo-Wood, G., Brown, C. G., Knobf, M. T., Lyon, D., Mallory, G., Mitchell, S. A.,. . . Fellman, B. (2014). Priorities for oncology nursing research: The 2013 national survey. *Oncology Nursing Forum, 41*, 67–76. doi:10.1188/14ONF.67-67

LoBiondo-Wood, G., & Haber, J. (2014). *Nursing research: Methods and critical appraisal for evidence-based practice* (8th ed.). St. Louis, MO: Mosby Elsevier.

Marvin, M. (1927). Research in nursing. *American Journal of Nursing, 27*, 331–335. http://www.nursingcenter.com/lnc/journalissue?Journal_ID=54030

Massive nurses' health study in seventh year, reports first findings on disease links in women. (1983). *American Journal of Nursing, 83*, 998–999. http://journals.lww.com/ajnonline/Citation/1983/83070/Massive_Nurses__Health_Study,_in_Seventh_Year,.8.aspx

Melnyk, B. M. (2014). Speeding the translation of research into evidence-based practice and conducting projects that impact healthcare quality, patient outcomes and costs: The "So What" outcome factor. *Worldviews on Evidence-Based Nursing, 11*, 1–4. doi:10.IIII/wvn.12025

Newhouse, R., Barksdale, D. J., & Miller, J. A. (2014). Patient-Centered Outcomes Research Institute: Research done differently. *Nursing Research, 64*, 72–77. doi:10.1097/NNR.0000000000000070

Oman, K. S., Krugman, M. E., & Fink, R. M. (2003). *Nursing research secrets*. Philadelphia: Hanley & Belfus.

Polit, D. F., & Beck, C. T. (2012). *Nursing research: Generating and assessing evidence for nursing practice* (9th ed.). Philadelphia: Wolters Kluwer | Lippincott Williams & Wilkins.

Pullen, L., Tuck, I., & Wallace, D. C. (1999). Research priorities in mental health nursing. *Issues in Mental Health Nursing, 20*, 217–227. http://informahealthcare.com/loi/mhn/

Rittenmeyer, P. (1982). The evolution of nursing research. *Western Journal of Nursing Research, 4*, 223–225. http://wjn.sagepub.com/

Sabourin, H. (2009). The last word: Getting on with the job of supporting research. *Canadian Nurse, 105*, 40. http://www.canadian-nurse.com/

Salmond, S. W. (1994). Orthopaedic nursing research priorities: A Delphi study. *Orthopaedic Nursing, 13*, 31–45. http://journals.lww.com/orthopaedicnursing/pages/default.aspx

Schultz, C. M. (Ed.). (2009). *Building a science of nursing education: Foundations for evidence-based teaching–learning*. New York: National League for Nursing.

Sedlak, C., Ross, D., Arslanian, C., & Taggart, H. (1998). Orthopaedic nursing research priorities: A replication and extension. *Orthopaedic Nursing, 17*(2), 51–58. http://journals.lww.com/orthopaedicnursing/pages/default.aspx

Simmons, L. W., & Henderson, V. (1964). *Nursing research—A survey and assessment*. New York: Appleton-Century-Crofts.

Stevens, K. R. (2013). The impact of evidence-based practice in nursing and the next big ideas. *Online Journal of Issues in Nursing, 18*(2), Manuscript 4. doi:10.3912/OJIN.Vol18No02Man04

Tucker-Allen, S. (2003). Nursing education as a respected area of research [Editorial]. *Association of Black Nursing Faculty Journal, 14*, 115. http://tuckerpub.com/abnf.htm

Chapter 2
Evidence-Based Nursing Practice

Rose Nieswiadomy, PhD, RN, and Catherine Bailey, PhD, RN

Objectives

On completion of this chapter, you will be prepared to:

1. Summarize the importance of evidence-based practice in the field of nursing.
2. Differentiate between research utilization and evidence-based nursing practice.
3. Discuss the importance of the Cochrane Collaboration and the Cochrane Nursing Care Field to evidence-based practice.
4. Explain the role of the Agency for Healthcare Research and Quality in evidence-based practice.
5. Summarize the roles of evidence-based nursing practice centers.

Defining Evidence-Based Practice

Have you heard the term "evidence-based practice"? If your answer is, "No," then you must be living on another planet. If your answer is, "Yes," you may also reply that you are tired of hearing the term. However, this term is vital for the future of nursing care.

Everyone is talking about evidence-based practice, best practice, evidence-based nursing, and evidence-based nursing practice. You have probably heard the old adage "In God we trust; all others bring data." Nursing's goal of evidence-based practice (EBP) must be based on data, especially data gained from nursing research. However, often there aren't the research results or data, or data that is not available or does not yield strong enough results to support adoption into day-to-day practice (Dougherty, 2014, p. S3).

In April 2015, a search of the term *evidence-based nursing practice* in the online search engine Google came up with about 24,800,000 results. Of course, many of these hits were duplicates, and others were only closely related. ProQuest Nursing & Allied Health Source revealed 40,775 documents, mostly from scholarly and trade journals, dissertations, and theses, on evidence-based nursing practice (EBNP).

Why we use evidence-based practice

Why are we so concerned with the use of evidence in nursing practice? Have we not always searched for and used the best evidence when seeking answers to clinical questions? Unfortunately, we have not. Although much has been done to support the activities of EBP in nursing, there are more challenges that must be overcome before EBNP is well established in nursing practice (Stevens, 2013).

The term *evidence-based practice* originated in the field of medicine. Most people credit the beginning of the movement toward evidence-based practice to Archie Cochrane (1909–1988), a British medical researcher and epidemiologist. In 1972, Cochrane published a book titled *Effectiveness and Efficiency: Random Reflections on Health Services*. His book pointed out the lack of solid evidence about the effects of healthcare. Cochrane suggested that because healthcare resources would always be limited, these resources should be used to provide the most effective healthcare. He emphasized the importance of using evidence from randomized controlled trials (RCTs), also called randomized clinical trials. This type of study is considered the gold standard or strongest evidence that can be used as a basis for practice decisions.

When Cochrane's book was published in 1972, the medical profession did not seem ready for Cochrane's ideas about the need to examine the effectiveness of medical interventions. Physicians may not have wanted to hear that their care might not be effective. It took another 20 years before the evidence-based practice movement really began to flourish.

In 1996, Sackett et al. wrote an editorial, "Evidence Based Medicine: What It Is and What It Isn't," that was published in the *British Medical Journal*. This editorial caught the attention of the medical profession, and the idea of evidence-based medicine became accepted by many physicians.

You will encounter many terms in the literature that relate to the use of evidence in the practice decisions of healthcare professionals, including:

Evidence-based medicine (EBM)

Evidence-based practice (EBP)

Evidence-based care (EBC)

Evidence-based healthcare (EBHC)

Evidence-based nursing (EBN)

Evidence-based nursing practice (EBNP)

Sackett et al. (1996) initially defined evidence-based medicine as "the conscientious, explicit, and judicious use of current best evidence in making decisions about the care of individual patients" (p. 71). Later, clinical expertise and patient values were included as additional determinants for EBP clinical decision making (Sackett, Straus, Richardson, Rosenberg, & Haynes, 2000). Ideally speaking, this definition of an EBP would result from the synthesis of quality research about a specific practice problem by experienced clinicians who incorporate the values and expectations of their patients in the management of their healthcare.

As the Honor Society of Nursing, Sigma Theta Tau International (STTI) supports the dissemination of knowledge to improve nursing practice, STTI defined EBP in a way that is specific to nursing. One of the roles that is specific to nurses is that of a patient advocate. Therefore evidence-based nursing (EBN) is defined as "an integration of the best evidence available, nursing expertise, and the values and preferences of the individuals, families, and communities who are served" (STTI, 2005). This position statement, which is located on the SSTI website, assumes that optimal nursing care will be provided when healthcare decision makers and nurses have access to the synthesis of current research. Before proceeding with more discussions about EBP, you may need to know how an EBP differs from research utilization.

Research Utilization versus Evidence-Based Practice

Research utilization (RU) is a more narrow term than evidence-based nursing practice. In the past, RU referred to the use of research knowledge for clinical practice (Ciliska et al., 2011). RU involves the use of results from specific research studies that focused on one clinical problem and had good results. The knowledge from RU accumulates over time and works its way into practice. For example, we no longer routinely irrigate urinary drainage systems or clamp and disconnect the tubing when the patient ambulates. This research-driven recommendation is now widely accepted for clinical practice because research showed that interrupting the closed system increased the likelihood of a urinary tract infection (Harris, 2010). This example of research utilization was supported by a federally funded demonstration project, the Conduct and Utilization of Research in Nursing (CURN) project. The CURN project was one of the earliest attempts to encourage registered nurses to improve their practice, which had depended on customs, opinions, and authority, with research findings (Schmidt & Brown, 2009).

Evidence-based practice is broader in scope than RU because the clinician is expected to consider more than evidence during the clinical decision-making process (Ciliska et al., 2011). In addition to using the synthesis of the best evidence from multiple studies, expert clinicians are expected to consider the patient's circumstances, as well as the results generated from outcomes management or quality improvement projects, the patient's preferences and the available resources for clinical decision making (Ciliska et al., 2011). In other words, the creation of an EBP depends on a systematic approach that enables clinicians to identify best practices and determine if and how these practices can be introduced into the healthcare for a relevant patient population (Poe & White, 2010).

Evidence-Based Nursing Practice

Although the idea of EBP has been in existence since the 1970s, it has become very important in all areas of healthcare in a short period of time. Overall, the goal of EBP in nursing is to introduce current knowledge into common care decisions that will improve both the effectiveness of processes and the patient outcomes associated with healthcare (Stevens, 2013). In the presence of escalating healthcare costs EBP has also been promoted by public and professional desires for accountability in safety and quality improvement in healthcare services. As nurses have always wanted what is best for their patients/clients, it is appropriate that nurses incorporate EBPs into everyday nursing care practices.

Benefits of EBP

The most celebrated benefits of EBPs are the improved patient outcomes that have been shown through the synthesis of many research studies (Grove, Burns, & Gray, 2013). Other benefits associated with the use of EBPs relate to the way the Joint Commission (JC) and the American Nurses Credentialing Center (ANCC) have recognized them as the best treatment plans or standards of care for those who are maintaining accreditation and seeking Magnet Hospital recognition (Grove et al., 2013).

The JC is an independent, not-for-profit organization that accredits and certifies more than 20,500 healthcare organizations and programs in the U.S. The JC is the nation's oldest and largest standards-setting and accrediting body in healthcare. According to the information on the JC website, an organization must undergo an on-site review by a survey team at least every three years in order to acquire and maintain The Joint Commission's Gold Seal of Approval™. Magnet Recognition (MR) is a program that was developed by the ANCC to recognize healthcare organizations for quality patient care, nursing excellence and innovations in nursing practice. According to the information on the ANCC website, a focus on quality/safety nurse-sensitive clinical indicators, such as falls with injury and catheter-associated urinary tract infections, are examples of patient outcomes used to measure nursing excellence within an agency seeking Magnet Recognition.

Asking Clinical Questions

Now that you understand the importance of EBP, are you wondering how you might begin the work of implementing an EBP? First, you need to identify a clinical problem that suggests there is a better way to provide care that will promote improved healthcare in a cost-effective way. A popular approach is to create a clinical question in PICOT format then follow a systematic literature review to discover the available research evidence (Hain & Kear, 2015).

The acronym PICOT is a format for writing clinical questions that was developed by Fineout-Overholt and Johnston (2005). The five letters stand for:

P = Patient or population
I = Intervention or interest area
C = Comparison intervention or current practice
O = Outcome(s) desired
T = Time to achieve outcome (optional)

A discussion of this format can be found in an article titled "Using Evidence-Based Practice to Move Beyond Doing Things the Way We Have Always Done Them" (Hain & Kear, 2015). The authors describe the steps of developing an evidence-based project that could address a patient- or organizational-focused clinical problem. The following PICOT format was established to assess adults with chronic kidney disease, questioning how attending an exercise program compared to attending no exercise program affects participation in regular exercise within three months (Hain & Kear, 2015, p. 13). The population (P) was "adults with chronic kidney disease." The intervention of interest (I) was "exercise program." The comparison intervention (C) was "no exercise program." The outcome (O) was "affect participation in regular exercise." Finally, the time (T) was "within three months." After the clinical question is created, a search of the relevant research-based literature that addresses the clinical issue and patient care question ensues (Hain & Kear, 2015).

Sources for Evidence for Practice

According to Hain and Kear (2015), research evidence can be classified as translational literature, evidence summaries, and primary evidence. *Translational research* refers to evidence that has been incorporated into guidelines that are used in clinical settings. Standards of practice, protocols, and critical pathways are examples of translational research, which can be found in the Cumulative Index to Nursing and Allied Health Literature (CINAHL), PubMed, and the National Clearinghouse databases, or the Best Practice Information Sheets of the Joanna Briggs Institute.

Evidence summaries such as systematic reviews are described as summaries of the literature that appraise research that is appropriate for the research question (Hain & Kear, 2015). Evidence summaries are typically found in nursing and non-nursing online databases, such as PubMed, CINAHL, the Cochrane Library, the Joanna Briggs Institute, and library catalogs.

Primary evidence may be collected directly from the patient or from clinical trial information, peer-reviewed research articles in journals, conference proceedings, and large data sets from organizations (Hain & Kear, 2015). Databases from primary evidence may be found in PubMed, CINAHL, Excerpta Medical Medica Database (EM-BASE), and institutional sources.

The Cochrane Collaboration

The Cochrane Collaboration (CC) is an international nonprofit organization that supports efforts to make well-informed decisions about healthcare. The contributors of the Cochrane Collaboration are from more than 120 countries and they work together to produce credible, accessible health information that is free from commercial sponsorship and other conflicts of interest. The Cochrane Collaboration was established in 1993 and named after Archie Cochrane.

There are 53 Cochrane Review Groups. Each group focuses on a specific topic area, such as breast cancer, drugs and alcohol, multiple sclerosis, and sexually transmitted diseases. These review groups provide authors with methodological and editorial support to prepare *Cochrane Reviews*. They also manage the editorial process, which includes peer review. Funding may be provided by the government, universities, hospital trusts, charities, and personal donations. More information on this topic can be obtained from the Cochrane Collaboration's website.

Cochrane Reviews are based on the best available information about healthcare interventions. These reviews provide evidence for and against the effectiveness and appropriateness of treatments such as medications, surgery, and educational programs. Systematic reviews of healthcare interventions have become popular sources of support for EBPs. A **systematic review**, also called an integrative review, is a rigorous scientific approach that combines results from a group of original research studies and looks at the studies as a whole. While focusing on a single area of interest, a systematic review may provide a summary of many studies at once.

Interventions for Preventing Falls in Older People Living in the Community is an example of a systematic review that might be of interest to nurses (Gillespie et al., 2012). The results of this review identified which interventions helped to reduce falls among older people in the community. The investigators looked at 159 clinical trials with a total of 79,193 participants. They found that group and home-based exercise programs that included balance and strength training exercises effectively reduced falls. While some medications were linked to increased risks of falling, one study showed that gradually reducing a particular medication that was prescribed for improving sleep and reducing anxiety actually reduced falls. The reviewers also found that falls were reduced among those who were receiving cataract surgery in the first affected eye, and among people who had pacemakers inserted for sudden changes in their heart rate and blood pressure.

The Cochrane Library

The *Cochrane Library* is the medium used to publish the work of the Cochrane Collaboration. It consists of six databases that contain evidence to promote decision making in healthcare. These six databases are: (1) *Cochrane Database of Systematic Reviews (CDSR)*, (2) *Cochrane Central Register of Controlled Trials (CENTRAL)*, (3) *Cochrane Methodology Register (CMAR)*, (4) *Database of Abstracts of Reviews of Effects (DARE)*, (5) *Health Technology Assessment Database (HTA)*, and (6) *NHS Economic Evaluation Database (EED)*. A seventh database provides information about the groups in the Cochrane Collaboration.

Cochrane Database

The main output of the Cochrane Collaboration, the *Cochrane Reviews*, is found in the *Cochrane Database of Systematic Reviews*, which is published electronically as part of the Cochrane Library archives. As new information is located, *Cochrane Reviews* are updated regularly and published online monthly, with quarterly DVDs. More than 6,300 reviews and 2,400 protocols were available in the Cochrane Database in May 2015. The protocols for *Cochrane Reviews* describe the research methods and objectives for reviews that are in progress. Abstracts of *Cochrane Reviews* are also available free online to everyone. These summaries are provided in easily understandable terms.

Cochrane Centers

Cochrane Centers are located throughout the world, including locations in Australia, Brazil, Canada, China, Denmark, France, Germany, Italy, the Netherlands, South Africa, Spain, the United Kingdom, and the United States. All Cochrane Centers help to coordinate and support the members of the Cochrane Collaboration. Some of the common responsibilities include helping people to find out about the Cochrane Collaboration and its reviews, providing training for people who will do reviews, fostering collaboration among people with similar research interests, and organizing workshops, seminars, and colloquia to support the Cochrane Collaboration. In addition, each center reflects the interests of the individuals associated with that particular center. A special mission of the Cochrane Center in the United States is to support a partnership with health and consumer advocacy groups who are interested in using evidence-based healthcare practice findings to assist their advocacy activities, to strengthen the voices of consumers in healthcare research, and to provide leadership in those areas.

Cochrane Nursing Care Field

The website for the Cochrane Nursing Care Field (CNCF) is one of twelve fields in the Cochrane Collaboration (CC). The purpose of the CNCF is to support the development of systematic reviews and the dissemination and utilization of systematic reviews that are relevant to the field of nursing. Some core functions include (a) identifying topics related to nursing care that are not covered in existing Cochrane reviews, (b) identifying primary studies in nursing care by searching databases, relevant journals, and conference proceedings, (c) promoting the field's perspectives across the CC, (d) raising awareness of the resources that the CC offers to nursing, (e) disseminating the findings of relevant Cochrane reviews to the nursing community, and (f) identifying sources of funding to undertake or complete Cochrane reviews of interest.

The activities of the CNCF are coordinated from a dedicated unit within the School of Translational Science at the University of Adelaide in Adelaide, South Australia, and six Cochrane Nursing Care (CNC) field groups from 35 countries around the world with over 1200 members. The CNC field groups are designed to promote a geographical spread of activities internationally, and each group is responsible for a substantive field activity. Membership is open to consumers of nursing care, nurses, formal and informal caregivers, other healthcare professionals, researchers, and others involved in the delivery of nursing care.

When you explore the CNCF website, you will discover a number of resources that relate to nursing care. Some of the resources include information about becoming involved with a nursing care review support group, Cochrane Reviews in Nursing Care and Review Summaries, podcasts for nursing care, monthly CNCF newsletters, and online and face-to-face involvement of its members in preparing summaries and other materials. Volunteers are needed to help with all of these projects, and visitors of the CNCF website are asked to register their interests.

Agency for Healthcare Research and Quality

To help understand how the notion of evidence-based practice in healthcare has been evolving in the United States, it is necessary to provide an abbreviated account of the mission and activities of the Agency for Healthcare Research and Quality (AHRQ). The AHRQ is the health services research branch of the U.S. Department of Health and Human Services (HHS). The website for the AHRQ has vast amounts of information about EBP topics for professionals as well as consumers.

The AHRQ, formerly known as the Agency for Healthcare Policy and Research, began an initiative to improve the quality, effectiveness, and appropriateness of healthcare delivery in the United States. In 1997, the AHRQ promoted the idea of evidence-based practices through the leadership of Evidence-Based Practice Centers (EPCs). In 1998, the AHRQ began to sponsor the work of an independent panel of private-sector experts (the U.S. Preventive Services Task Force [USPSTF]) in the area of primary care and preventive services. Then, in 2010, the Patient Protection and Affordable Care Act (PPACA) directed the Secretary of the HHS to establish a national strategy to improve healthcare delivery services, patient health outcomes, and population health (HHS, 2014). On behalf of the HHS, the AHRQ delivered the National Quality Strategy (NQS) publication to Congress in 2011.

The NQS served as a vehicle to focus nationwide attention on quality improvement efforts and a common approach to measuring quality healthcare (HHS, 2014). The aims of the strategy were to improve the overall quality of healthcare, to support interventions that aided in improving health, and to reduce the cost of quality healthcare. The priorities were: (a) to reduce the harm caused in the delivery of care; (b) to ensure that each person and family engaged as partners in their care; (c) to promote communication and coordination of care; (d) to promote the most effective prevention and treatment practices for the leading causes of mortality; (e) to work with communities to promote wide use of best healthcare practices to enable healthy living, and (f) to make quality care more affordable.

After embracing the NQS, the AHRQs mission was expanded to produce evidence to make healthcare safer, of a higher quality, more accessible, equitable, and affordable, and to work with the HHS and other partners to make sure that the evidence is understood and used (HHS, 2014). Thus, the AHRQ identified four priorities to promote an evidence-based improvement of healthcare services and outcomes. The priorities are: (1) to improve healthcare quality through the implementation of Patient-Centered Outcome Research (PCOR), especially within small-to-medium-sized primary care practices; (2) to make healthcare safer not only in hospital settings, but also in primary care settings and nursing homes; (3) to increase accessibility of healthcare by studying the effects of health insurance expansion (following the passage of the PPACA) in access to care, use of healthcare, healthcare spending, and health outcomes, and the labor market, and; (4) to improve healthcare affordability, efficiency, and cost transparency.

The activities of fulfilling the above priorities were supported by a budget of $465,004 million in 2015 and managed through seven offices or centers that fall under the authority of the AHRQ and other entities that are supported by the AHRQ. Some notable entities that support the AHRQ mission include Evidence-Based Practice Centers (EPCs), the U.S. Preventive Services Task Force (USPSTF), the National Guideline Clearinghouse, and the National Quality Forum.

Evidence-Based Practice Centers

The EPCs are responsible for developing evidence reports and technology assessments on topics related to clinical, social science/behavioral science, economic, and other healthcare organization and delivery issues. Topics for consideration are nominated by such groups as professional societies, insurers, employers, and patient groups. In May 2014, 13 EPCs were funded by the AHRQ. Twelve of these centers were located in the United States, and one was located in Canada:

    Evidence-Based Practice Centers Brown University, Providence, RI

    Duke University, Durham, NC

    ECRI Institute-Penn Medicine, Plymouth Meeting, PA

    John Hopkins University, Baltimore, MD

    Kaiser Permanente Research Affiliates, Portland, OR

    Mayo Clinic, Rochester, MN

    Pacific Northwest Evidence-based Practice Center-Oregon Health & Science University, Portland, OR

    RTI International-University of North Carolina at Chapel Hill, Chapel Hill, NC

Southern California Evidence-based Practice Center-Rand Corporation, Santa Monica, CA
University of Alberta, Alberta, Canada
Minnesota Evidence-based Practice Center, Minneapolis, MN
Vanderbilt University, Nashville, Tennessee
University of Connecticut, Hartford, Connecticut

U.S. Preventive Services Task Force

The USPSTF is supported by the 13 EPCs previously mentioned. The EPCs conduct systematic reviews on clinical preventative services, and the results of their reviews are used to make recommendations for use in primary care settings. The USPSTF then reviews the evidence and determines the benefits and harms (or unintended consequences) for each preventive service. Despite the ways in which the AHRQ supports the work of the USPSTF, it operates as an independent body and its work does not require AHRQ or HHS approval.

The USPSTF grades its recommendations as follows: (A) Recommends the service; there is high certainty that the net benefit is substantial; (B) Recommends the service; there is high certainty that the net benefit is moderate or there is moderate certainty that the net benefit is moderate to substantial; (C) Recommends the service; there is at least moderate certainty that the net benefit is small; (D) Recommends against the service; there is moderate or high certainty that the service has no net benefit or that the harms outweigh the benefits; (I) The current evidence is insufficient to assess the balance of benefits and harms of the service.

At least once every 5 years, a decision is made to either update a recommendation or inactivate a topic. Topics may be inactivated when they are no longer relevant to clinical practice.

The PPACA of 2010 has additionally charged the USPSTF to make an annual report to Congress that identifies gaps in the evidence base for clinical preventive services and recommends priority areas that deserve further examination. In 2014, the Task Force's *Fourth Annual Report to Congress on High-Priority Evidence Gaps for Clinical Preventive Services* identified evidence gaps related to the care of children and adolescents. According the USPSTF, more research in these areas would result in important new knowledge that may improve the health and healthcare of young Americans, with lasting benefits through adulthood.

National Guideline Clearinghouse

The National Guideline Clearinghouse (NGC) is a database of evidence-based clinical practice guidelines and related documents. The NGC is sponsored by the AHRQ, U.S. Department of Health and Human Services. In May 2015, the NGC contained 2,401 summaries of guidelines with 87 guidelines in progress.

Every nurse should know about the practice guidelines that are specific for her or his area of practice. Although most guidelines are developed through the work of physician groups, many nurses have been involved in developing practice guidelines. Diane Langemo, a nurse expert in the field of pressure ulcers, was the chairperson of the National Pressure Ulcer Advisory Panel (2014) that authored the *Prevention of Pressure Ulcers. In Prevention and Treatment of Pressure Ulcers: Clinical Practice Guidelines*. The University of Texas at Austin School of Nursing Family Nurse Practitioner Program (2014) was recognized for developing guidelines for the *Evaluation of Vertigo in the Adult*. The Registered Nurses' Association of Ontario (RNAC) (2013) developed guidelines for the *Assessment and Management of Pain*. More examples associated with the NGC can easily be accessed through their online services.

NATIONAL QUALITY FORUM The National Quality Forum (NQF) is a not-for-profit, nonpartisan, membership-based organization that works to support the AHRQ goals of improving health and healthcare quality through measurement. The NQF's vision is to assist in the establishment of national priorities and goals to achieve healthcare that is safe, effective, patient-centered, timely, efficient, and equitable. Another NQF vision is to endorse standards that will facilitate the ongoing quality improvement (QI) of American healthcare quality.

Stated more simply, the NQF works to create **measures** or strategies that show whether the standards for prevention, screening, and managing health conditions are met. They may be (a) *structural measures*, which assess the healthcare infrastructure, (b) *process measures* that assess the steps that should be followed to provide good care, (c) *outcome measures* that assess the results of healthcare that are experienced by patients, (d) *patient engagement or experiences measures* that may be collected as surveys in order to gain feedback from the recipients of healthcare, or (e) *composite measures* that combine multiple measures to produce a single score. As you may have guessed, the works of the NQF complement the ways in which an EBP may become standardized and evaluated. For a more in depth understanding of how the NQF supports an EBP, visit the NQF website. While you are there, review the definitions of terms and lists of measures that may be useful to you as you learn more about clinically based research.

AHRQ-Funded Nursing Study

A qualitative case study evaluation approach was used to identify the experiences of staff members during the implementation of a quality improvement (QI) project that focused on pain reduction strategies among residents in eight nursing homes (Abrahamson, DeCrane, Mueller, & Davila, 2014). Semistructured interviews with open-ended questions were used to gain an understanding of the processes that supported the project from the staff member participants. The respondents identified interdisciplinary communications between physical therapists and nurses, accessibility to leadership, pain management training, and nursing assistant participation as characteristics that facilitated the success of the project. Notable challenges of the project included perceptions that increased documentation related to the management of pain was burdensome and time-consuming.

The fact that some families of the residents did not want to go along with all of the pain control strategies was a serious barrier that had to be overcome. Abrahamson et al. (2014) concluded that an interdisciplinary approach to pain management strategies that include pharmaceutical and nonpharmaceutical strategies may support different expectations for pain outcome measures during the day when mobility is encouraged and at night when it is important for the nursing home residents to rest.

Evidence-Based Nursing Practice Centers

The introduction of EBP onto the notion of QI has generated a major paradigm shift within healthcare in the United States (Stevens, 2013). As nurses are an integral part of healthcare, the AHRQ supported NQS is a call for nurses to redesign their care to strategies that promote evidence of healthcare that is also safe and effective as well as efficient. Rather than employ research utilization as a strategy to support their practices, nurses are encouraged to incorporate new forms of evidence (such as those from systematic reviews), new interprofessional team efforts, and new fields of science to complement their own fields of EBP.

To assist with the implementation of these goals, there has been a proliferation of journals, books and websites devoted to this topic. Two journals that focus on evidence-based nursing practice are *Evidence-Based Nursing* and *Worldviews on Evidence-Based Nursing*. Two of the more recent books are *Evidence-Based Practice in Nursing & Healthcare: A Guide to Best Practice*, by Melnyk and Fineout-Overholt (2011) and *Johns Hopkins Nursing Evidence-Based Practice: Implementation and Translation*, by Poe and White (2010). The Joanna

Briggs Institute, the ACE Center for Advancing Clinical Excellence, and Cole Hirsch Institute for Best Nursing Practices are examples of centers that promote EBP for nursing.

Joanna Briggs Institute

The Joanna Briggs Institute (JBI), established in 1996, is an international not-for-profit collaboration involving nursing, medical, and allied health researchers; clinicians; academics; and quality managers. The JBI collaborates internationally with over 70 entities around the world. The JBI institute was named after Joanna Briggs (1805–1880), the first Matron (Head Nurse) of the Royal Adelaide Hospital in Australia and it is housed in the Faculty of Health Sciences at the University of Adelaide, South Australia.

The JBI coordinates the efforts of a group of self-governing collaborative centers. The goals of the institute are to promote and support the improvement of healthcare outcomes globally by identifying feasible, appropriate, meaningful, and effective healthcare practices through the synthesis of research findings. There are three collaborating nursing centers in the United States: (a) Indiana Center for Evidence-Based Nursing Practice (Purdue University Calumet in Hammond, IN); (b) the Northeast Institute for Evidence Synthesis and Translation (Rutgers, the State University of New Jersey School of Nursing in Newark, NJ); and (c) Texas Christian University Center for Evidence Based Practice and Research (Texas Christian University in Fort Worth, TX).

An example of a Best Practice Recommendation from the Joanna Briggs Institute website is titled, *Blood pressure: Sodium Chloride (Salt) Intake* (Swe, 2014). The recommendation is in response to identifying what the best available evidence is regarding the effect of salt intake on blood pressure in normotensive and hypertensive adults (Swe, 2014, p. 1). The Best Practice Recommendation includes a discussion about the conclusions from different sources of evidence, the characteristics of the evidence (such as a Cochrane systematic review and meta-analysis), the resulting recommendations, and references. The recommendation states that there is evidence that supports a reduction of salt intake to decrease blood pressure, especially among people with hypertension.

ACE Center for Advancing Clinical Excellence

The ACE Center is located at the School of Nursing of the University of Texas Health Science Center at San Antonio. The ACE Center was established in 2000 and originally named the Academic Center for Evidence-Based Practice. The purpose of this center is to advance cutting edge, state-of-the-art evidence-based nursing practice, research, and education within an interdisciplinary context. Ultimately the goal is to translate research-based findings into clinical actions that will improve healthcare through the evaluation of the impact that an evidence-based practice (EBP) has on patient health outcomes, satisfaction, efficacy and efficiency of care, and health policy (Stevens, 2013). In other words, the ACE Center is focused on conducting research on every facet of the translational science model. More information about the UT Health Science Center San Antonio can be assessed by going to the School of Nursing's website.

Sarah Cole Hirsh Institute

The Sarah Cole Hirsh Institute (SCHI) for Best Nursing Practices Based on Evidence is a Center for Excellence located at the Case Western Reserve University Frances Payne Bolton School of Nursing in Cleveland, Ohio. The SCHI conducts evidence syntheses, provides consulting services on evidence-based practice across healthcare settings, and offers certificate programs to educate nurses on the best practice based on evidence. The SCHI also facilitates and mentors others in the transfer of research knowledge into practice and searches for and synthesizes current research on specific topics. A search of the literature suggests that many authors who have published EBP articles have acknowledged receiving assistance from the SCHI. Two examples of those articles are titled *Manual Turns in Patients receiving Mechanical Ventilation*

(Winkelman & Chiang, 2010) and *Group Visits for Chronic Illness Management: Implementation Challenges and Recommendations* (Jones, Kaewluang, & Lekhak, 2014). For more information about the consulting services of SCHI, go to Case Western Reserve University Sarah Cole Hirsh Institute website.

Summary

The term *evidence-based practice* (EBP) originated in the field of medicine. Most people credit the beginning of the movement toward EBP to Archie Cochrane, a British medical researcher and epidemiologist. In 1972, Cochrane published a book titled *Effectiveness and Efficiency: Random Reflections on Health Services.* His book pointed out the lack of solid evidence about the effects of healthcare.

Sackett et al. (1996) initially defined evidence-based medicine as "the conscientious, explicit, and judicious use of current best evidence in making decisions about the care of individual patients" (p. 71). Later, clinical expertise and patient values were included as determinants for EBP clinical decision making.

Sigma Theta Tau International, the Honor Society for Nursing defined EBP as "an integration of the best evidence available, nursing expertise, and the values and preferences of the individuals, families, and communities who are served" (STTI, 2005). Research utilization (RU) should not be confused with EBP. RU is the use of evidence (or results) from a specific research study that focused on one clinical problem. EBP involves using evidence from the synthesis of the best evidence from multiple studies, while considering the patient's circumstances, outcomes management or quality improvement projects, the patient's preferences and the available resources for clinical decision making (Ciliska et al., 2011).

The work of implementing an EBP begins with identifying a clinical problem that suggests there is a better way to provide care that will promote improved health in a cost-effective way. The acronym PICOT is a format for writing a clinical question. After the clinical question is created, a search of the relevant literature is used to assess the evidence that addresses the clinical issue and patient care question. The evidence for practice may be classified as translational research evidence, evidence summaries, and primary evidence.

The Cochrane Collaboration is an international nonprofit organization that supports efforts to make well-informed decisions about healthcare. The main output of the Cochrane Collaboration, the *Cochrane Reviews*, is found in the *Cochrane Database of Systematic Reviews*, which is published electronically as part of the Cochrane Library archives. A systematic review is a rigorous scientific approach that combines results from a group of original research studies and looks at the studies as a whole.

The Agency for Healthcare Research and Quality (AHRQ) is a branch of the U.S. Department of Health and Human Services. In 1997, the AHRQ promoted the idea of evidence-based practices through the leadership of Evidence-Based Practice Centers (EPCs). The EPCs conduct systematic reviews on clinical preventative services, and the results of the reviews are used to make recommendations for use in primary care settings. As of 1998, The USPSTF became responsible for reviewing and rating the recommendations submitted by the EPCs.

In 2010, the Patient Protection and Affordable Care Act (PPACA) directed the Secretary of the HHS to establish a national strategy to improve healthcare delivery services, patient health outcomes, and population health (HHS, 2014). On behalf of the HHS the AHRQ delivered the National Quality Strategy (NQS) publication to Congress in 2011.

The *National Guideline Clearinghouse* (NGC) is an AHRQ-sponsored database of evidence-based clinical practice guidelines and related documents. The National Quality Forum (NQF) is a not-for-profit, nonpartisan, membership-based organization that works to support the AHRQ goals of improving health and healthcare quality through measurement. The NQF works to create **measures** or strategies that show whether the standards for prevention, screening, and managing health conditions are met.

There are an increasing number of evidence-based practice centers in nursing. Three of these centers are: the Academic Center for Evidence-Based Nursing, located at the University of Texas Health Science Center at San Antonio; Joanna Briggs Institute, in Australia; and Sarah Cole Hirsh Institute for Best Nursing Practices Based on Evidence, based at the Case Western Reserve University Frances Payne Bolton School of Nursing in Cleveland, Ohio.

Self-Test

Circle the letter before the best answer.

1. What person or organization is generally credited with starting the movement toward evidence-based practice?
   A. Archie Cochrane
   B. David Sackett
   C. Cochrane Collaboration
   D. Agency for Healthcare Quality and Research
2. Identify the professional role of the person who introduced the concept of using evidence as a basis for practice decisions.
   A. an American Nurse
   B. a British epidemiologist
   C. one of the earliest male nurses
   D. an Australian who started the Cochrane Library
3. Which type of evidence is considered the gold standard for practice decisions?
   A. survey evidence from patients following discharge from the hospital
   B. responses from a patient during his or her history and physical assessment
   C. evidence from randomized clinical trial research studies
   D. evidence from the clinician's clinical experiences
4. Identify which concept within Sigma Theta Tau International's definition of EBP, seems most sensitive to the nurses' role as patient advocate.
   A. the patient's values
   B. the best available evidence
   C. a conscientious use of the best evidence
   D. cost-effectiveness
5. Complete the statement that best describes an evidence-based practice (EBP). An EBP is based on evidence
   A. and changes to practice over time.
   B. from multiple studies that agree with the clinician's expert opinion.
   C. from combinations of research studies and the patient's needs and desires.
   D. from a synthesis of studies and expert decisions that consider the patient's circumstances and values.
6. What is the overall goal of an evidence-based practice for nurses?
   A. to improve patient outcomes with traditional nursing knowledge
   B. to improve the effectiveness of processes and patient outcomes with the introduction of current knowledge into common care decisions
   C. to explore how nursing expertise supports the best healthcare for patients
   D. to introduce the knowledge gained from patient surveys into clinical decision making
7. Identify which two entities recognize EBP in nursing as the best treatment plans for patient care.
   A. Cochrane Library and the National Guideline Clearinghouse
   B. David Sackett and Florence Nightingale
   C. Joint Commission and the American Nurses Credentialing Center
   D. AHRQ and the National Quality Strategy

8. Select the outcome for the following PICOT statement. Among patients with migraine headaches in the emergency room, how does the administration of an opioid medication compared with the administration of music therapy affect patient satisfaction at the time of discharge?
   A. patients with migraine headaches
   B. administration of opioid medication
   C. administration of music therapy
   D. patient satisfaction
9. Select two websites that would provide examples of translational research.
   A. CINAHL and primary research studies
   B. National Guideline Clearinghouse and the Best Practice Information sheets of the JBI
   C. PubMed and the Cochrane Library
   D. PubMed and patient databases
10. The National Quality Forum (NQF) works to create measures that show how standards for prevention, screening, and managing health conditions are met. Which type of measure would help to assess the results of healthcare?
    A. structural
    B. process
    C. outcome
    D. composite

See answers to Self-Test in the Answer Section at the back of the book.

References

Abrahamson, K., DeCrane, S., Mueller, C., & Davila, H. W. (2014). Implementation of a nursing home quality improvement project to reduce resident pain. *Journal of Nursing Care Quality, 0*, 1–8. doi:10.1097/NCQ.0000000000000099

Ciliska, D., DiCenso, A., Melnyk, B., Fineout-Overholt, E., Stetler, C., Cullen, L.,... Newhouse, R. (2011). Models to Guide Implementation of Evidence-Based Practice. In B. Melnyk & Finout-Overhold, E. (Eds.), *Evidence-Based Practice in Nursing & Health Care* (2nd ed., pp. 241–275). Philadelphia: Wolters Kluwer | Lippincott Williams & Wilkins.

Dougherty, L. (2014). (Editorial) Evidence-based practice requires research and data. IV Therapy Supplement. *British Journal of Nursing, 23*, S3. http://info.britishjournalofnursing.com/

Fineout-Overholt, E., & Johnston, L. (2005). Teaching EBP: Asking searchable, answerable clinical questions. *Worldviews on Evidence-Based Nursing, 2*, 157–160. doi:10.1111/j.1741-6787.2005.00032.x

Gillespie, L. D., Robertson, M. C., Gillespie, W. J., Sherrington, C., Gates, S., Clemson, L. M., & Lamb, S. E. (2012). Interventions for preventing falls in older people living in the community. Cochrane Database of Systematic Reviews 2012, Issue 9. Art. No.:CD007146. doi:10.1002/14651858.CD007146.pub2.

Grove, S. K., Burns, N. & Gray, J. R. (2013).*The practice of nursing research: Appraisal, synthesis, and generation of evidence* (7th ed.). China: Elsevier.

Hain, D. J. & Kear, T. M. (2015). Using evidence-based practice to move beyond doing things the way we have always done them. *Nephrology Nursing Journal, 42*, 11–20. https://www.annanurse.org/resources/products/nephrology-nursing-journal

Harris, T. A. (2010). Changing practice to reduce the use of urinary catheters. *Nursing 2010, 40*, 18–20. doi:10.1097/01.NURSE.0000367857.98069.ad.

Jones, K. R., Kaewluang, N., Lekhak, N. (2014). Group visits for chronic illness management: Implementation challenges and recommendations. *Nursing Economic$, 32*(3), 118–147. http://www.nursingeconomics.net/cgi-bin/WebObjects/NECJournal.woa

Melnyk, B. M. & Fineout-Overholt, E. (2011). *Evidence-Based Practice in Nursing & Healthcare: A Guide to Best Practice* (2nd ed.). China: Wolters Kluwer Health | Lippincott Williams & Wilkins.

National Pressure Ulcer Advisory Panel, European Pressure Ulcer Advisory Panel, Pan Pacific Pressure Injury Alliance. (2014). Prevention of pressure ulcers. In *Prevention and treatment of pressure ulcers: Clinical practice guideline* (p. 42–78). Washington, D.C,: National

Pressure Ulcer Advisory Panel. http://www.guideline.gov/content.aspx?id=48864

Poe, S. S. & White, K. M. (2010). *Johns Hopkins nursing evidence-based practice: Implementation and translation.* Indianapolis: Sigma Theta Tau International.

Registered Nurses' Association of Ontario (RNAO). (2013). *Assessment and management of pain.* Toronto: Registered Nurses' Association of Ontario. http://www.guideline.gov/content.aspx?id=47796

Sackett, D. L., Rosenberg, W. M., Gray, J. A., Haynes, R. B., & Richardson, W. S. (1996). Evidence based medicine: What it is and what it isn't. *British Medical Journal, 312,* 71–72. http://dx.doi.org/10.1136/bmj.312.7023.71

Sackett, D. L., Straus, S. E. Richardson, W. S., Rosenberg, W., & Haynes, R. B. (2000). *Evidence-based medicine: How to practice & teach EBM* (2nd ed.). London: Churchill Livingstone.

Schmidt, N. A. & Brown, J. M. (2009). *Evidence-Based Practice for Nurses: Appraisal and Application of Research.* Sudbury, UK: Jones and Bartlett.

Stevens, K. (2013). The impact of evidence-based practice in nursing and the next big ideas. *Online Journal of Issues in Nursing, 18,* 2. doi:10.3912/OJIN.Vol18No02Man04

Stillwell, S. B., Fineout-Overholt, E., Melnyk, B. M., & Williamson, K. M. (2010). Asking the clinical question: A key step in evidence-based practice. *American Journal of Nursing, 110,* 58–61. doi:10.1097/01.NAJ.0000368959.11129.79

Swe, K. K. (2014). Blood pressure: Sodium Chloride (Salt) Intake, 1–3. Joanna Briggs Institute. http://joannabriggs.org/

University of Texas at Austin School of Nursing, Family Nurse Practitioner Program. (2014). Evaluation of vertigo in the adult patient. Austin: University of Texas at Austin, School of Nursing. http://www.guideline.gov/content.aspx?id=48220

U.S. Department of Health and Health Services (HHS). (2014). National Quality Strategy. Better Care. Healthy People/Healthy Communities. Affordable Care. *National Strategy for Quality Improvement in Healthcare 2014 Annual Progress Report to Congress.* http://www.ahrq.gov/workingforquality/reports/annual-reports/nqs2014annlrpt.pdf

Volante, M. (2008). Qualitative research. *Nurse Researcher, 16*(1), 4–6. http://journals.rcni.com/doi/abs/10.7748/nr2004.07.12.1.7.c5927

Winkelman, C. & Chiang, L. (2010) Manual turns in patients receiving mechanical ventilation. *Critical Care Nurse, 30*(4), 36–44. doi:10.4037/ccn2010106

Windle, P. E. (2010). The systematic review process: An overview. *Journal of PeriAnesthesia Nursing, 25,* 40–42. doi:10.1016/j.jopan.2009.12.001

Chapter 3
Research Evidence in Nursing Practice

Catherine Bailey, PhD, RN, and Stephanie Huckaby, MSN, RN

 Objectives

On completion of this chapter, you will be prepared to:

1. Explain how the concept of evidence-based practice (EBP) is evolving in nursing
2. Describe models that promote the implementation of EBP in nursing practice
3. Identify barriers that could challenge the effective implementation of an EBP
4. Incorporate ideas into a plan for facilitating the success of an EBP
5. Develop a plan for implementing an EBP for nurses in a clinical setting

The Evolving Nature of Evidence-Based Practice

With the changes in expectations associated with outcomes among the leaders of healthcare, the definition of evidence-based practice (EBP) for clinical purposes has evolved to include the concepts of quality and efficiency. Thus, Grove, Burns, and Gray (2013) have redefined EBP as the "conscientious integration of best research evidence with clinical expertise and patient values and needs in the delivery of quality, cost effective health care" (p. 17). However, Titler (2014) has warned that an emerging field of research called translation science has been used interchangeably with EBP.

To clarify the differences between EBP and translation science, Titler (2014) defines EBP as the application of "the conscientious and judicious use of current best evidence in conjunction with clinical expertise and patient values to guide health care decisions" (p. 270). However, Titler considers best evidence to include more than the results from randomized controlled clinical trials (as have been promoted by the medical profession), but also descriptive and qualitative research as well as knowledge from case studies and scientific principles. With this understanding in mind, **translation science** is described as "the study of implementation interventions, factors, and contextual variables that affect knowledge uptake and use in practices and communities" (Titler, 2014, p. 270). This description suggests that the implementation of

EBPs is an ongoing process that entails studying the different circumstances that influence the value of the EBP in practices as well in communities. Based on a review of the literature, it could be said that the profession of nursing is *in the process* of using EBP interventions that rest on the best research knowledge available. However, researchers are being called to demonstrate that these interventions are effective in producing the desired outcomes in clinical practice through what is called the application of EBP or **translational research**. These efforts are being supported by a variety of conceptual models that have been introduced to promote an EBP in nursing.

Models to Promote Evidence-Based Practice in Nursing

The Stetler Model of Research Utilization to Facilitate EBP (Stetler Model) (Stetler, 2001) and the Iowa Model of Evidence Based Practice to Promote Quality of Care (Iowa Model) (Titler et al., 2001) are two popular examples of models that have been used to implement evidence-based guidelines in clinical settings. The Stetler Model provides a framework to facilitate the use of research evidence in practice for individual nurses or healthcare institutions. The Iowa Model provides direction for the development of an EBP in a clinical agency with a built-in focus toward informing quality improvement (QI) after the practice is established (Titler et al., 2001; Shirey et al., 2011).

The Stetler Model

The Stetler Model (2001) lists five phases of activities that guide the nurse through the process of implementing EBPs. They include (1) preparation, (2) validation, (3) comparative evaluation and decision making, (4) translation and application, and (5) evaluation. The preparation phase includes the collection of information that provides the reason to change the practice as well as the strength of research evidence that will be used for the anticipated change. The validation phase includes a critical analysis of the research related to the potential practice. The comparative evaluation and decision-making phase deals with the fit of the evidence to the clinical setting, the feasibility of using the research findings, and the decision that a new practice activity would make a positive difference to patient outcomes. The translation and application phase involves the actual implementation of the practice. Finally, the evaluation phase includes both informal and formal evaluations, which could be presented as case studies, audits, and quality assurance or outcomes research projects. The National Collaborating Center for Methods and Tools website provides more information about the Stetler Model.

The Iowa Model

The Iowa Model (Titler et al., 2001) suggests that the implementation of an EBP protocol rests on a continuum of activities that advance from (1) identifying either problem-focused or knowledge-focused triggers; (2) to forming a team; (3) to assembling, synthesizing, and critiquing the research associated with a practice that would provide a solution for the trigger; (4) to piloting the new practice; (5) to evaluating the structure, processes, and outcomes of the practice (with a potential possibility of modifying the practice before it is officially adopted); (6) to disseminating the results; and then (7) to returning to the first steps of identifying triggers that may indicate a need for a revision of the EBP. A visit to the Iowa Model of Evidence Based Practice to Promote Quality of Care at the Iowa University Hospital website will provide much more information on this topic.

Discussion of Iowa Model Concepts

The following section provides a literature-based discussion of some of the concepts described within the Iowa Model. A problem-focused trigger could include information from a clinical problem or data that relates to risk management, process improvement, benchmarking, and financial issues. In order to reduce the incidence of a problem-focused trigger, Harris (2010) described a project to implement a Center for Disease Control and Prevention (CDC) recommendation of an EBP care bundle to reduce catheter-associated urinary tract infections (CAUTIs). The care bundle included a combination of five practice interventions that consisted of (1) toileting dependent and incontinent patients every two hours, (2) inserting only justified urinary catheters, (3) enforcing the use of proper and aseptic techniques for the insertion of catheters, (4) collecting specimens properly, and (5) maintaining the catheters according to CDC guidelines.

Knowledge-focused triggers relate to new research findings or changes in agency standards (such as federal regulations or standards committee decisions). Glowacki (2015) reported on the implementation and evaluation of best practice pain management strategies. This effort was introduced in response to a Joint Commission (JC) requirement to focus on knowledge-based improvements in quality pain management and a Centers for Medicare and Medicaid program that mandated hospitals to participate in public reporting of overall patient satisfaction surveys.

Titler et al. (2001) recommend that the success of the implementation of an EBP depends on a team effort. However, Fisher and Sheeron (2014) believe that it is important to build a cultural environment for the implementation of transferring research evidence into clinical practice before a team can become a sustainable reality. From an organizational perspective an agency could begin by (1) recognizing staff members who actively work toward improving their practice with EBPs on annual nursing performance evaluations, (2) creating a novice-to-expert competency framework for nurses who wish to eventually guide EBP projects, and (3) offering educational opportunities from experts from local universities to help nurses search databases and critique sources of information. For example, journal clubs designed to provide nurses opportunities to discuss articles relevant to clinical practice topics have been shown to help nurses critically appraise those articles (Dovi, 2015).

On the unit level an agency could arrange for time allotments and shared governance committees for nurses who wish to enhance their EBP skills and knowledge and also provide built-in coaching supports with the nurses' daily responsibilities (Fisher & Sheeron, 2014). After a project team is assembled, Spruce (2015) advises that it is important to achieve buy-in from all of the disciplines involved in the practice then (ideally speaking) the team should agree on the scope, aim, and objectives of the anticipated project.

The need to assemble, synthesize, and critique the research that addresses a specific trigger stems from the fact that not all interventions are appropriate for all clinical settings (Titler et al., 2001). The assembled research evidence must be evaluated for its strengths, limitations, and value to the practice setting in terms of expected outcomes (O'Mathuna, Fineout-Overholt, & Johnston (2011). These concerns could also relate to the purpose of the study, the importance of the clinical issue, the reliability of the concepts that were used to measure the effectiveness of an intervention, and the validity of the findings (Makic, Rauen, Jones, & Fisk, 2015). All of these needs suggest that nurses must be active learners with the constantly evolving information that influences the effectiveness of care interventions.

An important consideration for appraising the evidence rests on an understanding about the hierarchy or the level of evidence of the studies. This means that different levels of evidence provide various types of confidence to support the implementation of a particular intervention (O'Mathuna et al., 2011). For example, there is a hierarchy of evidence that ranks the results from a systematic review of randomized controlled trials (RCT) as the highest to the least high level of evidence, which is a consensus opinion. A RCT is the best type of an interventional research design that provides knowledge for a cause-and-effect relationship, while a systematic review of RCTs is a synthesis of a collection of RCT studies with similar interventions (O'Mathuna et al., 2011). Other research designs with lesser strengths of evidence associated with the findings are listed as single comparative experimental or descriptive quantitative designs or those from qualitative research.

Speaking from a critical care nurse's perspective, Makic et al. (2015) believe that nurses need to understand more than just the essential elements of the quality of an EBP. They also need to combine their clinical expertise with their knowledge of a patient's preferences, values, and engagement in care decisions. As discussed earlier, these challenges should also be shared with other experts who are experienced at appraising and synthesizing research findings from the literature.

Theoretically speaking, implementing or piloting research-based evidence into nursing practices promotes high-quality patient care, reduced practice variations, greater patient safety strategies, and reduced healthcare costs (Stephens, 2013; Baird & Miller, 2015). Chambers (2015) claims that this activity should also include plans for sustaining quality improvement efforts for the practice over time. Some factors that support the sustainability of practice innovations include strong leadership, support from stakeholders, nurse champions, and modifiable projects that support the agencies' vision, mission, and goals.

LEADERSHIP RESPONSIBILITIES Leadership responsibilities include (1) aligning the project with the agency's goals, (2) allocating funds for improvement, (3) assigning teams who will assist with staff education and monitoring the processes and outcomes of the project, (4) assigning managers who will inform the unit staff members of quality improvement projects, and (5) appointing frontline managers who will encourage peers to monitor and record unit-based achievements (Chambers, 2015). Key stakeholders are individuals who have a vested interest in new projects and are in positions to affect the project. In healthcare, key stakeholders could be chief nursing officers, chief financial officers, nurse directors, medical directors, staff nurses, support staff, and patients (Chambers, 2015). Nurse champions are individuals who are clinically knowledgeable and committed to improve quality and patient safety within their agency. One responsibility of a nurse champion is to ensure that the EBP becomes deeply rooted in the agency's culture. Prior to the implementation of the pilot of the EBP, the plans for the project should be reviewed by the institutional review board for approval and integrated into the electronic health record for prompts for computerized decision support for clinical care (Makic et al., 2015).

EVALUATION The evaluation of the structure, processes, and outcomes of the EBP provides the developers with evidence to modify the practice before it is adopted throughout the entire agency (Chambers, 2015). This type of plan helps improve both the delivery of care and a longstanding potential of successful outcomes. For example, it is important to identify how the EBP is expected to benefit the facility with the standardized care of patients, its anticipated patient outcomes, and value-based healthcare (Spruce, 2015). Arming healthcare providers with an EBP gives them confidence that they are providing the best healthcare possible, which may also be tied to reimbursement for their performance. Patient-associated benefits of an EBP promote the belief that patients' treatment decisions are based on knowledge associated with what works and does not work. Ultimately, patients will become more informed healthcare consumers about their treatment options.

APPLICATION The EBP should be introduced across all of the applicable areas (Chambers, 2015). As the project evolves, Spruce (2015) recommends that the outcomes should be continually monitored and communicated to the entire team affected by the EBP. This type of planning also supports the suggestion that a review be performed every two years or as needed when the evidence or the practice needs change.

IMPLEMENTATION Finally, it is critical that the outcomes associated with the implementation of EBP initiatives are disseminated or published. It is also important to include the essential elements of the EBP initiative so readers can either replicate the studies or evaluate the findings for their potential use in other settings (Oermann, Turner, & Carman, 2014). Generally, the manuscript should provide the reasons that led to the project, a report on the processes associated with the search, the selection, and critique of the literature, and a report on the evidence-based factors that supported the ultimate clinical decision to implement the EBP with the resulting outcomes. Oermann et al. also believe that the characteristics of the setting (including adopters, stakeholders, implementation, fidelity, and sustainability) and the EBP model that guided the project as well as the PICOT statement should be included. Others recommend that the successes and lessons learned should also be published (Carman et al., 2013).

Barriers Associated with EBP

Although nursing research has generated evidence, there are many barriers associated with the advancement of an EBP in nursing. Understanding these barriers, either real or perceived, to the facilitation or implementation of EBP affects care at all levels of healthcare. Identifying and overcoming these barriers will improve not only nursing education and practices, but also patient outcomes (DeBryun, Ochoa-Marin, & Semenic, 2014). A significant barrier is that there are inadequate numbers of research studies from clinical trials that have compared patient outcomes from new innovative strategies with usual care (Grove et al., 2013). Another concern relates to the fact that most EBP guidelines (sometimes considered the gold standard of care) have been generated from population-based data. This means that some of the guidelines may not be considered practical for many patients who require individualized healthcare plans because of their unique needs.

Although barriers to EBP vary from setting to setting, some may be described from an organizational perspective. Some examples are associated with workloads, management that is not supportive of EBP, lack of resources, lack of authority to change practices, and a workplace culture that is resistant to change (Williams, Perillo, & Brown, 2014). One universal barrier is the complaint of not enough time due to workload issues or time constraints among nurses. Implementing an EBP project can be a lengthy, time-consuming process and during fast-paced, busy shift work, EBP often takes a backseat to the more demanding need for the provision of task-oriented patient cares for a population facing increases in acute illnesses. Understanding and navigating the internal organizational climate of healthcare systems can even be tricky for experienced administrators who also have priorities that compete with the implementation of EBP. Part of these competing priorities could be related to budgetary expenditures and reflected by an inadequate accessibility to current best evidence, journal articles with research reports, or point-of care EBP guidelines (Williams et al.; Grove et al., 2013). Needless to say, organizational support is critical in driving EBP practices down to the staff level.

From the individual nurse's perspective, some barriers could be due to a personal lack of knowledge, such as insufficient skills in finding and reviewing the relevant evidence (Baird & Miller, 2015). Other barriers could include a lack of time to access the new knowledge for practice, a perception that EBP is too time-consuming and burdensome, and resistance to changing practices among coworkers and leaders (Makic, Rauen, Jones, & Fisk, 2015). Barriers may vary according to the ages and experiences of the nurse. For example, a mature nurse, who demonstrates expert nursing skills, may have low computer skills and lack formal EBP knowledge or research training. Other nurses may not find value in taking the time to undertake an EBP project. Unfortunately, the idea of making time and understanding the value of EBP is absolutely critical for nurses who aspire to be leaders and active change agents in the design and delivery of healthcare strategies.

Facilitators of Evidence-Based Practice

Melnyk and Fineout-Overholt (2011) believe that champions at all levels of practice and strategies that support EBP are necessary to facilitate an EBP. Thus, an organizational culture that encourages improved clinical outcomes through the promotion of clinical inquiry and evidence-based changes is an important place to begin (Hall & Roussel, 2014). Some facilitating strategies include: (1) the support and encouragement of EBP projects from the leadership, (2) the sponsorship of relationships with mentors with excellent EBP skills, (3) the promotion of the use of the proper tools, such as computer-based best practice guidelines at the point of care, (4) the implementation of evidence-based clinical policies and procedures, and (5) the establishment of journal clubs (Melnyk & Fineout-Overholt, 2011).

Tapping into a nurse's expressed desire to participate in an EBP project can be viewed as an opportunity for administrators to facilitate EBP. By aligning the nurse's professional goals with those of the skills necessary for the advancement of EBP, the nurse could be introduced to doing systematic reviews of the literature and project management skills. As nurses become more skilled in the implementation of EBPs and recognized as nurse champions, they will realize that their activities have served as career-building opportunities.

Another strategy that has shown to facilitate an EBP within hospital departments of nursing has been the creation of committees or councils that focus primarily on nurse-led research and EBP. According to Giomuso et al. (2014), the committee should be comprised of members who can help facilitate and translate EBP into practice. To impact nursing at the bedside the committee should also be composed of frontline staff who have expressed a desire to participate in the committee and agreed to be the nurse champion for their departments. The additional provision of freeing up time for the members to participate in EBP and mentoring other nurses is essential to the success of these groups.

Providing resources to the nursing staff is another important piece of facilitation within a hospital setting. One such resource includes providing the services of a librarian who can assist with the acquisition of relevant literature from dedicated nursing databases. Budgeting and allotting times when frontline staff can work to become mentors and work on EBP projects is a key to eliminate the barrier of time constraints. Offering EBP training classes in traditional classroom settings or during unit-based shift changes or staff meetings helps reduce some of the anxiety frequently associated with taking on a new EBP project.

A work environment that encourages bedside providers to participate in journal clubs or independent article reviews of current literature tends to stimulate thought and questions about current practices. In one case, a nurse's review of an article at the end of a staff meeting led to a change in care delivery for the entire hospital system. After the nurse presented the latest American Society for Parenteral and Enteral Nutrition (A.S.P.E.N.) guidelines related to recommendations for enteral feedings, the staff realized that there were disparities between their practice and those of the recommended guidelines. This knowledge-based trigger eventually led to a hospital-wide policy change that reflected the recommendations of the guidelines. The nurse in this case demonstrated how one who succeeded in developing a skill set for EBP could also contribute to the overall nursing care and improvement in patient care.

Building partnerships and affiliations with schools of nursing can further enhance and support the nurse-led EBP and research within a hospital. The goal in forming these alliances is to provide support in an institution that may not have internal resources to support and mentor the nursing staff in the practice environment. Schools of nursing have professors who can partner with councils and committees to support the nursing staff and serve as mentors or EBP facilitators. These facilitators can be available to evaluate the current support structures and help the nurses to find, evaluate, and apply new evidence into practice. The benefits for both parties can be a partnership to further develop and implement research into a practice setting and the knowledge sharing can help to enhance the EBP capacity within a hospital.

Application of the Iowa Model

Policies and procedures in hospitals are examples of action plans that address concerns for daily nursing practice; however, those practices must evolve to reflect current knowledge. As nurses are responsible for providing quality healthcare within a safe environment, nurses must remain current with evidence-based practices (Blankenship, Lucas, & Sayre, 2013). The following discussion describes how Blankenship et al. reported on the creation of a seven-step process entitled Policy Development Seven (PD7) to construct a new policy.

Many of the steps of this project were similar to those described in the Iowa Model. For example, step one occurred following an encounter with an unfamiliar patient situation that lacked a procedural policy for care. Blankenship et al. (2013) gave the committee that reviews hospital policies a detailed explanation of the concerns and requested the resources necessary to develop a new EBP policy. Step two was dedicated to establishing a team approach with a clear description of role expectations that included key stakeholders to ensure the policy fit within the organization. Step three included searching databases that were popular with nurses (Cumulative Index of Nursing and Allied Health Literature [CINAHL], MEDLINE, the Education Resources Information Center, and PsychINFO), clinical practice guidelines, and information from a leading professional authority, the Association of Critical Care Nurses. They also reviewed their state practice act for limitations, compared policies from other hospitals, and polled their own hospital's preceptor committee (Blankenship et al., 2013).

Step four of the project entailed a review of the existing policy and brainstorming sessions with the planning team. The team used a conference room where they projected their typed suggestions onto a monitor then emailed themselves the results immediately after the meeting (Blankenship et al., 2013). Step five was dedicated to consulting with experts who helped transform a rough draft of the new policy into a workable plan for practice. Step six included submission of the final policy with references to the adult practice council of their hospital for approval and also to everyone who might have been affected by the policy. The seventh and final step of the project included educating the staff with hospital intranet to the human resources department so that the policy would be included in monthly education and leadership meetings. Those who were to be directly affected by the policy received hands-on information and experienced practice on the unit as well as during mandatory annual skills day.

Summary

The definition of evidence-based practice (EBP) for clinical purposes has evolved to include the concepts of quality and efficiency. Grove, Burns, and Gray (2013) have redefined EBP as the "conscientious integration of best research evidence with clinical expertise and patient values and needs in the delivery of quality, cost effective health care." Titler (2014) defines EBP as the application of "the conscientious and judicious use of current best evidence in conjunction with clinical expertise and patient values to guide health care decisions." Titler (2014) describes translation science as "the study of implementation interventions, factors, and contextual variables that affect knowledge uptake and use in practices and communities." This description suggests that the implementation of EBPs is an ongoing process that entails studying the different circumstances that influence the value of the EBP in practices.

The Stetler Model of Research Utilization to Facilitate EBP (Stetler Model) and the Iowa Model of Evidence Based Practice to Promote Quality of Care (Iowa Model) are two popular examples of models that have been used to implement evidence-based guidelines in clinical settings. Although nursing research has generated evidence, there are many barriers associated with the advancement of an EBP in nursing. Some examples are associated with workloads, management that is not supportive of EBP, lack of resources, lack of authority to change practices, and workplace culture that is resistant to change.

Some facilitating strategies for EBP include: (1) the support and encouragement of EBP projects from the leadership, (2) the sponsorship of relationships with mentors with excellent EBP skills, (3) the promotion of the use of the proper tools, such as computer-based best practice guidelines at the point of care, (4) the implementation of evidence-based clinical policies and procedures, and (5) the establishment of journal clubs. Policies and procedures in hospitals are examples of action plans that address concerns for daily nursing practice; however, those practices must evolve to reflect current knowledge. As nurses are responsible for providing quality healthcare within a safe environment, nurses must remain current with evidence-based practices.

Self-Test

Select the best answer to the following multiple choice questions:

1. Which concepts have been responsible for revisions in the definitions of EBP?
   A. evaluation of the process and structure of an EBP
   B. cost-efficiency and quality of healthcare
   C. concerns about the patient and family desires
   D. promotion of outcomes related to hierarchy of evidence
2. Other than RCTs, what other type of research evidence should nurses consider for an EBP for clinical decisions?
   A. qualitative
   B. expert opinions
   C. cost-containment data
   D. traditional preferences
3. What is an example of a knowledge-focused trigger for a change to clinical practice?
   A. persistent incidence of pressure sores among hospitalized elderly patients
   B. increases in complaints among patients with urinary retention
   C. a Medicare-based refusal to reimburse for catheter-associated urinary tract infections care
   D. high incidence of fall rates among patients on antihypertensive medications
4. What is an example of a problem-focused trigger for a change to clinical practice?
   A. HIPPA regulation to keep patient data secure from computer hackers
   B. Medicaid and Medicare decision to collect patient satisfaction data
   C. increasing incidence of ventilator-associated pneumonia
   D. Center for Disease Control and Prevention regulation to follow hand-washing guidelines
5. Building a team to effectively implement a sustainable EBP should be supported by
   A. an organizational culture for EBP.
   B. individuals who enjoy utilizing research findings.
   C. leaders who are experienced at implementing EBP.
   D. stakeholders who enjoy the benefits of EBP.
6. Which of the following would not be included as a benefit for implementing an EBP?
   A. high-quality patient care
   B. less variation in practice standards
   C. introduction of a newly patented device
   D. reduced healthcare costs
7. Which type of evidence is most often considered as the highest of the hierarchy of evidence for practice decisions?
   A. meta-analysis of multiple randomized clinical trials
   B. a single well-controlled experimental study
   C. consensus of opinion from a group of experts on the topic
   D. case-control studies
8. Care bundles have been used
   A. to reduce a problem-focused trigger
   B. most often in critical care units.
   C. only in pilot studies.
   D. in emergency rooms.

9. Why are inadequate numbers of research studies considered to be a barrier to EBP?
   A. There are not enough literature reviews that explain the existence of specific disorders.
   B. Not enough studies have compared innovative strategies with usual care for patients.
   C. Epidemiological databases do not reflect that the intended EBP is important.
   D. There are no case studies about the problem in the literature.
10. Why could there be resistance or barriers associated with the implementation of some clinical guidelines (CGs)?
    A. CGs may fail to consider unique patient needs
    B. CGs could be based on old research studies.
    C. CGs are not examples of quality healthcare interventions.
    D. CGs are never challenged.
11. How could a librarian facilitate a committee that wishes to develop an EBP? A librarian could
    A. interpret the research literature for the sake of future publications.
    B. help access the research articles that the committee wishes to critique.
    C. create outlines for possible plans for the EBP.
    D. provide a rubric for evaluating the evidence for the EBP.
12. How could professors from schools of nursing assist as facilitators of EBP in clinical settings? Professors
    A. can function as mentors to practice-based nurses for EBP projects.
    B. can establish the budgets for the resources that will facilitate EBP projects.
    C. can make recommendations about the vision, mission, and goal of the agency.
    D. are necessary contributors for the agency-based journal clubs.

See answers to Self-Test in the Answer Section at the back of the book.

References

Baird, L. M. & Miller, T. (2015). Factors influencing evidence-based practice for community nurses. *British Journal of Community Nursing, 20*(5), 233–242. doi:10.12968/bjcn.2015. 20.5.233

Blankenship, S., Lucas, A., & Sayre, S. (2013). Anatomy of an evidence-based policy. *Nursing, 43*(6), 1–5. doi:10.1097/01.NURSE.0000429799.26483.64

Carman, M. J., Wolf, L. A., Baker, K. M., Clark, P. R., Henderson, D. Manton, A., & Zavotshi, K. E. (2013). Translating research to practice: Bringing emergency nursing research full circle to the bedside. *Emergency Nurses Association, 39*, 657–659. http://dx.doi.org/10.1016/j.jen.2013.09.004

Chambers, L. L. (2015). Factors for sustainability of evidence-based practice innovations: Part 1. *Research and Theory for Nursing Practice, 29*(2), 89–93. http://www.springerpub.com/research-and-theory-for-nursing-practice.html

DeBruyn, R. R., Ochoa-Marin, S. C., & Semenic, S. (2014). Barriers and facilitators to evidence-based nursing in Colombia: Perspectives of nurse educators, nurse researchers and graduate students. *Investigacion & Educacion En Enfermeria, 32*(1), 9–21. doi:10.1590/S0120-53072014000100002

Dovi, G. (2015). Empowering change with traditional or virtual journal clubs. *Nursing Management*, 47–50. http://journals.lww.com/nursingmanagement/pages/default.aspx

Duffy, J. R., Culp, S., Yarberry, C., Stroupe, L., Sand-Jecklin, K., & Coburn, A. S. (2015). Nurses' research capacity and use of evidence in acute care: Baseline findings from a partnership study. *Nursing Administration, 45*(3), 158–164. doi:10.1097/NNA.000000000000176

Fisher, C. A., & Sheeron, J. (2014). Creating a culture of EBP: What's a manager to do? *Nursing Management, 45*(10), 21–23. http://journals.lww.com/nursingmanagement/pages/default.aspx

Giomuso, C., Chandler, T., Pulphus, D., Jones, L., Kresevic, D., Williams, T. & Long, D. (2014). A successful approach to implementing evidence-based practice. *Academy of Medical-Surgical Nursing, 23*(4), 4–9. http://www.prolibraries.com/amsn/?

Glowacki, D. (2015). Effective pain management and improvements in patients' outcomes and satisfaction. *Critical Care Nurse, 35*(3), 33–43. doi:http://org/org/10.4037/ccn2015440

Grove, S. K., Burns, N. & Gray, J. R. (2013). *The practice of nursing research: Appraisal, synthesis, and generation of evidence* (7th ed.). China: Elsevier.

Hall, H. R., & Roussel, L. A. (2014). Evidence-based practice: An integrative approach to research, administration, and practice. Burlington, MA: Jones and Bartlett.

Harris, T. A. (2010). Changing practice to reduce the use of urinary catheters. *Nursing 2010, 40*(2), 18–20. doi:10.1097/01.NURSE.0000367857.98069.ad

Makic, M. B., Rauen, C., Jones, K., & Fisk, A. C. (2015). Continuing to challenge practice to be evidence based. *Critical Care Nurse, 35*(2), 39–50. doi:http://dx.doi.org/10.4037/cnn2015693

Oermann, M. H., Turner, K. & Carman, M. (2014). Preparing quality improvement, research, and evidence-based practice manuscripts. *Urologic Nursing, 34*(3), 113–119. https://www.suna.org/unj

O'Mathuna, D. O., Fineout-Overholt, E., & Johnson, L. (2011). Critically appraising quantitative evidence for clinical decision making. In B. Melnyk & Fineout-Overholt, E. (Eds.), *Evidence-based practice in nursing and healthcare: A guide to best practice* (pp. 81–134). Philadelphia: Wolters Kluwer | Lippincott Williams & Wilkins.

Shirey, M. R., Hauck, S. L., Embree, J. L., Kinner, T. J., Schaar, G. L., Phillips, L. A., Ashby, S. R., . . . McCool, I. A. (2011). Showcasing differences between quality improvement, evidence-based practice, and research. *Continuing Education in Nursing, 42*(2), 57–68. doi:10.3928/00220124-20100701-01

Spruce, L. (2015). Back to basics: Implementing evidence-based practice. *Association of Operating Room Nurses, 101*(1), 107–106. http://dx.doi.org/10.1016j.aorn.2014.08.009

Stevens, K. (2013). The impact of evidence-based practice in nursing and the next big ideas. *Online Journal of Issues in Nursing, 18*, 2. doi:10.3912/OJIN.Vol18No02Man04

Stetler, C. B. (2001). Updating the Stetler model of research utilization to facilitate evidence-based practice. *Nursing Outlook, 49*(6), 272–279. http://dx.doi.org/10.1067/mno.2001.120517

Titler, M. (2014). Overview of evidence-based practice and translation science. *Nursing Clinics of North America, 49*, 269–274. http://dx.doi.org/10.1016/j.cnur.2014.05.001

Titler, M. G., Kleiber, C., Steelman, V., Rakel, B., Budreau, G., Everett, L. Q., . . . Goode. C. (2001). The Iowa model of evidence-based practice to promote quality care. *Critical Care Nursing Clinics of North America, 13*, 497–509. http://www.ccnursing.theclinics.com/

Williams, B., Perillo, S., & Brown, T. (2014). What are the factors of organizational culture in health care settings that act as barriers to the implementation of evidence-based practice? *Nurse Education Today, 35*, e34–e41. http://dx.doi.org/10.1016/j.nedt.2014.11.012

Chapter 4
Ethical Issues in Nursing Research

Rose Nieswiadomy, PhD, RN, and Catherine Bailey, PhD, RN

Objectives

On completion of this chapter, you will be prepared to:

1. Summarize the development of ethical codes and guidelines.
2. Describe the role of institutional review boards.
3. Cite examples for the elements of informed consent.
4. Discuss how integrity in research is promoted.
5. Analyze issues that threaten integrity in research among nurse researchers.
6. Explain the role of the nurse researcher as a patient advocate.

Development of Ethical Codes and Guidelines

The ethical aspects of a proposed research study take precedence over any other areas of the study. The rights of study participants must be protected in all research studies. Why, then, can everyone reading this book probably recall hearing about some unethical research?

Historical Overview

During 1942 and 1943, World War II prisoners' wounds were deliberately infected with bacteria. Infection was caused by forcing wood shavings and ground glass into the wounds. Sulfanilamide was then given to these prisoners to determine the effectiveness of this drug. Some subjects died, and others suffered serious injury. The so-called subjects for these experiments were prisoners in the German concentration camps. Many nurses participated in these unethical experiments; others found ways to avoid participation, such as becoming pregnant or asking for transfers to other assignments (Bonifazi, 2004).

Between June and September 1944, photographs and body measurements were taken of 112 Jewish prisoners. They were then killed, and their skeletons defleshed. One purpose of this study was to determine if photographs from live human beings could be used to predict skeletal size. The skeleton collection was to be displayed at the Reich University of Strasbourg (Nuremberg Military Tribunals, 1949). As other atrocities committed for the sake of research are too numerous and gruesome to list here, a more detailed record of these studies may be found by searching *Nuremberg Trials* from the home page of the Military Legal Resources in the Archives of the U.S. Library of Congress website.

How could such atrocities be committed in the name of science? Some of these studies were based on the rationale that the victims were not "real" people like the Germans. During that time in history, the leadership of the Third Reich viewed the German race as superior, and it was believed that this race would one day rule the world.

Widespread knowledge about unethical research conducted in Germany was obtained immediately after World War II. However, it was not until the early 1980s that the public became informed about the atrocities committed in Japan during that same period. It appears that a conspiracy between U.S. government leaders and the Japanese may have prevented this material from being made public (Shearer, 1982). To obtain the results of the Japanese experiments, immunity was granted to Shiro Ishii, commander of the Japanese biological warfare unit, and his subordinates. The silence was first broken in 1975 when a Japanese film producer, Haruko Yoshinaga, tracked down 35 people involved in the incidents. Japanese and American writers then began demanding information from the Pentagon under the Freedom of Information Act. Shearer revealed some of these horrible experiments:

1. Infecting women prisoners with syphilis, having them impregnated by male prisoners, then dissecting the live babies and mothers.
2. Draining the blood from prisoners' veins and substituting horse blood.
3. Exploding gas gangrene bombs next to prisoners tied to stakes.
4. Vivisecting prisoners to compile data on the human endurance of pain (p. 10).

In 1995, six former members of the Japanese biological warfare unit published a book, *The Truth about Unit 731*, to tell about the atrocities that they had seen or heard about (Japanese Book Details Scientific Atrocities, 1996).

Unethical Research in the United States

Because the United States has a strong Judeo-Christian background, it may seem unlikely that such heinous research could ever be conducted in this country. However, the following examples of research were, in fact, carried out in the United States.

One of the most widely known unethical studies was carried out in 1932 in Macon County, Alabama, by the U.S. Public Health Service. The study was titled "Tuskegee Study of Untreated Syphilis in the Negro Male." Of the 600 black male subjects, 399 had syphilis, and 201 did not have the disease. Subjects with active cases were given *no* treatment. Although all of the subjects were given free medical exams, free meals, and burial expenses, they were not told about the purpose of the study (Centers for Disease Control and Prevention [CDC], 2010). Even after penicillin was accepted as the treatment of choice for syphilis in 1945, subjects were still given no treatment. This unethical study became common knowledge 40 years after it was begun. On May 16, 1997, President Bill Clinton made a public apology on behalf of the nation. More about this study may be reviewed at the CDC website on the Tuskegee home page.

From 1963 to 1966, a group of children diagnosed with mental retardation were deliberately injected with the hepatitis virus in Willowbrook State Hospital on Staten Island, New York (Krugman, Giles, &

Hammond, 1971). The researchers defended the project by proposing that the vast majority of the children would acquire the infection anyway while at Willowbrook and that it would be better for them to acquire the disease under carefully controlled conditions. They then tried to treat them with gamma globulin antibodies. In order to learn more about this topic enter the search criteria *Willowbrook Hepatitis Study* in your internet browser.

In July 1963, doctors at the Jewish Chronic Disease Hospital in Brooklyn, New York, injected live cancer cells into 22 elderly patients. The study was designed to measure patients' ability to reject foreign cells. The patients were told that they were being given skin tests (Katz, 1972).

Ethical Research Guidelines

The need for ethical research guidelines becomes clear after reading accounts of unethical research projects. The development of appropriate guidelines is not simple. Ethics is concerned with rules and principles of human behavior. As human behavior is very complex, rules to govern the actions of human beings are difficult to formulate. Studies of recorded history show that people have always been interested in this topic. The biblical Ten Commandments are an example of a code of conduct that has endured through the centuries. Ethical principles frequently change with time and the development of new knowledge.

FOUNDING PRINCIPLES OF ETHICAL RESEARCH The present ethical standards used in nursing research, and in research conducted by other disciplines, are based on the guidelines developed after World War II. The atrocities committed in the German prison camps led to the Nuremberg Trials after the war. The 1947 Nuremberg Code resulted from the revelations of unethical human behavior that occurred during the war (Nuremberg Military Tribunals, 1949). This code seeks to ensure that several criteria for research are met, including the following:

1. Potential subjects must be informed about the study.
2. The research must be for the good of society.
3. Animal research should precede research on humans, if possible.
4. An attempt must be made by the researcher to avoid injury to research subjects.
5. The researcher must be qualified to conduct research.
6. Subjects or the researcher can stop the study if problems occur.

Many other ethical codes have been developed since the Nuremberg Code. On December 10, 1948, the General Assembly of the United Nations adopted the Universal Declaration of Human Rights. The full text of this document is available on the United Nations website under the title *Universal Declaration of Human Rights*.

The World Medical Association (WMA) adopted the Declaration of Helsinki Ethical Principles for Medical Research Involving Human Subjects during its General Assembly in Helsinki, Finland, in 1964. Revised several times, the latest revision was amended in 2013. This information may be found at the WMA website.

In 1978, the National Commission for the Protection of Human Subjects of Biomedical and Behavioral Research was formed. The goals of this commission were to (a) identify basic ethical principles that should guide the conduct of research involving human subjects, and (b) develop guidelines based on principles that had been identified. The report published by this commission in 1979 was titled the *Belmont Report* and named after the Belmont Conference Center where the document was drafted. The full text of this document is located at the U.S. Department of Health and Human Services (DHHS) website. The *Belmont Report* identified basic principles related to research subjects and how the principles to conduct research lead to considerations associated with informed consent of the participant, a risk/benefit assessment of the study, and the selection of the subjects of research. The three basic principles related to research subjects are:

1. *Respect for Persons.* Research subjects should have autonomy and self-determination.
2. *Beneficence.* Research subjects should be protected from harm.
3. *Justice.* Research subjects should receive fair treatment.

The U.S. Department of Health, Education and Welfare (HEW), now the DHHS, published general guidelines for research in 1981. The guidelines evolved into the Federal Policy for the Protection of Human Subjects or the "Common Rule" and then became codified in the Code of Federal Regulations (CFR) 45 Part 46. This CFR addresses the basic DHHS Policy as well as additional protections for pregnant women, human fetuses, neonates, children, and prisoners involved in research. Any institution that receives federal money for research must abide by the DHHS guidelines or risk losing federal money. The Office of Human Research and Protections (OHRP) operates under the authority of the DHHS and assists the research community in conducting ethical research that is in agreement with federal policy. On a local level, an institutional review board (IRB) or committee performs an ethical review of the proposed research studies. More information about this topic may be found at the home page of the OHRP, which is located at the DHHS website.

As most of you know, research has been conducted most often on men. This practice cannot continue. In the past, women typically were not included in research. Public Law 103-4, passed in 1993, requires that researchers recruit women and minorities for their studies. Consequently, the NIH now requires women and members of minorities to be included in federally funded research unless there is a compelling reason to exclude them based on threats to their health or the purposes of the research (Committee on Ethics, 2015). Despite the fact that there have been ethical concerns about research among fertile women, the committee-based representatives of the American College of Obstetricians and Gynecologists (ACOG) concluded that the potential for pregnancy should not automatically exclude a woman from participating in a study (Committee on Ethics, 2015). They remarked that the fact that men and women have biologic differences suggests that the findings of studies that have been generated from male-only studies might not be appropriately generalizable to women.

Institutional Review Boards

An **institutional review board** (IRB) is an administrative body that is established to review and approve research that is intended to study human subjects under the auspices of the institution with which the board is affiliated. According to federal policy, research is defined as "a systematic investigation, including research development, testing and evaluation, designed to develop or contribute to generalizable knowledge" (DHHS, 2009, 45 CFR 46.102d). Human subjects are defined as "living individual(s) about whom an investigator conducting research obtains (1) data through intervention or interaction with the individual, or (2) identifiable private information" (DHHS, 2009, 45 CFR 46.102f).

Note that the use of the term research *subjects* is decreasing. In today's literature, you may see the terms *participants, respondents*, and *informants*. The term *subject* is still used often in this text because it remains prominent in the literature. Also, subjects' rights is a very important issue. (The term *informants' rights* just does not seem to carry the same meaning. An informant sounds more like someone who is providing information to the police department.)

For the sake of discussions in this text, the term *human subjects* may be used interchangeably with the term *participants*.

It is also appropriate to note here that an investigative plan that does not fit the definition of research with human subjects may not need to be submitted for IRB review. One contested example of this notion relates to quality improvement (QI) initiatives that focus on ongoing and iterative efforts to provide the delivery of efficient and safe patient care in clinical settings (Ogrinc, Nelson, Adams, & O'Hara, 2013). Our current scope does not allow a detailed discussion on the differences between QI and clinical research with human subjects. However, Ogrinc et al. (2013) have developed an instrument that provides a way to compare and contrast the general attributes of each type of research activity for IRB review purposes. Some attributes associated with QI relate to (a) improvements in healthcare that are not consistently being implemented at a specific site, (b) plans for interventions and analysis within a specific system, (c) specifying a potential local institutional benefit, (d) risks that are limited to privacy or confidentiality of health information and not physical or psychological harm, and (e) system-level outcomes that are specific to the setting (Ogrinc et al., 2013).

Some attributes associated with clinical research with human subjects relate to a focus on (a) a proposal to develop new knowledge, (b) a plan for a protocol or intervention that is specifically defined and that may provoke minimal physical, psychological, or emotional risk as well as risk of confidentiality to the participants, (c) an analysis that depends on a comparison between the participants in the study, (d) a potential benefit to society in general, (e) an intervention that can inform future practices, and (f) results to be published through a peer-reviewed process (Ogrinc et al., 2013).

Members of Institutional Review Boards

According to federal regulations, each IRB should have at least five members whose backgrounds support an adequate review of the types of research activities usually conducted by the institution (DHHS, 2009). The IRB should be qualified through the expertise of its members, while considering race, gender, and cultural backgrounds to such issues as community attitudes, to promote respect for its counsel in safeguarding the rights and welfare of human subjects. If an IRB regularly reviews research studies that involve a vulnerable category of subjects, such as children, pregnant women, prisoners, or mentally disabled persons, one or more individuals who are experienced in working with these subjects should also be included in the membership.

Other membership-related regulations state the following: (a) no IRB may consist entirely of members of one profession, (b) at least one member must have primary concerns in scientific areas, (c) at least one member must have primary concerns in nonscientific areas, and (d) there should be at least one member who is not affiliated with the institution of record. For a more detailed review of the regulations associated with IRB membership and its functions, access the DHHS website for the Code of Federal Regulations for Protection of Human Subjects. You may also access the National Institute of Health (NIH) Office of Extramural Research website for a computer-based training module to learn how to protect human research participants.

IRB Review

IRB approval is a necessity for investigators who wish to do research with human subjects. The type of IRB review depends on the anticipated risk of potential harm to the human subjects during the research study. An IRB review may be identified as exempt, expedited, or a full review (DHHS, 2009). A research study could be identified as exempt from requiring IRB review when educational testing or survey procedures do not link the subjects' responses with their identities and the disclosure of their data could not reasonably place the subjects at risk of harm. An example of research that is exempt from the regulations that require IRB oversight could be a survey that asks the respondents to anonymously respond to questions about attitudes or opinions about some nonsensitive topic (DHHS, 2009).

An expedited review would include a research study protocol that might cause minimal risk to a participant who may identify one's self while responding to survey questions that may relate to somewhat sensitive material. An example of a study that qualifies for an expedited review could be a study that examines how a participant responds to a specific type of exercise to strengthen muscles. Finally, a full review with a quorum of the IRB voting for approval of the study would be expected for a research study that involves more than minimal risks to the participant. This type of IRB review would be necessary if the study included members from a vulnerable population such as pregnant women, children, fetuses, and infants.

Elements of Informed Consent

The principal means for ensuring that the rights of research participants are protected is through the process of informed consent. **Informed consent** concerns a participant's participation in research in which they have full understanding of the study before the study begins. Generally speaking, the following basic elements should be addressed within the informed consent. A more comprehensive explanation of this topic can be reviewed in 45 CFR Part 46 at the DHHS website. The basic elements of informed consent should include the following:

1. A statement that the study involves research with an explanation of the purposes of the research, a description of the procedures to be implemented, and the duration of the participant's activities
2. A description of any foreseeable risks or discomforts
3. A description of any benefits to the subject or to others
4. A disclosure of appropriate alternative procedures that might help the participant, in the case of a study with therapeutic interventions
5. A statement describing how confidentiality of the participant's records will be maintained
6. An explanation of how unforeseeable injuries will be handled
7. An explanation of whom to contact for answers to questions relevant to the study
8. A statement that participation is voluntary and that refusal to participate or the prerogative to withdraw from the study will be assured without negative consequences at any time.

Description of Purpose of Study and Study Procedures

While informing the participant of the purpose or the objectives of the study, the researcher should clearly present the information and all printed material in the participant's language and reading level. It is not always necessary, however, to describe the entire nature of the study. For example, if a study were being conducted to determine the difference between patients' satisfaction with nursing care given under a primary nursing or team nursing approach, subjects might be told that the study was examining patients' satisfaction with the type of nursing care that they were receiving. It would not be necessary to explicitly describe "primary nursing" to the potential participants. Ask yourself what information you would want to receive, or would want a close relative to receive, to make an informed decision about participation in a study.

All aspects of the study should be fully explained. This includes telling the potential participants when and where the study will take place. The researcher must emphasize the participant's time involvement and all activities that the subjects must perform. This part of informed consent is particularly important in experimental studies in which people will receive some type of treatment. Sometimes a so-called cover story is presented to participants rather than the true explanation of the study. Deliberate deception of this sort is unethical. Even if participants are later told of the deception, the use of false information is unethical.

Many researchers prefer not to conduct studies in which the researcher is not completely candid with subjects before the beginning of the study. Under these circumstances, subjects have the right to be fully informed at the conclusion of the study during debriefing, and to be given an opportunity to withdraw consent for their data to be included in the study results. **Debriefing** involves a meeting with research participants that ensures their understanding of the reasons and justification for the procedures that were used in the study.

Description of Unforeseeable Risks

It is the researcher's responsibility to ensure that no more than minimal risks are involved in the study. This also means the investigator is obligated to try to identify all possible risks or discomforts (either physical or psychological) that would surely influence the participant's decision to participate. Any invasion of privacy must also be discussed. It is difficult at times for the researcher to identify all of the potential risk factors because of the variations in human responses to different situations. Many questions arise about what constitutes a risk. If a study is being conducted with healthy volunteers who will perform mild exercise, should these subjects be informed explicitly that they could experience a heart attack or a stroke during the exercise? The researcher might scare off all prospective subjects. Consultation with experts in the research area should be held and then discretion exercised in presenting risks to potential subjects. One of the roles of IRBs is to assess the adequacy of consent forms.

Description of Benefits

The Nuremberg Code set the requirement that research must be for the good of society. All research, even basic research that is conducted primarily to obtain new knowledge, must have the potential to benefit society. In describing benefits to potential subjects, the investigator should describe both those applicable to the people involved in the study as well as how the results could benefit others. In a study involving the use of play therapy before physical examinations of preschool children, the mothers of the potential subjects were told that the potential benefits included possible reductions in anxiety of the children during the physical examinations, better cooperation during the procedures, and, therefore, more accurate results from the examinations (Simpson, 1985). Mothers also were told that these results would help nurses in the future to better prepare preschool children for physical examinations.

Monetary compensation, or any other type of compensation, should be described to potential subjects. Any time compensation is being provided in a study, the possibility exists that biased results may be obtained. Participants may try to perform in a manner that they believe will fulfill the researcher's expectations. Nevertheless, researchers frequently use small monetary incentives as enticements for potential subjects. One good example of this is seen in the various types of market research that are conducted around the United States. To control for biased responses, participants are usually not told which of the comparison products is the focus of the study. In nursing research, the researcher should avoid monetary compensation, if possible. Participant compensation should come from those items listed under potential benefits. However, it is acceptable for the researcher to cover the cost of such items as laboratory tests and travel expenses for the participants.

Disclosure of Appropriate Alternative Procedures

Potential subjects should be informed of any alternative procedures that may be followed, such as "You may fill out the questionnaire here or take it home." More important, they must be given an explanation of alternative procedures or treatments that may be received by others in the study. For example, a control group of subjects in an experimental study must be made aware that other subjects will be receiving some type of treatment. If potential subjects have a choice of groups, this option must be presented to them.

The **Hawthorne effect** is a phenomenon that brings about changes in subjects because they are aware that they are participants in a study. For this reason, it is becoming increasingly common to provide some type of alternative activity for the control group to make them feel they are actually study participants. Frequently, as part of the explanation given before the study, the researcher tells the control group that the experimental treatment will be available to them on completion of the study. If the control group is really a comparison group, in that these subjects are receiving some alternative or routine treatment, the subjects in the experimental group could also be offered this alternative or routine treatment at the conclusion of the study.

Description of Maintenance of Confidentiality or Anonymity

Anonymity occurs when no one, including the researcher, can link subjects with the data they provide. If subjects can be linked to data, the researcher has the obligation to address confidentiality. **Confidentiality** involves protection of the subjects' identities by the researcher. In many studies, it is not possible to maintain anonymity. The researcher will usually come face to face with subjects in an experimental study. To maintain confidentiality, data are coded and subjects' names and code numbers are kept in a separate location that is accessible only to the researcher or members of the research team. Any list that links subject names with data should be destroyed at the conclusion of the study.

To assure anonymity or confidentiality, subjects and the site where the study was conducted should be described in general terms in the description of the sample and the setting. If either the subjects or the study location can be identified by this general description, confidentiality has been violated. For example, the setting might be identified as a 1000-bed psychiatric institution in a small southwestern city. If there is only one such institution in that area, you have identified the institution as surely as if you had included the name. The identities of hospitals, schools, and other institutions should be kept confidential unless these agencies have given permission to be identified in the study.

Confidentiality can be assured by the deletion of any identifying information that would allow subject identification. Subjects should always be assured that they are free to omit information from their responses if they believe the data will identify them in any way. If subjects are being assured of anonymity, which is frequently done in survey research, instructions should clearly inform subjects to refrain from including their names or other identifying information on the questionnaires.

Plans for Unforeseeable Injuries

For research that involves more than minimal risk, there should be an explanation of what the participant would expect if an injury related to the study occurs. This type of information would include whether or not the participant would be entitled to monetary compensation or medical treatments. The extent of compensation and medical treatments should also be identified.

Contact Information for Questions Relevant to the Study

Prior to receiving informed consent it is important for researchers to identify themselves and describe their qualifications to conduct the study. If a sponsor or sponsoring agency is involved, subjects should be given this information. Frequently, a sentence will be included in the study explanation such as: "I am a nursing student at _____ University and am conducting a research study as part of the requirements for _____."

Potential subjects must always be given the opportunity to ask questions they may have about the study. It is almost impossible for the researcher to include every aspect of the study in a oral or written explanation. Subjects frequently have questions about the study, and an opportunity should be presented for these questions during the oral explanation of the study. The researcher is obligated to be available (by phone, postal mail, or email) if questions arise at a later time, or if subjects have questions when reading the written explanation of a study. Many potential research subjects are concerned with the use of study findings. Will their employers get a copy of the results? Will the study results be published? How can they find out the results? Although the researcher probably does not know for sure if the study results will ever be published, the researcher's publication plans (and desires) must be indicated.

Research subjects should always be given the opportunity to obtain the study results. This does not mean that a copy must be sent to all participants. In fact, many participants are not interested in the results. It is, therefore, appropriate for the researcher to place some of the responsibility for obtaining results on the study subjects. A comment such as the following may be included in the consent information: "A copy of the study results may be obtained by writing or calling the researcher." Of course, this would necessitate the inclusion of a phone number or a mailing address or email address where the researcher could be reached at the conclusion of the study. The approximate date when results will be available should also be provided.

Assurance of Freedom to Volunteer for or Withdraw from the Study

All participation in nursing research must be voluntary. No form of coercion should be involved. There must be no penalty involved for nonparticipation. For example, patient care should not be affected by a patient's participation or nonparticipation in a study. Students' grades in a course should not be influenced by research participation. Potential research subjects must also be informed that they may withdraw from a study at any time, and for any reason. This is particularly important in experimental studies in which a treatment is involved. As you may remember, the Nuremberg Code stated that a subject might withdraw from a study if any problem occurred. Today, subjects may withdraw for *any* reason.

Documentation of Informed Consent

The researcher must document that informed consent was obtained. This is usually provided when the participant signs an IRB-approved written consent form that states that the participant has willingly given permission and is aware of the risks and benefits of the study. In some cases, when there is no need to identify the participant's name and a self-report questionnaire is used, documentation of the informed consent is unnecessary. However, a statement that is similar to the following should be added to the questionnaire: RETURN OF THIS QUESTIONNAIRE WILL INDICATE YOUR CONSENT TO PARTICIPATE IN THIS STUDY.

Oral permission without the participant's signature may be obtained, but this must be witnessed by a third person. If the subject is a minor or is not able to give informed consent because of mental or physical disability, that subject may provide what is called *assent* to participate in the study. However, there must also be documentation of consent from a legally authorized representative, such as a child's parent, and in some circumstances both parents.

One circumstance to which this waiver would apply relates to a situation in which a principal risk of the study would be a potential harm resulting from a breach of confidentiality because of the record of informed consent linking the subject with the research. Specifically, 45 CFR 46.117 titled *Documentation of informed consent* states if the subject does not want documentation that links the subject to the research, the subjects wishes will govern this decision. More information on this topic may be found by searching for the Code of Federal Regulations at the DHHS website.

One frequently cited study by Milgram (1963) examined obedience to authority. The study was done in a laboratory setting and described to potential subjects as a learning experiment. Subjects were told to administer electrical shocks when the so-called learners gave incorrect responses, but the learners were actually actors. These actors, who were out of sight, groaned and screamed during the experiment. Twenty-six of the subjects, or 65% of the group, continued to administer shocks throughout the experiment, even when they thought they were administering lethal shocks. Responses of discomfort among the subjects who were administering the supposed electrical shocks included sweating, trembling, and stuttering. One subject had a convulsive seizure. This study demonstrates deception by the researcher and this type of misinformed consent is a morally unacceptable breach of trust (Baumrind, 2015). In the case of this study, volunteers were recruited to participate in a study of memory and learning; once recruited, they were told they would be teachers who would punish the learners with increasingly powerful electric shocks when the learner made mistakes. During debriefing, the volunteers were told that the shocks were not as painful as they seemed despite the fact that there were no shocks delivered (Baumrind, 2015).

Integrity in Research

The Office of Research Integrity (ORI) is supported by the U.S. Public Health Services (PHS). This organization promotes integrity in biomedical and behavioral research among institutions that receive research funds from the PHS. The ORI has jurisdiction over allegations of research misconduct that are deemed to be credible and significant. Research misconduct consists of fabrication of the data or results, falsification of data and results, or plagiarism. Research misconduct can occur at any stage of the research project from the time of submission of the proposal to dissemination of the findings (Bierer & Barnes, 2014). Once an allegation of research misconduct is reported, the ORI is charged to investigate the researcher and report its findings. For example, a recent ORI 2012 Annual Report listed 423 allegations of misconduct from 6714 funded institutions with 14 ORI findings of investigator-related research misconduct. More details about this topic may be viewed at the Office of Research Integrity website.

A review of the ORI files for research misconduct indicates that there are not many recorded cases of scientific misconduct among nursing research studies. However, in January 2010 a former professor at a school of nursing was issued a final notice of debarment based on falsified data on a research study that involved an intervention to reduce sexual risk behaviors in high risk, impaired populations of homeless men with mental illness (ORI Annual Report 2010). More recently in Great Britain, the Nursing and Midwifery Council suspended a specialist nurse for fabricating data for a research study that compared the effectiveness of different catheters that were used for patients receiving chemotherapy. Instead of reporting on data associated with 300 different catheter insertions, the nurse reported on the effects found in 300 different patients (Stephenson, 2015).

Following a review of the literature that focused on the promotion of research integrity, Fierz et al. (2014) also discovered a lack of published examples of research misconduct (RM) in the field of nursing science. However, based on the prevalence and risks of RM that were identified among other fields of health professionals, the authors concluded that there was reason to raise awareness of the ways in which scientific integrity could be compromised in nursing research. The authors described the major forms of RM as data fabrication, data falsification, and plagiarism.

Data fabrication refers to making up data for the purpose of deception, while data falsification refers to the willful distortion of the results of the study or the reported collection of the data (Fierz et al., 2014). Plagiarism refers to the near or verbatim copying of texts or ideas without identifying the original source of the citation (Fierz et al., 2014). Other forms of misconduct that could compromise the integrity of nursing science relate to the inappropriate management of data; publication-related misconduct; and failure to disclose conflicts of interest, ghostwriting, and authorship issues (Fierz et al., 2014). Authorship issues relate to the criteria that qualify a person to be included as an author in the publications associated with the research. A ghostwriter is someone who authors a text that is credited to another person.

In this day of promoting evidence-informed practice protocols, corporations may be interested in certain projects that may match their companies' interests with products associated with healthcare interventions. Conflicts of interest (COI) in research may occur when nurses receive payments from companies that also sponsor their research (Lach, 2014). When the research is associated with the use of a company's product, there is a risk that this type of relationship could create a bias that relates to the results and dissemination of the findings of the study. In response to this risk, federal regulations now require universities to obtain disclosures from researchers about any financial relationships that they may have with industry and to also manage the requirements that will mitigate the possible effects of bias (Lach, 2014).

There are situations where researchers may want to conduct a study in which their own patients will be the subjects, or the patients' charts are necessary for data collection. In this case, the researcher must approach the research setting as a complete stranger. If research is being conducted, permission must be obtained to use patients' records, even if the nurse has full access to the record in clinical practice. For cases such as this, the Health Insurance Portability and Accountability Act (HIPAA) Privacy Rule provides federal protections for individually identifiable health information held by covered entities and their business associates, and gives patients an array of rights with respect to that information. This provides for the unauthorized use and disclosure of a person's medical and health information. Authorization for use and disclosure must be obtained in writing from the person involved. This requirement pertains both to healthcare and to research conducted in a healthcare setting. Researchers may be required to obtain the person's signature on a separate document or integrate the information into the research informed consent document that potential research subjects must sign. A summary of the HIPPA Privacy Rule may be found on the U.S. Department of Human and Health Services website.

Research Guidelines for Nurses

In 1968, the American Nurses Association (ANA) Research and Studies Commission published a set of guidelines for nursing research. These guidelines, revised in 1975 and 1985, are titled *Human Rights Guidelines for Nurses in Clinical and Other Research*. They address the rights of research subjects and nurses involved in research. Subjects must be protected from harm, their privacy ensured, and their dignity preserved. Nurses who are asked to participate in research should be fully informed about the research and be included on the IRB applications of the research proposals. Later in 2015, the ANA published the *Code of Ethics for Nurses with Interpretative Statements*. Provision 3.2 of the document on Protection of Human Participants in Research stems from concerns related to the principles of respect for autonomy, respect for persons, and respect for self-determination (ANA, 2015). The code affirms that the research nurse's role as a patient advocate should include assurances of the fulfillment of human rights through the process of ongoing informed consent, continual assessment of risk versus benefit for research participants, and the prevention of harm. **Advocacy** is defined as "the act or process of pleading for, supporting or recommending a cause or a course of action" (ANA, 2015, p.41). The code also states that nurses have a duty to question and, if necessary, to report to the appropriate oversight bodies any researcher who violates a participant's rights or is involved in research that is ethically questionable, and advocate for anyone who wishes to decline from participating in a study before completion of the study.

Nurse Researcher as a Patient Advocate

In cases in which research nurses assist clinicians to run clinical trials, they have a central role as patient advocates (Pick, Berry, Gilbert, & McCaul, 2013). **Clinical trials** are research studies conducted to evaluate new treatments, new drugs, and new or improved medical equipment. Thousands of people participate in clinical trials each year in the United States. These studies are sponsored and funded by a number of organizations such as medical institutions. The purposes of the studies are often related to discovering a cure or a new strategy to manage a disease or improve health. In this type of case, a potential participant may be in an extraordinary situation of dependency on the researcher and be at risk of exploitation (Schrems, 2014).

Nurses should consider protecting the interests of the patients who have agreed to be in the studies (Pick et al., 2013). Although the lead investigator often acquires informed consent, nursing advocacy entails an ethical obligation to also evaluate and communicate the participant's understanding of the study as well as answer questions that will support the needs of the patient (Bristol & Hicks, 2014; Pick et al.). Additionally, nurses who are in dual roles of healthcare provider and researcher must be especially careful of risks associated with conflicts of interest between the participant's care and the needs of the research intervention (Bristol & Hicks, 2014). Bristol and Hicks have also stated that nurses who are not a part of the research team should also familiarize themselves with any clinical trials that are being conducted in their work setting in order to be aware if a participant should want to withdraw from participating in the study.

Bristol and Hicks (2014) state that successful clinical research outcomes are an important part of improving patient care. This idea implies that nurse researchers are equipped with the knowledge necessary to develop and implement quality research projects. A significant concern with this goal rests on becoming informed about the ethical issues associated with clinical research. This chapter provides an overview of some of the issues surrounding the development of an ethical approach to the promotion of clinical research.

Critiquing the Ethical Aspects of a Study

It may be difficult to critique the ethical aspects of a research report. Little space is usually given to this part of the study in published reports. Most journal articles contain one or two sentences that mention subjects' rights were protected and informed consent was obtained. It is understandable that little is printed about the ethical issues of the study. Much of this information would be repeated in each study report that is published. However, the reader of a research report may be able to determine the ethical nature of the study. For example, if the report states that permission to conduct the study was obtained from an IRB, the subjects' rights were likely protected. Also, if the study has been federally funded, there is some assurance that the researcher had to provide evidence of protection of subjects' rights before funds were awarded. Box 4–1 lists guidelines for critiquing the ethical aspects of a study.

Box 4–1 Guidelines for Critiquing the Ethical Aspects of a Study

1. Was the study approved by an Institutional Review Board (IRB)?
2. Was informed consent obtained from the subjects?
3. Is there information about provisions for anonymity or confidentiality?
4. Were vulnerable subjects used?
5. Does it appear that subjects might have been coerced into acting as subjects?
6. Is it evident that the benefits of participation in the study outweighed the risks involved?
7. Were subjects provided the opportunity to ask questions about the study and told how to contact the researcher if other questions arose?
8. Were the subjects told how they could obtain the results of the study?

Summary

Many unethical studies were conducted during World War II, particularly in the prison camps in Germany. Unethical research studies have also been revealed here in the United States.

Because of the public outcry against the atrocities committed in Germany in the 1940s, the Nuremberg Code was developed in 1947. This code calls for voluntary subjects and qualified researchers. Other ethical codes have been formulated since World War II. Many professional groups have developed codes for their members.

The federal government developed research guidelines in the early 1970s, and these guidelines have been revised several times. The original guidelines called for the creation of institutional review boards (IRBs) to be established in all agencies that receive federal money for research. IRBs review research proposals and set standards for research conducted in their agencies.

In 1968, the American Nurses Association developed a set of guidelines for nursing research. These guidelines, *Human Rights Guidelines for Nurses in Clinical and Other Research*, were revised in 1975 and 1985. The American Nurses Association published another set of guidelines in 1995, *Ethical Guidelines in the Conduct, Dissemination, and Implementation of Nursing Research*.

The principal means for ensuring the rights of research subjects is through informed consent.

Informed consent means that subjects agree to participate in studies about which they have complete understanding before the study begins. The major elements of informed consent concern the researcher's qualifications, subject selection process, purpose of the study, study procedures, potential risks and benefits to subjects, compensation, alternative procedures, anonymity and confidentiality, right to refuse to participate, offer to answer questions, and means of obtaining study results. Debriefing involves a meeting with research participants after the study is completed. The purpose is to ensure subjects' understanding of the reasons and the justification for the procedures used in the study.

Anonymity means that no one can identify the subjects in a study. Confidentiality means that the researcher will protect the subjects' identities.

The nurse researcher must act as a patient advocate, particularly in clinical trials. This advocacy involves protecting patients' privacy and dignity and ensuring that there are no undue physical or psychological risks to subjects. Particular attention should be given to the rights of certain vulnerable groups, such as children, geriatric clients, prisoners, and unconscious or sedated patients. If a child is older than 7 years, the child must give assent to participate in a study.

Self-Test

1. What activities committed during World War II triggered the need for the Nuremberg Trials?
   A. atrocities committed for the sake of research
   B. abuses committed on military prisoners in Japan
   C. atrocities committed in the labor camps in Germany
   D. the need to establish guidelines for researchers

2. Which publication revealed the various types of experiments on biological warfare in Japan during World War II?
   A. the Tuskegee Study
   B. *The Truth about Unit 731*
   C. the Nuremberg Code
   D. the Universal Declaration of Human Rights

3. Which popularly named principles for research subjects evolved from the Belmont Report?
   A. to promote informed consent, risk assessments, and voluntary consent
   B. conflict of interest, to avoid injury, and to promote benefit
   C. the Universal Declaration of Human Rights
   D. respect for persons, beneficence, and justice
4. Who must abide by the U.S. Department of Health and Human Services federal policies (Code of Federal Regulations 45 Part 46) for conducting ethical research?
   A. any researcher who receives scholarship money
   B. any institution that receives federal money for research
   C. researchers who study vulnerable human subjects
   D. the Office of Human Research and Protections
5. According to federal policy, what characteristics of a research proposal need IRB review?
   A. a systematic investigation with an intervention on an object that provides generalizable knowledge
   B. an investigation with a research protocol that may change to provide safe care for patients
   C. a systematic investigation with an intervention with identifiable information from a human subject that will contribute to generalizable knowledge
   D. an investigation with a protocol that rests on best practice from unit to unit with a focus on outcomes that are collected by the electronic health record
6. When compared to a research study, quality improvement project findings would more likely be focused on
   A. outcomes within a specific clinical setting.
   B. new knowledge that can be translated to other populations of patients.
   C. each of the human subjects and their families' concerns.
   D. curing a patient with a complex situation.
7. Which type of IRB review would be appropriate for research that focuses on a newborn patient?
   A. exempt review
   B. expedited review
   C. full review
   D. regular review
8. Which is a required element of informed consent for a research subject?
   A. a statement that provides a description of the corporate rewards associated with the study
   B. a statement that provides a clear understanding of all of the rationales for the study
   C. a promise of the expected results from the research intervention
   D. a statement that describes how their information will be kept confidential
9. A questionnaire is being used to gather data from the participants of the study. Identification numbers on the corner of the questionnaires correspond to the researcher's master list of names and numbers. Respondents are assured that this information will not be shared with anyone. The researcher is trying to ensure
   A. confidentiality
   B. informed consent
   C. anonymity
   D. data security
10. Which of the following is least likely to be provided for subjects?
    A. informed consent
    B. anonymity
    C. confidentiality
    D. privacy
11. What is the name of the process used to obtain a child's agreement for participation in a study?
    A. assent
    B. consent of a minor
    C. minor agreement
    D. informed consent
12. A friend has agreed to participate in a research study. She thinks she should automatically be sent a copy of the study results. You tell her:
    A. The researcher *should* automatically send a copy of the study results to all participants.
    B. Federal regulations require researchers to send a copy of the study results to all participants.

C. Study participants should be provided with the researcher's contact information if a copy of the study results is desired.
D. A copy of the study abstract should be mailed to all participants within 6 weeks of completion of the study.

13. What principle should guide nurses who are involved in research in the practice setting?
    A. Assure human rights of participants throughout the research study.
    B. Continue to encourage participation in the study.
    C. Document any adverse events during the study.
    D. Make certain that IRB has approved of the study.

14. The researcher added answers to the places where there is missing data on the research subject's questionnaire. Which term best describes this type of research misconduct?
    A. plagiarism
    B. data fabrication
    C. data falsification
    D. ghostwriting

15. There are suspicions of research misconduct in a study that is being carried out in a nurse's clinical setting. What agency is responsible for investigating this type of activity?
    A. the federal agency for the HIPPA Privacy Rule
    B. the American Nurses Association
    C. the Nursing and Midwifery Council
    D. the Office of Research Integrity

16. Which situation could place a nurse researcher at risk of research misconduct?
    A. when a nurse is funded by the manufacturer to test a device for healthcare
    B. when a nurse waits for authorization from the patient to use his health data
    C. when the researcher invites a colleague with mutual responsibility for the study to be a co-author of the written report.
    D. when the researcher discloses a financial relationship with an industrial manufacturer

17. What situation is an example of nurse advocating for the research participant?
    A. The nurse reports the noncompliant behaviors of the participant.
    B. The nurse tells the participant how others have had problems with the study.
    C. The nurse takes extra time to explain more about the details of the study.
    D. The nurse treats the subject as a personal friend.

18. How would a nurse who is not on the research team advocate for a research participant in the clinical setting?
    A. Make the care of the patient be a priority over the research intervention.
    B. Be prepared to evaluate the patient for any adverse effects of the research intervention.
    C. Take responsibility of witnessing the informed consent.
    D. Offer to collect data if the research team member is absent.

See answers to Self-Test in the Answer Section at the back of the book.

References

American Nurses Association. (2015). Code of ethics for nurses with interpretive statements. http:/www.nursingworld.org

Baumrind, D. (2015). When the subjects become objects: The lies behind the Milgram legend. *Theory & Psychology, 25*(5), 690–696. doi:10.1177/0959354315592062

Bierer, B. E. & Barnes, M. on behalf of the IRB/RIO/IO Working Group. (2014). Research misconduct involving noncompliance in human subjects research supported by the Public Health Service: Reconciling separate regulatory systems, the intersection of research fraud and human subjects research: A regulatory review. *Hastings Center Report* 44(4), S2–S26. doi:10.1002/hast.336

Bonifazi, W. L. (2004, November 1). Cruelty and courage: Nurses in the Nazi era. *Nurseweek*, pp. 24–26. https://news.nurse.com/

Bristol, S. T., & Hicks, R. W. (2014). Protecting boundaries of consent in clinical research: Implications for improvement. *Nursing Ethics, 21*(1), 16–27. doi:10.1177/0969733013487190

Centers for Disease Control and Prevention. (2010). The Tuskegee timeline. http://cdc.gov/nchstp/od/tuskegee/time.htm

Committee on Ethics. (2015). Committee opinion: Ethical considerations for including women as research participants. *American College of Obstetricians and Gynecologists, 646*, 1–8. http://www.acog.org/

DHHS. (2009). Code of federal regulations: Title 45 public welfare. http://www.hhs.gov/ohrp/humansubjects/guidance/45cfr46.html

DHHS. (1993). Institutional Review Board guidebook: Chapter 1 institutional administration. http://www.hhs.gov/ohrp/assurances/irb/

Fierz, K., Gennaro, S., Dierickx, K., Van Achterberg, T., Morin, K. H., DeGeest, S., & for the editorial board of Journal of Nursing Scholarship. (2014). Scientific misconduct: Also an issue in nursing science? *Nursing Scholarship, 46*(4), 271–280. doi:10.1111/jnu.12082

Japanese book details scientific atrocities. (1996, February 5). *Dallas Morning News*, p. 24A.

Katz, K. (1972). *Experimentation with human beings*. New York: Russell Sage.

Krugman, S., Giles, J., & Hammond, J. (1971). Viral hepatitis, type B (MS-2 strain): Studies on active immunization. *American Medical Association, 217*, 41–45. doi:10.1001/jama.1971.03190010023005.

Lach, H. W. (2014). Financial conflicts of interest in research: Recognition and management. *Nursing Research, 63*(3), 228–232. doi:10.1097/NNR.0000000000000016

Milgram, S. (1963). Behavioral study of obedience. *Abnormal and Social Psychology, 67*, 371–378. http://dx.doi.org/10.1037/h0040525

Nuremberg Military Tribunals. (1949). *Trials of war criminals before the Nuremberg Military Tribunals under Control Council Law No. 10* (Publication No. 1949–841584, Vol. 2). Washington, D.C.: U.S. Government Printing Office.

Ogrinc, G., Nelson, W. A., Adams, S. M., & O'Hara, A. E. (2013). An instrument to differentiate between clinical research and quality improvement. *IRB: Ethics & Human Research, 35*(5), 1–8. http://www.thehastingscenter.org/Publications/IRB/

ORI Annual Report 2010. (2010). Office of Research Integrity, U.S. Department of Health and Human Services. https://ori.hhs.gov/images/ddblock/ori_annual_report_2010.pdf

ORI Annual Report 2012. (2012). Office of Research Integrity, U.S. Department of Health and Human Services. https://ori.hhs.gov/images/ddblock/ori_annual_report_2012.pdf

Pick, A., Berry, S., Gilbert, K., & McCaul, J. (2013). Informed consent in clinical research. *Nursing Standard, 27*(49), 44–47. http://journals.rcni.com/journal/ns

Schrems, B. M. (2014). Informed consent, vulnerability and the risks of group-specific attribution. *Nursing Ethics, 21*(7), 829–843. doi:10.1177/0969733013518448

Shearer, L. (1982, October 17). Now it can be told. *Dallas Morning News*, pp. 10–11.

Simpson, M. (1985). *Therapeutic play and cooperation of preschoolers during physical examinations*. Unpublished master's thesis, Texas Woman's University, Denton.

Stephenson, J. (2015). NMC suspends specialist nurse over fabricated research report. *Nursing Times, 111*, 6. htpp://www.nursingtimes.net

Chapter 5
An Overview of Quantitative and Qualitative Research

Donna Scott Tilley, PhD, RN, CNE, CA SANE

Objectives

On completion of this chapter, you will be prepared to:

1. Differentiate between qualitative and quantitative research.
2. Summarize the steps in quantitative research.
3. Describe a nursing problem that could be addressed through a qualitative study.
4. Explain the use of both qualitative and quantitative research methods in a single study.

Introduction

There are many ways to get answers to important questions. In research, there are some general approaches one might take to answer important questions: the quantitative approach, the qualitative approach, or a combination of the two. In all cases, the research question should lead the researcher to the method instead of the researcher having a particular affinity for a specific method and fitting the question to the method. This chapter provides a general overview of two approaches to research: quantitative and qualitative, and introduces the concept of mixed methods research.

Comparison of Qualitative and Quantitative Research

Quantitative research is a systematic empirical approach to understanding phenomena. The data, or individual pieces of information produced in a quantitative study, are often numeric, observable, and measurable. Although quantitative research is not completely unbiased, it provides a level of objectivity that makes

Table 5-1 Comparison of Qualitative and Quantitative Research

Quantitative	Qualitative
Objective data	Subjective data
Explanation	Discovery
Parts are equal to the whole	Whole is greater than the parts
One truth	Multiple truths
Large sample sizes	Small sample sizes
Random samples	Deliberately selected samples
Participants or subjects	Participants or informants
Results presented as numbers/statistics	Results presented as narrative data
Researcher separate from the study	Researcher part of the study

it easier for us to conclude that results are based on the nature of what was studied, rather than the personality, beliefs, or values of the researcher. Quantitative research is based on the concepts of manipulation and control of phenomena and the verification of results, using empirical data gathered through the senses.

Qualitative research focuses on gaining insight into a phenomenon or understanding about an individual's perception of events. Qualitative research does not rely on manipulation and control but, instead, focuses on observing and describing things as they naturally occur. Often, the researcher is most interested in the person's interpretation of events and how those events shaped the person's beliefs or behaviors.

These approaches, while very different, can both inform nursing care. Table 5-1 compares some of the characteristics of the quantitative and qualitative research approaches.

The nature of nursing lends itself well to both quantitative and qualitative research, depending on the problem of interest. When there is a problem about which little is known or that is poorly understood, collecting qualitative data that provide a rich and deep description of the problem is ideal. Having this rich and deep perspective about a problem can help the researcher develop research hypotheses that are amenable to study using quantitative methods. For example, researchers started systematically observing social spaces and bystander reactions to abandoned cars in the early 1990s. Based on this qualitative work, they developed a theory about how things like broken windows in a neighborhood could lead to crime in the area. These researchers are now doing quantitative work to assess pathways to violence in neighborhoods using large-scale digital records (O'Brien & Sampson, 2015). Once the researchers had rich and deep qualitative data they were able to move to a quantitative approach that allowed them to collect objective data, often involving assessment of the effectiveness of interventions to prevent neighborhood violence.

Both quantitative and qualitative research methods share some commonly accepted steps in the research process. Most quantitative studies follow similar steps in the research process. As you progress through this book, you will find that these steps become clearer. Each of the steps in conducting both quantitative and qualitative study is elaborated upon in other chapters in this book.

Steps in Quantitative Research

Though different authors describe steps in quantitative research in different ways, nearly every author refers to the identification of the problem as the first step, and the communication of research findings or the utilization of research findings as the final step. There is some variation in the steps between. There can be some overlapping of the steps in the research process and some shifting back and forth between the steps. In general, however, the scientific research process proceeds in an orderly fashion, and consists of the steps identified in Box 5-1.

> **Box 5–1 Steps in the Quantitative Research Process**
>
> Identify the research problem
> Determine the purpose of the study
> Formulate the research question
> Review the literature
> Develop a theoretical/conceptual framework
> Identify the study assumptions
> Acknowledge the limitations of the study
> Formulate the hypothesis
> Define the study variables/terms
> Select the research design
>
> Identify the population
> Select the sample
> Conduct a pilot study
> Collect the data
> Organize the data for analysis
> Analyze the data
> Interpret the findings
> Communicate the findings
> Utilize the findings

Identify the Research Problem

The first, and one of the most important steps, in the research process is to clearly identify the problem that will be studied. In a nursing study, the **research problem** is an area where knowledge is needed to advance the practice of nursing. Generally, a broad topic area is identified, then the topic is narrowed down to a specific problem to be studied. This step of the research process is often the most difficult of all and may take a great deal of time.

Study problems can be identified from suggestions published in the literature, from recommendations made following previous studies, through the testing of theories, or from personal experiences. The problem should be of interest to the researcher and be significant to nursing.

An example of a problem area is "managing intraoperative hypothermia." The researcher has observed the problem of patients experiencing chilling during and after surgery in her area of practice, and wonders whether there are things nurses can do to prevent intraoperative chilling. The specific problem to be studied relates to keeping patients as close to their normal body temperature as possible during surgery, and possible interventions for nurses to accomplish this. In an introductory section, such as "Background" or "Literature Review," there would be a broad discussion of the problem area, including the number of people who have complications from chilling during surgery each year, and then a narrowing down to the specific causes of intraoperative hypothermia.

The terms *goals, objectives, problem area, problem statement, purpose,* and *research question* are sometimes used interchangeably, even though each term means something different. The problem statement (or problem area) is the broad identification of a problem that leads the researcher toward a research question. A research question is an interrogative sentence that asks a specific question about the topic of interest. A good research question is clear and specific. In this text, all examples of research problems are written in the interrogative form, as research questions.

Determine the Purpose of the Study

Although the term *purpose* is sometimes used interchangeably with *problem*, there is a distinction between these two terms. The research problem addresses *what* will be studied; the purpose provides *why* the study is being done. In most published nursing research studies, the purpose of the study is presented rather than a problem statement or a research question. The following is an example of a purpose statement for the study concerning prevention of intraoperative hypothermia: "This study seeks to determine if warmed IV fluids are effective in preventing intraoperative hypothermia."

Formulate the Research Question

A **research question** is the specific question that the researcher expects to be answered in a study. The research question should specify the variables and the population that are being studied. A **variable** is a characteristic or attribute that differs among the persons, objects, events, and so forth being studied (e.g., age, blood type). The population is the group that will be studied. Here is an example of a research question: "Is there a difference in core body temperature of surgical patients who receive warmed IV fluids, and those who receive room temperature IV fluids?"

Review the Literature

Research should build on previous knowledge. Before beginning a quantitative study, it is important to determine what knowledge exists of the study topic. There are few topics about which there is no existing knowledge base. There are many routes of access to the published literature. Literature sources can be located through indexes, abstracts, and computer-assisted searches. Besides determining the extent of the existing knowledge related to the study topic, the review of the literature also helps develop a theoretical or conceptual framework for a study. Finally, the review of the literature can help the researcher plan study methods. For example, instruments or tools may be discovered that can be used to measure the study variables. By reviewing the literature, a researcher will be able to profit from the successes and failures of other researchers.

The literature review should be continued during the course of the investigation until the time of data collection. This ensures the researcher that she or he has as much information as possible, and the most up-to-date information on the study topic.

Occasionally, the initial review of the literature may actually occur before the identification of the problem. The problem area may be determined from the suggestions or recommendations of researchers who have conducted previous studies in the area of interest.

Develop a Theoretical/Conceptual Framework

The goal of research is to develop scientific knowledge. Research and theory are closely intertwined. Research can test theories as well as help develop and refine theories. Thus, theoretical frameworks are a valuable part of scientific research. The theoretical or conceptual framework assists in the selection of the study variables and in defining them. The framework also directs the hypothesis(es) and the interpretation of the findings. In a classic editorial in *Nursing Research*, Florence Downs (1994) stated that a "study that lacks a theoretical rationale lacks substance and fails to answer the 'so what' question" (p. 195).

Some research of a purely descriptive nature may not require a theoretical framework. Most nursing studies can profit, however, from the identification of a framework for the study. An examination of recently published nursing studies reveals that increasing numbers of these studies are based on a clearly identified theoretical framework. For example, Ramey et al. (2015) applied the Preconception Stress and Resiliency Pathways model in their community-based research to improve intergenerational health. In this case, the model guided the researchers to include all family members and engage the community at multiple levels to promote resilience, reduce chronic and acute stressors, and expand individualized healthcare that integrated health promotion and prevention strategies. Research conducted within the context of a theoretical framework, compared to research that is not theory based, is more valuable in providing understanding and knowledge that can be used in the future. Research without theory provides a set of isolated facts.

Identify the Study Assumptions

Assumptions are beliefs that are held to be true, but have not necessarily been proven. Each scientific investigation is based on assumptions. These assumptions should be stated explicitly. Frequently, however, the assumptions are implicit. This means that the study was based on certain assumptions, but the researcher did not openly acknowledge or list these assumptions.

Assumptions are of three types: universal assumptions, assumptions based on theory or research findings, and common sense assumptions that are necessary to carry out the study. Universal assumptions are beliefs that are assumed to be true by a large percentage of society, such as, "All human beings need love." Assumptions also can be derived from theory or previous research. If a study is based on a certain theory, the assumptions of that theory become the assumptions of the study based on that particular theory. In addition, the results of previous studies can form the basis for assumptions in the present research investigation. Finally, certain commonsense assumptions must be made to carry out a study. For example, if an investigator were conducting a study to examine behaviors of fathers toward their children, it would be necessary to assume that the men in the study were actually the fathers of the children in the study.

Consider an example in which nurses are trying to determine the most appropriate means to teach patients to operate an insulin pump. A universal assumption might be that uncontrolled diabetes is a threat to the physical well-being of individuals. An assumption based on research might be that the insulin pump is an effective means of delivering medication to diabetics. Finally, a commonsense assumption might be made that the participants are interested in controlling their diabetes, and that they have the mental capacity to understand the material being taught.

Acknowledge the Limitations of the Study

The researcher should try to identify limitations or weaknesses of their study in advance. **Limitations** are uncontrolled variables that may affect study results and limit the generalizability of the findings. In nearly every research study, including nursing studies, there are variables over which the researcher either has no control or chooses not to exercise control. These variables are called *extraneous variables*. For example, the educational level of participants would be a study limitation if the researcher could not control this variable and thought that it might influence the study results. In experimental studies, uncontrolled variables are referred to as threats to internal and external validity.

As much as possible, the researcher should openly acknowledge the limitations of a study before data are collected. Other limitations may occur while the study is in progress (such as malfunctions of equipment and participant dropout). The limitations must be taken into consideration when the conclusions of a study are formulated, and when recommendations are made for future research.

Formulate the Hypothesis

A researcher's expectation about the results of a study is expressed in a hypothesis. A **hypothesis** predicts the relationship between two or more variables. The hypothesis furnishes the predicted answer to the research question. The hypothesis contains the population and variables, just as does the research question. In addition, the hypothesis proposes the relationship between the independent and the dependent variables. In experimental studies, the **independent variable** is the cause or the variable thought to influence the dependent variable. The **dependent variable** is the effect or the variable influenced by the researcher's manipulation (control) of the independent variable. A hypothesis must be testable or verifiable empirically, which means that it must be capable of being tested in the real world by observations gathered through the senses.

Consider this research question: "Is there a correlation between body image and self-esteem levels of women who have experienced a mastectomy?" After the review of the literature on the topic, a theory might be located that predicts a positive relationship between body image and self-esteem levels. The following hypothesis might then be formulated: The more positive the body image of women who have experienced a mastectomy, the higher is their self-esteem level. This type of hypothesis is referred to as a *directional research hypothesis*. It contains the direction of the researcher's expectations for the study results.

Although the null hypothesis (which predicts that no relationship exists between variables) is tested statistically, the directional research hypothesis is the preferred type for nursing studies. This type of hypothesis is derived from the theoretical/conceptual framework for the study and should, therefore, indicate the expected relationship between variables.

Experimental, comparative, and correlational studies call for hypotheses. In qualitative studies and some descriptive studies, a hypothesis is not needed. In those studies that do not require hypotheses, the research is guided by the research question(s). The following are examples of research questions that would not call for hypotheses: "What are the adjustment behaviors of family members when the husband/father has experienced a myocardial infarction?" "Do family members become closer or more distant in their interpersonal relationships with each other?" "What is the greatest adjustment difficulty reported by family members?" "Do different families report similar or dissimilar adjustment problems?"

Define the Study Variables/Terms

The variables and terms contained in the study hypothesis or research question need to be defined so their meaning is clear to the researcher and to the reader of a research report. Terms should be defined both conceptually and operationally. A **conceptual definition** is a dictionary definition or theoretical definition of an abstract idea that is being studied by the researcher. An **operational definition** indicates how a variable will be observed or measured. Operational definitions frequently include the instrument that will be used to measure the variables. If anxiety were being measured, the theoretical definition might be taken from a certain theorist's description of anxiety. The operational definition would then be indicated by the identification of the tool or behavior that would be used to measure anxiety.

The operational definition allows replication of a study. If a researcher would like to replicate a study using another group of participants or another setting, it would be necessary to know exactly how the variables were measured in the previous study.

Besides defining the variables in a hypothesis or research question, the population for the study should be defined or narrowed down to the specific group that will be studied. If the population were identified as myocardial infarction patients, this group could be further defined as men between the ages of 35 and 55 years who have experienced a first myocardial infarction and are patients in a large teaching hospital in the northeastern United States.

Select the Research Design

The **research design** is the plan for how the study will be conducted. It is concerned with the type of data that will be collected and the means used to obtain these data. For example, the researcher must decide if the study will examine cause-and-effect relationships or only describe existing situations. The researcher chooses the design that is most appropriate to test the study hypothesis(es) or answer the research question(s).

Research designs can be categorized as quantitative or qualitative. They also can be categorized as experimental or nonexperimental. Experimental designs can be further divided into true experimental, quasiexperimental, and pre-experimental designs. Nonexperimental designs include survey studies, correlational studies, comparative studies, and methodological studies.

In experimental research, the investigator plays an active role and has more control over the research situation than in a nonexperimental study. More control can be exercised over the extraneous variables that might influence research results. In experimental nursing studies, a nursing intervention is usually introduced. The nurse researcher manipulates this variable by randomly assigning people to groups that will and will not receive an intervention. Frequently, one group (the control group) receives the usual intervention, while another group (the treatment group) receives some new intervention that is hoped to be more effective. Usually, placement in the control or treatment group is randomized—that is, each participant or subject has an equal chance of being placed in either group.

In nonexperimental research, the investigator collects data without actively manipulating any variable. It is appropriate to discuss cause-and-effect relationships only when experimental designs are used. However, because of ethical reasons, it is sometimes difficult to conduct experimental research with human beings.

Identify the Population

The **population** is a complete set of individuals or objects that possess some common characteristic of interest to the researcher. The researcher must specify the broad population or group of interest as well as the actual population that is available for the study. The first type of population is identified as the target population, and the second type is called the accessible population. The **target population**, also called the *universe*, is made up of the group of people or objects to which the researcher wishes to generalize the findings of a study. The **accessible population** is the group that is actually available for study by the researcher. The term *population* does not always mean that human beings will be studied. A nurse researcher might study a population of charts or a population of blood pressure readings, for example.

By identifying the population, the researcher makes clear the group to which the study results can be applied. Scientific research is concerned with generalizing research results to other participants and other settings. Populations are always of interest in scientific research, even when only a small group of participants is being studied.

Although the researcher would like to assert that the study results apply to a wide target population, this population must be similar to the accessible population for such an assertion to be made. For example, the accessible population might be pregnant women in one clinic setting. These women are in their first pregnancy and their ages vary from 25 to 35 years. The target population would be 25-to-35-year-old women in their first pregnancy. It might also be necessary to further delineate the target population according to ethnicity or income levels of the accessible population in the clinical setting of the study. In other words, the target population to which the researcher wishes to generalize study results must be similar to the accessible population.

Select the Sample

Although researchers are always interested in populations, usually a subgroup of the population, called a **sample**, is studied. The sample is chosen to represent the population, and is used to make generalizations about the population. Obtaining data from an entire population is costly and time consuming, and it may even be impossible, at times, to contact or locate every member of a given population. If the sample is carefully selected, the researcher can make claims about the population with a certain degree of confidence. The method of selecting the sample determines how representative the sample is of the population.

Probability samples are those chosen by a random selection process in which each member of the population has a chance of being in the sample. If nonprobability sampling is used, the researcher has less confidence that the sample is representative of the population. The investigator cannot estimate the probability that each element of the population has a chance of being selected for the sample, and the possibility of a biased sample is great. After considering the advantages and disadvantages of the various types of probability and nonprobability sampling methods, the researcher must determine which sampling method to use.

Nursing research is generally conducted with human beings; therefore, participants' rights must be considered and the proper permissions secured before participants are approached to participate in a study. All research with humans must involve voluntary participation of the participants.

Conduct a Pilot Study

It is advisable to conduct a pilot study before the study participants are approached and the actual study is carried out. A **pilot study** involves a miniature trial version of the planned study. People are selected for the pilot study with similar characteristics to those of the sample that will be used for the actual study. Sometimes, doing a pilot study can prevent the researcher from conducting a large-scale study that might have little value. Pilot studies are smaller studies that build the body of evidence to support a large study. The body of evidence collected from pilot studies might be related to study design, sampling plans or necessary sample size, data collection procedures, and data analysis processes.

A pilot study can be used to test a new instrument or to evaluate an existing instrument that has been altered. The researcher may think that the questionnaire is so simple that a 10-year-old could fill it out, but finds out in a pilot study that 30-year-olds have great difficulty in understanding some of the questions. The pilot study also can be used to evaluate the study procedures and, in general, help identify potential problems before the actual study is conducted. Factors can be examined, such as how long it will take to conduct the data collection and how participants can be expected to respond to the data collection methods.

After the pilot study is conducted, necessary revisions to the plan for a larger study should be made. It may be advisable to carry out another pilot study if changes have been made in the instrument(s) or the research procedures.

Collect the Data

The **data** are the pieces of information or facts that are collected in research. Although the data-collection step of the research process may be very time consuming, it is sometimes considered the most exciting part of research.

The variable or variables in a study must be measured. This is carried out through the data-collection procedures. Data collection should be a systematic process. These questions must be answered: Who will collect the data? When will the data be collected? Where will the data be collected? What data will be collected? How will the data be collected?

A multitude of data-collection methods are available to nurse researchers. The choice of methods is determined by the study hypothesis(es) or the research question(s), the design of the study, and the amount of knowledge available about the study topic. Many research projects use more than one data-collection method.

Organize the Data for Analysis

After the data are collected, it is necessary to organize the data for tabulation and evaluation. This task can be overwhelming at times. This step of the research process should have been carefully planned, ideally with a statistician, long before the data were collected. The researcher should have prepared dummy tables and graphs that could then be filled in with the data once they are obtained.

If questionnaires have been used, it will be necessary to determine if they have been completed correctly. Decisions will have to be made about missing data. If interviews have been recorded, the tapes will have to be analyzed and data then placed in some kind of written form.

A statistician should be consulted early in the planning phase of the research process, as well as in the data analysis phase of the study. Just as plans for organizing the data should be made before data collection begins, plans for analyzing the data also should be made before obtaining the data. It is frustrating for a statistician to be approached by a researcher with a mound of data and the plea "What should I do with this stuff?" The statistician can help determine what data are needed for a study and what statistical procedures will be appropriate to analyze the data.

Analyze the Data

This stage of the research process—analyzing the data—may make some of you cringe, for you can quickly ascertain that statistics may be involved. An understanding of difficult mathematical principles is not necessary to conduct research or evaluate research results.

Data analysis has been simplified with a great number and variety of data analysis software programs. When data had to be analyzed by hand, or even when pocket calculators became available, data analysis was very time consuming. Today, if a study is well planned and data are well organized, a researcher can enter large amounts of data into a data analysis program and receive the results of the analysis almost instantaneously.

Interpret the Findings

After the data are analyzed, the findings should be interpreted in light of the study hypothesis(es) or research question(s). If a hypothesis was tested, a determination is made as to whether the data support the research hypothesis. Also, the framework for the study is discussed in light of the findings. If the data support the research hypothesis, then the theoretical or conceptual framework is also supported. Conversely, if the research hypothesis is not supported, the framework for the study is also not supported. Of course, the researcher should discuss any problems incurred in the course of the study or any limitations of the design that may have influenced the study results.

The results of the present study are compared with those of previous studies that investigated the same or similar variables. This is an important step because it allows the researcher to contribute to the existing body of knowledge on the study topic.

After the findings are interpreted, the researcher should indicate the implications for nursing. A consideration is made of changes that might be called for in nursing practice, nursing education, or nursing administration as a result of the study findings. These recommendations should be based on study findings rather than the researcher's personal opinion.

Often, researchers find that they are only able to answer a small part of a larger question, or that their research raised as many questions as it answered. Thus, recommendations for future research are proposed.

Communicate the Findings

This step of the research process may be the most important one for nursing. No matter how significant the findings may be, they are of little value to the nursing profession if the researcher fails to disseminate the results to other colleagues. Even studies with nonsignificant findings should be published so that other researchers know the question was asked and studied. The results of many nursing studies never get published or shared with other nurses.

Research findings can be communicated through many different mediums. The most effective method of reaching a large number of nurses is through publication in research journals such as *Applied Nursing Research, Biological Research for Nursing, Clinical Nursing Research, Nursing Research, Advanced Nursing, Research in Nursing and Health*, and *Western Journal of Nursing Research*. Research results also may be published in clinical journals such as *Heart & Lung, Issues in Mental Health Nursing*, and *Obstetric, Gynecologic, and Neonatal Nursing*.

Nurses should also present their research results in person to colleagues at national, regional, state, and local nursing conferences. Research findings can be presented at conferences in an oral presentation, sometimes called a podium or paper presentation, or in a poster format. Oral or paper presentations are often limited to about 20 minutes. Poster presentations are usually displayed for a longer period of time, and the presenter is not expected to make a formal spoken presentation. Whether doing an oral presentation or presenting a poster, the presenter should plan to describe the major areas of the research, such as the problem area, hypotheses, and findings.

Utilize the Findings

The researcher should take an active part in implementing the findings of his or her study. The researcher may not actually implement the findings, but he or she can make recommendations about how the findings could be integrated into nursing practice. For example, the researcher could act as a consultant to nurses in healthcare agencies who want to use the study findings. Additionally, the researcher is actually helping promote utilization of study findings by disseminating these findings in as many ways as possible.

Qualitative Nursing Research

Nursing has traditionally focused on the individual and the holistic nature of the person. This value system is more consistent with qualitative research philosophy than with quantitative research philosophy. In qualitative research, the individual's perspective is very important, whereas in quantitative research, the focus is on the group or population of interest, rather than the individual.

Qualitative research is an important source of knowledge about nursing. Here is a list of some of the many qualitative studies published in 2014 and 2015:

- Activity Engagement: Perspectives from Nursing Home Residents with Dementia (Tak, Kedia, Tongumpun, & Hong, 2015).
- Lived Experience in Teaching Mental Health Nursing: Issues of Fear and Power (Happell, Bennetts, Harris, Platania-Phung, Tohotoa, Byrne, & Wynaden, 2015).
- Understanding Patient-to-Worker Violence in Hospitals: A Qualitative Analysis of "Documented Incident Reports" (Arnetz, Hamblin, Essenmacher, Upfal, Ager, & Luborsky, 2015).
- Comparison of Meaningful Learning Characteristics in Simulated Nursing Practice After Traditional Versus Computer-Based Simulation Method: A Qualitative Videography Study (Poikela, Ruokamo, & Teras, 2015).

Were you able to detect that these studies were qualitative based on the wording in some of the titles? Such terms as "Perspectives of . . ." and "Lived Experience of . . ." provide clues that these articles would present the results of qualitative studies.

Table 5–2 Types of Qualitative Research

Action research	Ethnography	Grounded theory
Case study	Ethnology	Hermeneutics
Critical social inquiry	Ethnomethodology	Historical
Discourse analysis	Ethnonursing	Phenomenology
Ecological psychology	Ethnoscience	Philosophical inquiry
Ethical inquiry	Feminist inquiry	Symbolic interaction

Box 5–2 Steps in the Qualitative Research Process

Identify the problem of the study	Protect the rights of participants
State the purpose	Collect the data
Select the research design	Analyze the data
Review the literature	Interpret the data
Select the sample	Communicate the study results
Gain entry to the research site	

Types of Qualitative Research

There are many different types of qualitative research; Table 5–2 lists some of these.

Like quantitative studies, qualitative studies also have generally accepted steps in the research process. These generally accepted steps are listed in Box 5–2. However, depending on the qualitative design chosen, the steps may vary. It's also important to note that in most qualitative designs, the research process is not linear. The researchers are often analyzing data while they are collecting data. They may even be mentally formulating new interview questions for the next participants as they are interviewing someone. This process is called constant comparison, and it's a feature of many qualitative designs.

Identify the Problem of the Study

Just as the identification of the problem is the first step in quantitative research studies, the identification of the problem or phenomenon of the study is also the first step in the qualitative research process. In quantitative research, the researcher generally begins with a broad general area of study, then narrows the focus to a small area of study before data collection begins. In qualitative research, the problem area or phenomenon of study may remain general until the researcher actually enters the field setting. Then, the topic area may be narrowed down. The problem to be examined in a qualitative study may indicate the general nature of the phenomenon to be studied and the group or community that will be studied.

State the Purpose

In an article reporting on a qualitative study, the reader might see a one-sentence statement of purpose. For example, a purpose statement might be: "To describe the experiences of victims of sexual assault during the criminal justice process."

Select the Research Design

The research design in a qualitative study depends on the phenomenon that will be studied. For example, in a purpose statement about the victims of sexual assault, the researcher would be interested in a description of what people experienced during that criminal justice process. This study would probably call for a phenomenological approach to data collection. If the researcher were interested in the processes that the victims used to cope with this experience, a grounded-theory approach might be used. If the researcher were interested in how nurses could facilitate a better experience for sexual assault victims during the criminal justice process, an action research approach might be used.

Review the Literature

Qualitative researchers debate about the timing of the review of literature. Some believe that a review of the literature prior to conducting research may help identify the gaps in knowledge and focus the study, but some qualitative researchers do not begin with a review of the literature.

While a quantitative study always begins with an extensive review of the literature, some qualitative research may not. A very few qualitative researchers believe that extensively reviewing the literature before conducting a qualitative study, particularly a phenomenological study, will bias the study results. They do not want to know what other researchers think or believe about the phenomenon of interest prior to collecting their own data. In these rare cases, the researchers believe that the review of the literature should be conducted at the conclusion of the study. The purpose of the literature, then, is to obtain information that will enable researchers to inform readers of their research study results, and how the findings of their particular study fit into the existing body of knowledge on the topic of interest.

Select the Sample

One of the main ways qualitative studies differ from quantitative is that the sample sizes are generally smaller. There are no set rules about the necessary sample size for a qualitative study. Sandelowski's classic (1995) article "Sample Size in Qualitative Research" is an excellent source on this topic. She claims that the quality of information obtained from each respondent is more important than the amount of data obtained. The data produced in qualitative studies are often deeper and richer than in quantitative studies and, at some point, collecting more data does not lead to a better understanding of the phenomenon of interest. The guiding principle when considering sample size in qualitative research is quality of data and whether adding more participants will increase understanding.

Frequently, sample sizes are small in qualitative research. In a study by Snellgrove, Beck, Green, and McSweeney (2015), 11 certified nurse assistants participated in semi-structured interviews to learn more about how they prevent and manage resident-to-resident violence in nursing homes. Rodger, Neill, and Nugent (2015) described the lived experience of 6 informal caregivers of elders. Braaten (2015) conducted interviews with 12 medical surgical nurses to learn more about how nurses make decisions about when to activate a rapid response team. Given the depth of this data and the volume such data collection methods would generate, sample sizes much larger than 6, 11, or 12 might generate more data than a researcher could reasonably analyze and interpret.

Saturation is an important concept in qualitative studies regarding sampling. **Saturation** occurs when the researcher hears a repetition of themes or salient points as additional participants are interviewed. No new information is obtained; the data become redundant. This can happen after interviewing 10 people, or not until after 100 are interviewed. Sieverdes et al. (2015) asserted that saturation occurred after they had interviewed 22 patients on kidney transplant waiting lists regarding their attitudes toward a mobile health-delivered physical activity program.

Saturation

A group of researchers studied the perceptions of labor and delivery nurses caring for women in persistent vegetative states with viable pregnancies (Fedorka, Heasley, & Patton, 2014). Using the constant comparison method, the researchers simultaneously collected and analyzed data from interviews with nurses. When they reached saturation after interviewing 13 nurses, they presented their results to the participants for corroboration.

Gain Entry to the Research Site

Qualitative researchers conduct their research in the field or place where the research participants live or work. However, before approaching potential research participants, the researcher must obtain permission from the IRB where she or he is employed, as well as the location from where the data are being collected. Additionally, to receive research funding, the researcher has to demonstrate that the study proposal has been approved by an IRB.

Generally, the qualitative researcher tries to contact key people in the area of interest. These people may be known as gatekeepers. In ethnographic research, these individuals are called *key informants*. They may be able to help the researcher get in touch with potential research participants who would be able to provide valuable insight into the phenomenon of interest.

Protect the Rights of Participants

In qualitative research, the researcher interacts very closely with the study participants. Therefore, ethical issues may be even more important in qualitative research than in quantitative research. Because of the close relationship between the researcher and the study participants, these people tend to share personal and private information with the researcher.

Anonymity is generally not a consideration in qualitative research because the researcher knows the identity of the study participants. However, confidentiality is very important. The researcher must take particular care to protect the identity of study participants. The sample size is usually small and, because of the rich descriptive information presented in study results, it might be easy to identify study participants. The researcher may have to omit the usual demographic information that is presented on study participants in a quantitative research report. For example, the qualitative researcher may want to omit such information as the age, educational level, and occupation of study participants.

Collect the Data

Interview is probably the most common type of data-collection method used in qualitative studies. An **interview** is a method of data collection in which an interviewer obtains responses from a participant in a face-to-face encounter or through a telephone call. The interviews used in qualitative research are generally semistructured rather than structured, as might be the case in quantitative research. In a structured interview, the researcher has a structured list of questions that are answered in order, and deviation from the questions does not occur. In contrast, a semistructured interview is one in which some general questions are constructed, but the interviewer is open to allowing new ideas or topics to be introduced by the interviewee. While nurses may be comfortable talking with patients, the research interview is different and requires a different set of skills. The interviewer must be able to keep the interview on topic while allowing the participant to introduce new material that may be important. It is important for the novice interviewer to practice the method repeatedly, preferably under the guidance of an experienced interviewer.

Interviews and observation allow for the flexibility that is needed in qualitative research. Other types of data-collection methods include open-ended questionnaires, diaries, life histories, official documents, letters, and photographs. A less common type of data-collection method in qualitative research is participant observation. **Participant observation** involves the direct observation and recording of information and requires that the researcher become a part of the setting in which the person, group, or culture is being observed.

In qualitative research, the amount of time for data collection is generally not specified when a study begins. In most types of qualitative research, such as grounded theory methodology, data collection continues until the data are saturated. Even with a with a small number of participants, the data are usually voluminous.

The use of focus groups has increased in nursing studies. A **focus group** consists of a small group of individuals meeting together and being asked questions by a moderator about a certain topic or topics. The advantage of this approach is that it is a time-saver compared to individual interviews. However, there may not be equal participation by group members. Some people may be reluctant to express their views to others in a group setting. Côté-Arsenault and Morrison-Beedy (2005) noted in an article in *Research in Nursing & Health* that the cornerstones for successful focus groups are a well-defined purpose, carefully planned environment, and well-trained personnel. Many examples are found in the literature in which a focus group has been used.

Focus Group

Focus groups were used to understand how healthcare professionals assess and manage procedural pain for preterm infants who undergo repeated therapeutic procedures while in the Neonatal Intensive Care Unit (Gibbins et al., 2015). The researchers identified four themes from the content analysis: (1) subtlety and unpredictability of pain indicators, (2) infant and caregiver attributes and contextual factors that influence pain response and practices, (3) the complex nature of pain assessment, and (4) uncertainty in the management of pain. The researchers reported that this study was helpful in identifying gaps in knowledge and informing strategies to improve pain management for preterm infants.

While quantitative researchers think about reliability and validity of their research, qualitative researchers tend to think about the **rigor** of their research. There is no one way to assess or assure rigor in a qualitative study. One of the most widely used frameworks for assessing or assuring rigor in a qualitative study was proposed by Lincoln and Guba in 1985. Lincoln and Guba talked about the rigor of a qualitative study in terms of trustworthiness. To assure trustworthiness, the researcher should demonstrate (1) credibility, (2) transferability, (3) dependability, and (4) confirmability. Credibility, or truth value, is comparable to validity in a quantitative study and can be demonstrated through spending sufficient time with participants and collecting sufficient data. Transferability, or showing that the findings can be applied in other contexts, is comparable to external validity in a qualitative study and can be demonstrated through thick and rich description of data. Thick description is a detailed account of all elements of the research and provides context to the data. Dependability is comparable to reliability in a quantitative study and can be demonstrated by audit. An audit is a process where an outsider to the study can review the study, challenge the processes used, assess the adequacy of data, and provide feedback to improve the study. Confirmability is being as objective as possible. Confirmability can be demonstrated in a number of ways, including creating a clear audit trail so another researcher can reasonably follow the steps taken in the study, using multiple data sources to ensure robust data, and systematically planning and attending to each step of the study to avoid researcher bias.

Analyze the Data

Data analysis in qualitative research begins once data collection begins. The researchers begin looking immediately for themes in the data and adjust their data collection (for instance, who they interview or the questions they ask participants) slightly as themes emerge. Analysis of data in qualitative studies usually involves an examination of words rather than numbers, as is the case in quantitative studies. Generally, a large number of direct quotes made by the participants are included in study reports. The task of analyzing all of these data can be overwhelming. One large study might involve the analysis of several thousand pages of notes. Qualitative researchers may spend months analyzing their data.

Though specific steps of **content analysis** differ among qualitative designs, qualitative studies involve content analysis procedures. In general, content analysis involves creating categories of data and developing rules for coding data into these categories. The use of content analysis varies according to the type of qualitative study that is conducted. Grounded theory, ethnography, and phenomenological research are based on the specific techniques developed from the three disciplines that developed these methods: sociology, anthropology, and psychology, respectively. More information on specific content analysis methods can be found in other sources.

Coding is the basic data analysis tool of qualitative researchers. Statements made by study participants are grouped and given a code. Coded data are clustered together into themes. The qualitative researcher is then presented with the challenge of conveying the study findings to the reader. Data can be analyzed manually or through the aid of computer software programs. With the advent of these software programs, data analysis has been greatly enhanced for qualitative researchers. Qualitative data analysis software (QDAS) can store data, edit data, retrieve segments of text, and assemble data according to themes or categories.

A number of software programs are helpful in analyzing qualitative data. The programs do not analyze the data—only the researcher can do that. Rather these programs store and manage the large volumes of data and facilitate analysis by the researcher.

Interpret the Data

Interpretation of the data frequently occurs simultaneously with data collection. Interpretation is different from data analysis. In data analysis, the qualitative researcher is looking for themes and patterns. During interpretation, researchers pore over their data again and again, trying to find the meaning in the data. Perhaps there are relationships between themes and patterns that mean something. Although qualitative researchers generally do not try to make generalizations from their findings, they do try to determine how their study results can be applied and usually address this issue at the end of their study reports.

Communicate the Study Results

Where and how do qualitative researchers present their study results? Research findings can be communicated through many different mediums, including publication in peer-reviewed journals. Most nursing research journals contain qualitative research reports. In fact, some of the most prestigious nursing research journals publish only qualitative research reports. *Qualitative Health Research* is one example of such a journal.

Nurses who conduct qualitative research should present their research results to colleagues at national, regional, state, and local nursing conferences. Posters are a very effective means of presenting quantitative findings, and qualitative researchers may also present their results on posters.

Utilize the Study Results

The findings of qualitative research should be used in nursing practice, just like the results of quantitative studies. Implications for nursing practice are usually included at the end of a qualitative research report, just as is found in quantitative reports.

Lancaster et al. (2015) examined the interdisciplinary communication and collaboration among physicians, nurses, and unlicensed assistive personnel, using a phenomenological research approach. They identified that most of the time, physicians, nurses, and unlicensed assistive personnel operate as separate healthcare providers with little communication. At the end of their article in *Nursing Scholarship*, they called for organizations to improve patient safety by removing or reducing hierarchical structures that impede communication between and among healthcare professionals.

There is some confusion about the implementation of the results of qualitative studies. Morden et al. (2015) proposed that qualitative nursing research can be used to inform clinical nursing practice when it is aligned with theory. They stated that using qualitative research that is underpinned by theory can provide insight into the context and complex dynamics of healthcare decisions about interventions.

Combining Qualitative and Quantitative Methods

Although anthropologists and social scientists have used mixed methods in research since the early 20th century, using mixed methods research is a fairly new practice for nurse researchers (Pelto, 2015). Mixed method studies use a variety of methods in a single study to answer a question. Most commonly, a mix of qualitative and quantitative research methods are used, but researchers may also combine two different qualitative approaches in a single study (Morse & Cheek, 2015). Using a mixed method or multiple-methods approach allows the researcher to explore a problem from the most comprehensive point of view. Pelto (2015) asserted that combining methods is often the most efficient and cost-effective way to get answers to specific problems in research. Morse and Cheek (2015) propose that mixed method and multiple-method designs open up the possibility for new and exciting opportunities where thick descriptions, theory building, and reports of statistical findings provide a rich foundation for understanding.

Triangulation is a concept that is important in mixed methods studies. Triangulation most often indicates the use of two or more different sampling strategies, data collectors, data-collection procedures, or theories in one study. In trigonometry and geometry, triangulation is the process of determining the location of a point, indirectly, by measuring angles to it from known points. The term triangulation is used in many fields such as surveying and navigation. In the social sciences, it is used to indicate that an investigator is using more than one means of gaining understanding about the phenomenon under study. For example, a researcher interested in the role of alcohol use in situations of intimate partner violence might include a question about alcohol use in the interview, and use a quantitative alcohol use instrument.

Mixed Methods Study

To learn more about how health professionals assess and manage procedural pain in extremely low gestational age infants, Gibbins et al. (2015) conducted a mixed methods study. They utilized unstructured interviews and focus groups along with scales with a quantitative response about pain assessment and management. The themes derived from the qualitative data were reinforced by the quantitative data—specifically that healthcare professionals feel uncertainty about the management of pain in these tiny infants.

Summary

Quantitative research is an important source of information to inform nursing practice. Quantitative research emphasizes empirical evidence gained from tightly controlled experiments with manipulation of variables, though some experimental studies can be descriptive or quasi-experimental.

Qualitative research is an important way for nurses to better understand human experiences and processes. Qualitative research generally has fewer participants and produces richer data that is more subjective in nature than quantitative research. There are a number of different quantitative designs a researcher can use to answer their questions. In most of those designs, the researcher should work closely with a statistician beginning in the planning of the study through the analysis of data.

Both quantitative and qualitative methods have a place in nursing research, and can inform nursing practice as long as the steps of the research process are followed carefully and the researcher is careful to adhere to standards expected to assure rigor. There are many different types of qualitative research designs, each with its set of expected outcomes and guidelines.

Combining quantitative and qualitative methods is also known as mixed methods research. Mixed methods research is a respected research methodology and may provide the richest source of information to inform nursing practice.

The rigor of research is assessed differently in quantitative studies than in qualitative studies. Quantitative studies tend to look at things like internal and external validity and reliability. Similar constructs to assess rigor in qualitative studies may include credibility, transferability, dependability, and confirmability. These four traits are collectively known as trustworthiness.

Self-Test

Select True or False for the following statements:
1. Researchers should fit their research question to the research method they prefer to use.
2. The researcher exerts tight controls over the research situation in qualitative research.
3. The steps to follow in quantitative research are firmly fixed and cannot be changed.
4. Many research questions are appropriate for mixed methods research.
5. Qualitative researchers are very concerned with the generalizability of their study findings.
6. The number of participants is generally larger in qualitative research than in quantitative research.
7. Communicating study results is an important step in the research process.
8. Which statement is true when comparing qualitative research to quantitative research?
   A. Qualitative research is easier to conduct than quantitative research.
   B. The amount of data to be analyzed is usually greater in qualitative studies than in quantitative studies.
   C. The amount of time needed to conduct a qualitative study is usually less than in a quantitative study.
   D. Qualitative research focuses on an individual, whereas quantitative research focuses on a group.
9. Which data collection methods are the most appropriate for a qualitative study?
   A. closed-ended questions and nonparticipant observations

B. participant observations and semistructured interviews
C. structured interviews and physiological measures
D. closed-ended questions and structured interviews
E. All of these data-collection methods would probably be considered.

10. When both qualitative and quantitative research methods are used simultaneously in the same study, this procedure is called:
A. mixed methods
B. meta-analysis
C. multitrait/multimethod
D. methodological plurality

See answers to Self-Test in the Answer Section at the back of the book.

References

Arnetz, J. E., Hamblin, L., Essenmacher, L., Upfal, M. J., Ager, J., & Luborsky, M. (2015). Understanding patient-to-worker violence in hospitals: A qualitative analysis of documented incident reports. *Advanced Nursing, 71*(2), 338–348. doi:10.1111/jan.12494.

Braaten, J. S. (2015). Hospital system barriers to rapid response team activation: A cognitive work analysis. *American Journal of Nursing, 115*(2), 22–33. doi:10.1097/01.NAJ.0000460673.82070.af

Côté-Arsenault, D., & Morrison-Beedy, D. (2005). Focus on research methods. Maintaining your focus in focus groups: Avoiding common mistakes. *Research in Nursing & Health, 28*, 172–179. doi:10.1002/nur.20063

Downs, F. (1994). Hitching the research wagon to theory. *Nursing Research, 43*(4), 195. http://journals.lww.com/nursingresearchonline/pages/default.aspx

Fedorka, P. D., Heasley, S. W., & Patton, C. M. (2014). Perceptions of nurses caring for pregnant women in vegetative states. *MCN: American Journal of Maternal Child Nursing, 39*(2), 80–87. doi:10.1097/NMC0000000000000010

Gibbins, S., Stevens, B., Dionne, K., Yamada, J., Pillai Riddell, R., McGrath, P., & . . . Johnston, C. (2015). Perceptions of health professionals on pain in extremely low gestational age infants. *Qualitative Health Research, 25*(6), 763–774. doi:10.1177/1049732315580105

Happell, B., Bennetts, W., Harris, S., Platania-Phung, C., Tohotoa, J., Byrne, L., & Wynaden, D. (2015). Lived experience in teaching mental health nursing: Issues of fear and power. *International Journal of Mental Health Nursing, 24*(1), 19–27, CINAHL Complete, EBSCO*host*.

Lancaster, G., Kolakowsky-Hayner, S., Kovacich, J., & Greer-Williams, N. (2015). Interdisciplinary communication and collaboration among physicians, nurses, and unlicensed assistive personnel. *Nursing Scholarship, 47*(3), 275–284. doi:10.1111/jnu.12130

Lincoln, Y. S., & Guba, E. G. (1985). *Naturalistic inquiry*. Newbury Park, CA: Sage.

Morden, A., Ong, B. N., Brooks, L., Jinks, C., Porcheret, M., Edwards, J. J., & Dziedzic, K. S. (2015). Introducing evidence through research "push": Using theory and qualitative methods. *Qualitative Health Research, 25*(11), 1560–1575. doi:10.1177/1049732315570120.

Morse, J., & Cheek, J. (2015). Introducing qualitatively-driven mixed-method designs. *Qualitative Health Research, 25*(6), 731–733. doi:10.1177/10497323/5583299

O'Brien, D. T., & Sampson, R. J. (2015). Public and private spheres of neighborhood disorder: Assessing pathways to violence using large-scale digital records. *Research in Crime & Delinquency, 52*(4), 486–510. doi:10.1177/0022427815577835

Pelto, P. J. (2015). What is so new about mixed methods? *Qualitative Health Research, 25*(6), 734–745. doi:10.1177/1049732315573209

Poikela, P., Ruokamo, H., & Teräs, M. (2015). Comparison of meaningful learning characteristics in simulated nursing practice after traditional versus computer-based simulation method: A qualitative videography study. *Nurse Education Today, 35*(2), 373–382. doi:10.1016/j.nedt.2014.10.009

Ramey, S., Schafer, P., DeClerque, J., Lanzi, R., Hobel, C., Shalowitz, M., & Raju, T. (2015). The preconception stress and resiliency pathways model: A multi-level framework on maternal, paternal, and child health disparities derived by community-based participatory research. *Maternal & Child Health, 19*(4), 707–719. doi:10.1007/s10995-014-1581-1

Rodger, D., Neill, M. O., & Nugent, L. (2015). Informal carers' experiences of caring for older adults at home: a phenomenological study. *British Journal of Community Nursing, 20*(6), 280–285. doi:10.12968/bjcn.2015.20.6.280

Sieverdes, J. C., Raynor, P. A., Armstrong, T., Jenkins, C. H., Sox, L. R., & Treiber, F. A. (2015). Attitudes and perceptions of patients on the kidney transplant waiting list toward mobile health–delivered physical activity programs. *Progress in Transplantation, 25*(1), 26–34. doi:10.7182/pit2015884

Snellgrove, S., Beck, C., Green, A., & McSweeney, J. C. (2015). Putting residents first: Strategies developed by CNAs to prevent and manage resident-to-resident violence in nursing homes. *Gerontologist, 55*, s99–s107. doi:10.1093/geront/gnu161

Tak, S. H., Kedia, S., Tongumpun, T. M., & Hong, S. H. (2015). Activity engagement: Perspectives from nursing home residents with dementia. *Educational Gerontology, 41*(3), 182–192. doi:10.1080/03601277.2014.937217

PART II Preliminary Steps in the Research Process

Chapter 6
Identifying Nursing Research Problems

Rose Nieswiadomy, PhD, RN, and Vicki L. Zeigler, PhD, RN

Objectives

On completion of this chapter, you will be prepared to:

1. Identify and summarize sources of nursing research problems.
2. Describe factors to be considered when choosing an appropriate topic for a research study.
3. Compare the criteria to be considered when writing a research question.
4. Write research questions for proposed nursing studies.
5. Explain the guidelines for critiquing problem statements, purpose statements, and research questions in published research reports and articles.

Introduction

Many beginning or novice researchers believe that all the important nursing research studies have already been conducted. This is not true. Most of the studies that have been conducted have raised further questions that need answers.

How does a nurse determine what to study? Some nurse researchers have a clearly identified research problem area from the beginning of their research projects, but this usually is not the case. It is difficult to narrow down the broad problem area to a feasible study. A mistake of beginning researchers (and some experienced ones) is to try to examine too much in one study. The belief seems to be "If a little data are good, a lot of data are even better." It would be much more beneficial to nursing for a researcher to conduct a well-designed smaller study rather than a poorly designed larger study.

Bridges, McNeill, and Munro (2016) advocate studies that "lead to practice changes, address challenges at the bedside, and introduce new care studies" (p. 76). The studies that they report on are problems that frequently challenge the bedside critical care nurse. These issues that arise from clinical practice, and their associated findings that confirm their importance, are evidence that these issues arise repeatedly in critical care practice areas. Nancy Fugate Woods (2013), in an online presentation, states that there is "no substitute for passion about your work" (slide 6). She further suggests that researchers "care deeply" about the issues and phenomena being investigated and how they may ultimately effect the study/patient population.

The number of potential nursing studies is infinite. You may have read about some research priorities identified by various nursing leaders and nursing organizations. The excuse of "I can't think of anything to study" is not an acceptable reason for failing to conduct research.

The first step, and one of the most important requirements of the research process, is to be able to delineate the study area clearly and state the research problem concisely. This is also one of the most difficult tasks of the researcher, especially for the beginning researcher. Many hours may be spent on this part of the research project.

One of the expectations of undergraduate nursing students is that they will be able to identify problems that are appropriate for nursing research studies. Therefore, this chapter helps you determine how to identify a researchable problem and how to write a clear and concise research question. Also, information is provided on how to critique the problem statements, purpose statements, and research questions in published research reports and articles.

Sources of Nursing Research Problems

The sources for generating appropriate nursing research problems are numerous. Four of the most important ones are discussed here: personal experiences, literature sources, existing theories, and previous research.

Personal Experiences

There probably is not a nurse or nursing student among us who has not observed something in nursing practice that was a source of concern. You may have wondered why nurses dislike working with patients with a history of alcoholism, or why some nurses seem to make patients feel like criminals when pain medications are requested. You may also have experienced a nagging doubt about why a procedure is done in a certain manner. On the positive side, you may have observed that patients who are allowed unrestricted visiting hours seem to adjust better to hospitalization and that allowing patients to select special foods from a hospital menu seems to decrease their complaints about hospital food. Thus, from your personal experiences and observations, you may easily identify a topic for study.

Literature Sources

The existing nursing literature is an excellent source of ideas for new research. Nearly every published study concludes with recommendations for further studies. Unpublished theses and dissertations also contain suggestions for studies. Turn to the last page of the final chapter, and you probably will find the researcher's suggestions and pleas for needed future research. Responses to these suggestions could positively influence the direction of nursing research.

The call for future research is not limited to recommendations at the end of published and unpublished studies. Contemporary nursing leaders continually plead for nursing research in articles and books. Many speakers at nursing conventions and conferences address the need for specific areas of nursing research.

Existing Theories

One type of research that is desperately needed in nursing is the type of research that tests existing theories. Research is a process of theory development and testing. Nurses use many theories from other disciplines in their practices. Are these theories always appropriate for nursing? For example, is change theory as applicable in a hospital as it is in a manufacturing company? Are learning theories as predictive of the behavior of sick people as they are for the behavior of well people? For instance, Rose's father was an independent man from German ancestry. He was a "take-charge" kind of person. However, as a patient in a healthcare setting, such as a hospital or a doctor's office, he became as timid as a young child. His wife had to ask all of the questions of the healthcare personnel. Now, imagine if you tried to use a traditional learning theory while trying to teach him about some aspect of his healthcare. You might say to yourself, "This is an independent man who likes to take control." So, you might try to get him to direct his own learning. Wrong approach. He needed to be told, retold, and have demonstrated what he was supposed to do. As you can see, theories may need to be adapted for individual patients or patients in specific healthcare settings.

If an existing theory is used in a research study, a specific propositional statement or statements from the theory must be isolated. Generally, an entire theory is not tested; only a part or parts of the theory are subjected to testing in the clinical situation. For example, a learning principle from a theory of Carl Rogers (1969) might be chosen to guide a patient education program. This learning principle would be transformed into a propositional statement. Later, a hypothesis would be formulated from the propositional statement. Rogers has asserted that learning is facilitated when the student participates responsibly in the learning process. He calls for students to contract with the teacher about what the student should do in the pursuit of knowledge. The researcher would then ask, "Given this proposition from Rogers's theory, what hypothesis or research question would be needed to study this proposition?" For example you might hypothesize that "Nursing students who contract for a specific grade are more likely to obtain that grade than nursing students who do not contract for a specific grade."

The testing of an existing theory, or deductive research, is definitely needed in nursing. Most researchers, however, begin with a problem that has personal relevance in their immediate work environment. This is understandable because the motivation to conduct research is usually higher if the researcher feels some professional involvement and interest in the results of the study.

Previous Research

One disadvantage in using personal experiences as the source of research problems is that this practice frequently leads to a large number of small, unrelated studies, in which there is limited generalizability of the study results. Although "doing your own thing" is important in the motivation of researchers to conduct studies, the nursing profession needs researchers who are willing to replicate, or repeat, studies of other researchers. A body of knowledge should be developed on a sound foundation of research findings. If nursing practice is to be guided by research, the results of studies must be verified. Hypotheses must be tested and retested on adequate sample sizes. Replication studies, therefore, are needed. Replication studies involve repeating a study with all the essential elements of the original study held intact. Different samples and settings may be used. Replication studies in nursing have not been numerous, and the lack of these studies has hindered the development of a cumulative body of nursing knowledge. Although a cursory review of the titles of research reports in the CINAHL Complete database in 2016 uncovered few replications studies by nurses, more and more researchers are replicating earlier studies as evidenced in the literature.

For some reason, the idea of replication seems to carry a negative connotation. Students have asked, "Can a person copy someone else's study? Isn't that like cheating?" During the formative years in educational settings, the dire consequences of plagiarism are continually stressed. It is quite possible that nurses' reluctance to replicate studies is related to this earlier socialization process; however, replication of a previous study does not always imply plagiarism. Using another researcher's methodology, versus using that researcher's exact words to report the results of the replication study, does not constitute plagiarism, which is often referred to as a form of academic dishonesty (Broussard & Hurst, 2015).

The value of replication studies needs to be emphasized to beginning researchers and to experienced researchers as well. A researcher who avoids replication studies needs to ask the question, "Would I have more confidence in the results of a single study conducted with 30 subjects in one setting or the results of several similar studies using many subjects in different settings?"

In addition to exact replication studies, investigations are needed that address the shortcomings of previous research, often requiring minor deviations from the previous study. Different instruments may be used, refinements may be made in the experimental treatments, or more appropriate outcome measures may be identified.

Replication Study

Participants in a single site study were recruited for a study purposed to understand retention that is either supportive or restrictive in a sample of nursing students in a Midwestern RN-to-BSN nursing program (Kern, 2014). The students were asked to complete a 27-item survey assessing self-perceptions of domains related to retention. This study replicated a previous study conducted by Jeffreys (2007) with the only difference being that a single site versus a multisite setting was used. Results of the two studies were similar, in that all factors were found to be supportive, with environmental factors and support from family and friends to be least and most supportive respectively.

Research Problem Considerations

Many factors should be considered when trying to decide if a certain topic is appropriate for a scientific investigation. Some of these factors include ethical issues, significance of the study for nursing, personal motivation of the researcher, qualifications of the researcher, and feasibility of the study.

Ethical Issues

One of the most important considerations in a study concerns the ethical aspects of the project. Everyone is familiar with the terrible atrocities of World War II in which prisoners were subjected to many types of inhumane treatment under the guise of research. Although ethical guidelines for research were developed after World War II, many unethical studies have been conducted since then and continue today.

It is the responsibility of researchers to guarantee, to the best of their ability, that their research is conducted in an ethical manner. Investigators must be familiar with ethical guidelines of the federal government, professional organizations, and specific institutions where research is to be conducted. Any research conducted by most universities and institutions on human participants requires completion of human subjects protections training regarding the rights and protections of study participants.

Significance to Nursing

Every nursing study should have significance for nursing. This does not mean that the findings must have the capability of transforming the entire nursing profession and nursing practice. The researcher should ask questions such as these: Will patients or healthcare professionals benefit from the findings of this study? Will the body of nursing knowledge be increased as the result of this study? Can nurses use the results? Is there a gap in knowledge that this study will fill? If the answers to these questions are "Yes," the problem has significance for nursing.

Personal Motivation

Personal motivation may not be the single most important deciding factor in a researcher's decision to conduct a study, but it certainly ranks high on the priority list. If a person is not interested in the problem to be investigated, it will be difficult to work up enthusiasm for the project and conduct a worthwhile study. Remember the statement by Fugate Woods (2013) presented earlier in this chapter: Nurses should choose research questions that they "care deeply about."

Without personal interest, the research process may become very tedious, and the study may never be completed. But if a researcher is intrigued and curious about the problem, research can become fascinating. The steps can become a treasure hunt. When the data are being prepared for analysis, the excitement grows and the adrenaline flows. At this stage in your understanding and familiarity with the research process, you may be having difficulty believing this. Speak with a nurse who has conducted research. Even if her study was conducted as a course requirement and enthusiasm was not great at the beginning of the project, it is quite likely that excitement and curiosity increased as the study progressed.

Think of questions that have arisen during your clinical experiences. Also, you may have become intrigued by something you have read about in a professional journal or textbook. Many areas in nursing need further research. It is hoped that in the near future you will find an area that is not only significant to nursing but of personal interest to you.

Researcher Qualifications

Not every nurse is qualified to conduct research. Caution must be exercised when research skills are not well developed. Inappropriate designs may be chosen and inadequate data-collection methods used.

Research is generally conducted by nurses who have received advanced educational preparation concerning research design, methodology, and data analysis. However, beginning research skills should be learned at the undergraduate level. A class research project may be conducted in which the students design a survey study and act as the subjects. Enthusiasm for research seems to rise during the course of a class project. If several sections of a research course are being taught during the same semester, the students in the various sections may want to compare their results. A spirit of healthy competition may be fostered. If clinical research is planned, the beginning researcher should collaborate with a more experienced researcher such as a faculty member or an advanced practice nurse.

Feasibility of Study

Feasibility is an essential consideration of any research project. The researcher needs to be reasonably sure that the study can actually be carried out. Many questions need to be answered. How long will the project take? Are appropriate instruments available? Can subjects be obtained? What is the cost? Does the researcher have support for the project? These are only a few of the questions to determine whether a particular study is feasible or not.

TIME A nurse might be interested in studying sibling relationships among quintuplets. Knowledge of the incidence of quintuplet births would certainly discourage anyone considering research on this particular population unless the researcher planned to make this a lifetime project. Time is always a factor to be considered. It is wise to allow more time than seems to be needed because unexpected delays frequently occur.

COST All research projects cost money; some studies are much more expensive than others. The researcher must consider, realistically, the financial resources available. Many sources of outside funding exist, but not nearly enough to cover all of the needed resources to conduct the research.

EQUIPMENT AND SUPPLIES "The best laid plans of mice and men oft times go astray," to paraphrase a line in Robert Burns's poem *To a Mouse*. This saying is certainly true in the research situation. The researcher can devise a study that is significant to nursing and appears feasible to conduct, and suddenly find out that there is no equipment to measure the research variables accurately. Even if equipment is available, it may not be in proper working condition. All research projects require some types of resources. Making an accurate determination of the needed equipment and supplies before making the final decision to conduct a study is an essential component of the research planning process.

Some questions that should be asked (and answered) before beginning a research project include:

1. What equipment will be needed?
2. Is this equipment available and in proper working order?
3. Is there a qualified operator of the equipment?
4. Are the necessary supplies available or can they be obtained?

Some of the more common pieces of equipment that are used in nursing research are physiological data-gathering devices such as thermometers and stethoscopes. Also, office equipment such as computers and data analysis programs, which are not inexpensive, may be needed. Access to a computer is paramount today, even if the amount of data is rather small. Hardly any researcher hand analyzes data today. If the researcher takes into consideration equipment and supplies in the early phases of a research project, there is less likelihood that the project will have to be revised or discarded later because of lack of availability of appropriate equipment or because of supply problems.

ADMINISTRATIVE SUPPORT Many research projects require administrative support. Nurses working in healthcare institutions, such as hospitals, may seek release time to conduct research or ask for funds to support a proposed project. Research requires time, money, and supplies. The nurse researcher will find it very difficult to conduct research independently, without the support of colleagues, mentors, and administration.

Faculty research expectations and support for research by faculty members varies among educational institutions. Not only is financial support helpful, but also, in many cases, psychological support from the administration is even more helpful. Knowing that your superiors support your research efforts can be a very powerful motivating force.

PEER SUPPORT We never outgrow our need for peer support. Many research ideas have never been developed because potential researchers received no support for their ideas from their peers. A comment such as, "Why would you want to conduct a study like that?" could discourage a researcher from proceeding with a study. One of the best ways a nurse researcher can determine a researchable problem is through interactions and discussions with other nurses. This collegial relationship is very important for the researcher, especially for the beginning researcher who has not yet developed confidence in his research skills. A climate of shared interest in nursing research is essential among the members of the nursing profession.

AVAILABILITY OF SUBJECTS A researcher may believe that study subjects are readily available and anxious to participate in a proposed study. Much to the researcher's surprise, this may not be the case. Potential subjects may not meet the study inclusion criteria, may be unwilling to participate, or may already be participating in other studies.

Research Question Criteria

The important criteria for writing a research question are that it: (a) is written in interrogative sentence form, (b) includes the population, (c) includes the variable(s), and (d) is empirically testable.

Written in Interrogative Sentence Form

The use of a question format to narrow down the research problem seems to be the clearest way to identify the problem area of a study. When questions are asked, answers are sought. If a declarative sentence is used to describe the problem area, the desire to seek an answer to the problem does not seem as clear-cut.

Consider the following two ways of expressing the same study problem:

- *Declarative form:* This study examines the relationship between the number of hours that baccalaureate nursing students have studied and their anxiety levels before the midterm examination.
- *Interrogative form:* Is there a correlation (or relationship) between the number of hours that baccalaureate nursing students have studied and their anxiety levels before the midterm examination?

The question format seems to demand an answer more than the declarative form. However, many problem statements in the literature are written in the declarative form.

A research question should always be stated in a complete and grammatically correct sentence. It should be stated in such a manner that the research consumer can read it, understand it, and respond to it. To get all necessary information into the research question, the sentence may become rather long. Students have made comments such as, "You are asking me to write a run-on sentence" and "My English teacher would have given me a failing grade on a sentence like that." Although the research question may be long in some instances, it should always be grammatically correct. Otherwise, confusion will arise, and the research problem may be unclear.

Includes the Population

The population should be delimited (narrowed down) to the main group of interest. A population such as "nurses," "students," or "patients" is too broad to be examined. It would be better to identify these populations as "neonatal intensive care unit nurses," "baccalaureate nursing students," and "patients with a recent diagnosis of diabetes." This narrowing down of the population in the research question still does not identify the specific study population; the population within the study then becomes the sample. The specific population needs to be discussed in detail in another area of the research proposal or research report. This information is usually found in the "Methods" section.

Includes the Variable(s)

The research question should contain the variable(s) to be studied. There may be one, two, or many variables examined in a study.

ONE-VARIABLE STUDIES When a study is of an exploratory nature and contains only one variable, it may be called a **univariate study** or a single variable study. An example of a research question for such a study might be "What sources of work stress are identified by cardiac intensive care unit nurses?" The single variable in this question is "sources of work stress." It is considered a variable because it is expected that the reported sources of stress will vary among the different nurses surveyed. Single-variable, or univariate, studies are frequently the beginning step in a research project. In the example just given, sources of stress might be identified in a univariate study. Another study might then be conducted to determine if a correlation exists between the number of reported sources of stress and the nurses' desire to leave the cardiac intensive care unit as a place of employment. A further study might be conducted in which one of the common stressors was controlled to determine if the desire to leave cardiac intensive care nursing would differ between the experimental group members and the control group members. These last two study suggestions each focus on two variables, rather than just one.

TWO-VARIABLE STUDIES Generally, nursing research is concerned with more than one variable. It would be interesting to know what sources of stress are identified by cardiac intensive care unit nurses. However, it would be more important to know how these stressors affect these nurses, and whether anything could be done to decrease the stressors or reduce their impact on the nurses.

Research in nursing, as well as in other disciplines, is frequently concerned with two variables. When two variables are examined, the study may be called a **bivariate study**. Generally, one of the variables is called the independent variable, and the other is the dependent variable. Consider the example concerning stress among nurses in the cardiac intensive care unit. The research question might be "Is there a correlation between the number of sources of stress reported by nurses in a cardiac intensive care unit and the nurses' desire to leave employment in the cardiac intensive care unit?" In this question, the independent variable is "the number of reported sources of stress," and the dependent variable is "the desire to leave employment in the cardiac intensive care unit." The dependent variable if often referred to as the "outcome" variable as well.

Also, consider the previous example of the study in which an attempt might be made to control or decrease one of the stressors identified by cardiac intensive care unit nurses, to determine if their desire to leave this area of employment would decrease. The identified stressor might be the nurses' unfamiliarity with the equipment in the unit. The research question might be, "Is the level of desire to leave cardiac intensive care unit nursing different between a group of cardiac nurses who have attended a workshop on cardiac intensive care unit equipment and a group of cardiac nurses who have not attended the workshop?" Although the sentence is wordy, it is better to repeat words than to create any misunderstanding about what is being compared. The independent variable in this problem statement is "attendance or non-attendance at a workshop on cardiac intensive care unit equipment," and the dependent variable is "desire to leave cardiac intensive care unit nursing."

Occasionally, in a correlational study, an independent and dependent variable are not identifiable because it is not possible to determine which variable is influencing the other variable. For example, if you were examining the relationship between students' scores on a psychology test and their scores on a math test, it would not be appropriate to identify one as the independent and one as the dependent variable. You would not be able to label one of these variables as the cause and the other variable as the effect, so they would simply be described as *research variables*.

MULTIPLE-VARIABLE STUDIES Whenever more than two variables are examined in a study, the research can be considered a multiple-variable, or **multivariate study**. Multiple-variable research is becoming increasingly common in nursing. Frequently, it is the interaction of variables that is of interest. For example, a researcher might conduct a study to determine why patients do not take their medications as directed after they are discharged. Educational levels might be considered as an influential factor, and the researcher may believe that the patients with high levels of education will be more compliant with the medical regimen than patients with low levels of education. Quite likely the results of the study will not support this belief. Why? Many factors may be influencing the person's medication compliance behavior. People may consider themselves as weak and lacking control over their bodies if they have to take medications. Also, a relative of the patient may view the medicine favorably or unfavorably. The medication may be expensive and the person may not be able to afford having the prescription filled. The likelihood exists that a variety of factors may be influencing the patient's compliance behavior.

Why do nursing students pass or fail the national licensing examination? Is there just one factor involved, such as grade point average? Or could many factors be influential, such as the amount of time studied, the motivation to be a nurse, and the amount of time slept the night before the examination?

Empirically Testable

Testable research questions contain variables that can be measured by the researcher. For a research question to be empirically testable, empirical data must be available about the variable(s) of interest. As you remember, empirical data consist of data gathered through the sense organs. These data consist of observations that are made through hearing, sight, touch, taste, or smell. Additional equipment to aid our senses also may be used. This equipment might be thermometers, scales, or stethoscopes.

Ethical and value issues, or "right and wrong" decisions, are not appropriate for scientific research. Consider these research questions: "Should patients be allowed to have an unlimited number of visitors?" "What is the best way to teach nursing students about the research process?" These are not researchable questions. Most scientific studies do not concern values or ethical issues. A good way to detect a value question is to look for words like *should* and *better*. The two previous examples could be changed to testable research questions in the following manner: "Is there a difference in the anxiety levels of patients between those who are allowed an unlimited number of visitors, and those who are allowed visitors only at specified visiting hours?" and "Is there a difference between the final examination scores of nursing research students who are taught by a lecture method and those who are taught by a seminar method?"

It is also better to avoid words like *cause and effect*. Rather than writing a research question that says, "What is the effect of room temperature on the oral temperature measurements of children?" change this question to, "Is there a difference in the oral temperature measurements of a group of children in a room where the temperature is kept at 65°F in comparison to the oral temperature measurements of this same group of children when the room temperature is kept at 75°F?" Although investigators are interested in cause-and-effect relationships, causality is difficult to prove and, therefore, it is better to avoid using this word or similar words in the research question statement or hypothesis of a study.

Research Question Format

The following material is presented to help you learn how to write research questions. Please do not consider these examples as the only way to present research questions. These examples reflect a combination of ideas and thoughts about research and other researchers' ideas and beliefs. You are reading our ideas and thoughts about research in this textbook, but others have ideas and beliefs that are equal or superior to ours.

Research questions for studies that examine more than one variable are usually written as correlational statements or comparative statements.

I. **Correlational Statement**

Format: Is there a correlation (or relationship) between X (independent variable) and Y (dependent variable) in the population?

Example: Is there a correlation (or relationship) between *anxiety* and *midterm examination scores* of baccalaureate nursing students?

II. **Comparative Statement**

A. Descriptive Study

Format: Is there a difference in Y (dependent variable) between people in the population who *have X* characteristic (independent variable) and those who *do not have X* characteristic?

Example: Is there a difference in *readiness to learn about preoperative teaching* between preoperative patients who *have high anxiety levels* compared to preoperative patients who *have low anxiety levels?*

B. Experimental Study

Format: Is there a difference in Y (dependent variable) between Group A, who *received* X (independent variable) and Group B, who *did not receive* X?

Example: Is there a difference in the *preoperative anxiety levels* of patients who were *taught relaxation techniques* compared to those patients who were *not taught relaxation techniques?*

Practice substituting other variables for the X and Y in the examples. You will soon be able to formulate research questions with greater ease.

It may appear that there are two independent variables in the research question for the descriptive and experimental studies. Both of these research questions have only *one* independent variable, but the independent variable has two levels or subdivisions. In the descriptive study, the two levels of the independent variable are "high anxiety" and "low anxiety." In the experimental study, the two levels of the independent variable are "taught relaxation techniques" and "not taught relaxation techniques."

As you may have noticed, these research questions are written in a neutral, nonpredictive form. The descriptive study question could have been written, "Are preoperative patients who have high anxiety levels less ready to learn about preoperative teaching, than preoperative patients who have low anxiety levels?" There are several reasons for leaving the research question neutral or nonpredictive. The researcher may have very little information about the study area or little knowledge about the possible results of a study when the research question is written. It is advisable to conduct a review of the literature and then develop a theoretical or conceptual framework for the study. With this background, a hypothesis can then be written that predicts the expected study results. The prediction should be put in the hypothesis, not in the research question, although each may contain components of both.

Critiquing Problem Statements, Purpose Statements, and Research Questions

The initial task of the reader of a research article is to determine the problem of the study. The reader will need to locate the problem statement, purpose statement, or research question. The research report may also contain study objectives or goals. This information should be presented at the beginning of a research report. It is often found in the abstract, but also should be presented in the body of the article, usually at the end of the introductory section. If the problem statement, purpose statement, or research question is not clearly stated early in the research report, it will be difficult for the reader to proceed further in evaluating the study.

Problem Statement

Purpose statements and research questions are easily identifiable in a research report because they are labeled as such. Most recent research articles in *Nursing Research* contain a purpose statement. Problem statements may not be as easy to locate. A more general statement about the study problem may be located, such as this statement found in a study report by Read and Ward (2016): "despite widespread agreement that knowledge of genomics is a priority for all healthcare professionals, evidence exists that nurses and nurse faculty are not adequately prepared" (p. 6). Problem statements are designed to get the reader's attention to the problem being addressed by the research. They situate the problem in context so that the reader knows why the problem is important, and why it is significant to the body of knowledge of which it is intended to contribute. As stated previously, problem statements are often difficult to discern because they are either incomplete or absent. According to an editorial written nearly a decade ago by Hernon and Schwartz (2009) in *Library & Information Science Research*, four components of a problem statement were identified by David Clark of Indiana University. Those four components are: (a) lead-in; (b) declaration of originality; (c) Indication of the central focus of the study, and; (d) explanation of study significance (p. 308).

The lead-in is what we call the "hook." This is where you want to make sure that the reader clearly understands what the problem is and why it needs to be studied (declaration of originality). This would include brief background information for what has been done in the field, and what is lacking (the gap in knowledge) then this is followed by a description of the significance of the study which is intended to answer the question, "So what?" You have plenty of time to make your case later with supporting literature, so include the most compelling pieces here and expand on them later. Be clear and concise. You are the expert on your topic, so don't assume that the reader will know the topic as well as you do. Questions to ask yourself when critiquing a problem statement are: (a) Is the existing problem to be addressed clear to the reader?, (b) Is the problem supported by the literature? (c) Is the supporting rationale for the study evident and does it illustrate why the study is worthwhile? and (d) Are the existing gaps in knowledge addressed by the proposed research clear?

Purpose Statement

Questions to ask yourself when critiquing a purpose statement are: (a) Is the purpose of the study clearly stated? (b) Is the purpose of the study concisely stated? and (c) Does the purpose of the study logically flow from the problem previously described (the problem statement)?

Research Questions

Be as specific as possible with your question. If you have formulated a question involving quantitative variables, include those in the question. You should also include the targeted population as well.

Questions to ask yourself when critiquing the research questions in a study are: (a) Does/do the research question(s) follow directly from the study purpose? (b) Does the research question include the variables being studied and the population of interest? and (c) Is it empirically testable?

Once information about this area of a research report is located, certain guidelines may be used for evaluation purposes. First, the reader should determine if there is a problem statement, purpose statement, or research question early in the research report, and is the problem area narrowed down in one of these statements or questions? The scope of the problem is also considered. Is the problem area too narrow or too broad? It may appear that the researcher tried to study too many variables in one study. The problem statement, purpose statement, or research question should contain both the population and the variable(s) that will be studied. It should be apparent that the study was either quantitative or qualitative. The possibility of gathering empirical data on the topic of interest should be evident. Determination should then be made about the ethical nature of the study. Next, the reader must consider the significance of the problem area to nursing. Box 6–1 lists the questions to be asked while evaluating this area of a research report.

Box 6–1 Guidelines for Critiquing Problem Statements, Purpose Statements, and Research Questions

Based on the problem statement, purpose statement, or research question:

1. Is the research problem area clear?
2. Is there a succinct problem statement, purpose statement, or research question?
3. Are the study variables and the population included?
4. Can a determination be made as to whether the study was a quantitative or qualitative study?
5. Can a decision be made that empirical data were gathered on the topic of interest?
6. Does it appear that the study was ethical?
7. Is the feasibility of the study evident?
8. Is the significance of the study to nursing apparent?

Summary

The selection of a research problem is probably the most important and most difficult step in the research process. Some of the most common sources of research ideas are personal experiences, literature sources, existing theories, and previous studies. Nurses need to conduct replication studies based on previous nursing research investigations.

Several criteria should be considered in determining a problem to study. First, ethical issues must be considered. Second, the problem should be significant to nursing. Third, personal motivation to conduct the study should be present. Fourth, the researcher's qualifications must be considered. Finally, the feasibility of the study must be considered. How long will the project take? How much will it cost? Can the needed equipment and supplies be obtained? Does the researcher have administrative and peer support for the project? Is a study sample available?

The research problem area should be narrowed down to a research question. The question should contain the population and variables that are being studied, and be empirically testable. The use of a question format is a clear way to identify the problem area for a study. Questions demand answers. Another way to make a research question concise is by delimiting or narrowing down the population for the study. Also, the variables under study must be clearly identified. One, two, or many variables may be studied.

Studies may be referred to as univariate, bivariate, or multivariate studies, according to whether one, two, or many variables are being studied. There is an increasing emphasis on multivariate research because nursing is concerned with the relationships between many combinations of variables. Testable research questions contain variables that can be measured empirically. Empirical data consist of data gathered through the sense organs. Scientific research questions do not concern values or ethical issues. Research problems that examine more than one variable are usually written in the form of a correlational statement or comparative statement.

Self-Test

1. Evaluate this question for the presence of the necessary elements of an acceptable research question: Is there a difference in men and women who exercise daily?
   A. The population is missing.
   B. The dependent variable is missing.
   C. The independent variable is missing.
   D. All elements are present.

2. Evaluate this question for the presence of the necessary elements of an acceptable research question: Is there a correlation between body surface area in men who exercise regularly using weight training only, and those using weight training and aerobic exercise?
   A. The population is missing.
   B. The dependent variable is missing.
   C. The independent variable is missing.
   D. All elements are present.

3. Evaluate this question for the presence of the necessary elements of an acceptable research question: Is there a relationship between anxiety and quality of life?
   A. The population is missing.
   B. The dependent variable is missing.
   C. The independent variable is missing.
   D. All elements are present.

4. Evaluate this question for the presence of the necessary elements of an acceptable research question: Is there a difference in anxiety levels if the personal trainer is a female versus a personal trainer who is male?
   A. The population is missing.
   B. The dependent variable is missing.
   C. The independent variable is missing.
   D. All elements are present.

5. Evaluate this question for the presence of the necessary elements of an acceptable research question: Is there a correlation between personal trainers' experiences?
   A. The population is missing.
   B. The dependent variable is missing.
   C. Either the independent or dependent variable is missing.
   D. All elements are present.

6. Evaluate this question for the type of variable study being portrayed: Is there a difference in the quality of life in patients who receive peritoneal dialysis and those who receive hemodialysis?
   A. univariate study
   B. bivariate study
   C. multivariate study
   D. No variables are specified.

7. Evaluate this question for the type of variable study being portrayed: What are the infection rates among patients on hemodialysis?
   A. univariate study
   B. bivariate study
   C. multivariate study
   D. No variables are specified.

8. Evaluate this question for the type of variable study being portrayed: Are there correlations between weight, blood pressure, and type of dialysate in patients immediately following a dialysis session for patients undergoing peritoneal dialysis versus those undergoing hemodialysis?
   A. univariate study
   B. bivariate study
   C. multivariate study
   D. No variables are specified.

9. Evaluate this question for the variable that is missing: Are patients who receive hemodialysis different from those who receive peritoneal dialysis?
   A. The population is missing.
   B. The independent variable is missing.
   C. A univariate variable is missing.
   D. The dependent variable is missing.

10. Evaluate this question for the type of variable study being portrayed: Is there a correlation between fluctuations in blood pressure and level of fatigue in patients who undergo hemodialysis?
    A. univariate study
    B. bivariate study
    C. multivariate study
    D. No variables are specified.

See answers to Self-Test in the Answer Section at the back of the book.

References

Bridges, E., McNeill, M., & Munro, N. (2016). Research in review: Driving critical care practice change. *American Journal of Critical Care, 25*(1), 76–84. doi:10.4037/ajcc2016564

Broussard, L., & Hurst, H. (2015). Plagiarism prevention and detection a challenge. *Nurse Educator, 44,* 168–168. doi:10.1097/NNE.0000000000000147

Fugate Woods, N. (2013). Developing a research trajectory: Building on big ideas and small projects. http://www.advocatehealth.com/documents/pediatricresearch/WoodsPM.pdf

Hernon, P., & Schwartz, C. (2007). What is a problem statement? *Library & Information Science Research, 29,* 307–309. doi:10.1016/j.lisr.2007.06.001

Jeffreys, M. R. (2007). Nontraditional students' perceptions of variables influencing retention: A multisite study. *Nurse Educator, 32,* 161–167. doi:10.1097/01.NNE.0000282086.3564.

Kern, B. (2014). Factors that restrict or support retention among RN-to-BSN nursing students: A replication study. *Open Journal of Nursing, 4,* 296–302. doi:10.4236/ojn.2014.44034.

Read, C. Y., & Ward, L. D. (2016). Faculty performance on the Genomic Nursing Concept Inventory. *Nursing Scholarship, 48*(1), 5–13. doi:10.1111/jnu.12175.

Rogers, C. (1969). *Freedom to learn.* Columbus, OH: Charles E. Merrill.

Chapter 7
Review of the Literature

Rose Nieswiadomy, PhD, RN, and Connie Maxwell, BS, MLS

Objectives

On completion of this chapter, you will be prepared to:

1. Explain the purpose of a literature review.
2. Differentiate among primary and secondary sources and research articles and grey literature.
3. Construct an effectively designed search strategy that includes a concise research question.
4. Conduct a comprehensive literature search on a given topic.
5. Recognize differences in content and accessibility between nursing research databases.
6. Evaluate, analyze, and synthesize literature sources for inclusion in a literature review.

Introduction

Reviewing the literature relevant to a research topic is a standard part of doing research. A literature review provides an analysis and synthesis of information from research studies, scholarly articles, books, dissertations, conference proceedings, and other materials relevant to a particular topic. A literature review should foster new research by identifying the areas where extensive research has been completed, and by uncovering areas where more research is needed. In this chapter, we will discuss the importance and purposes of a literature review, types of literature sources, differences between primary and secondary sources, grey literature, research strategies, and guidelines for writing a literature review.

Purposes of the Literature Review

There are many purposes for reviewing the literature before conducting a research study. The most important one is to determine what is already known about the topic you are interested in. A search is made to locate previous studies in that area. There are very few topics so rare that they have never been investigated.

If previous research is found, the researcher must decide whether to replicate a study or to examine another aspect of the topic. The review of the literature is necessary, therefore, to specify the problem to be studied. Research is an ongoing process that builds on previous knowledge. Your ideas, based on what you learn and the things you question, will be the foundation for further research.

A comprehensive literature search is necessary to locate both classic and the most recent information sources. Once the researcher is familiar with the existing literature, a framework must be established in which to place the study results. In a quantitative study, this involves locating theoretical or conceptual formulations that will help guide the study. The research hypotheses or questions will be based on the theoretical or conceptual framework of the study, and the research findings will be interpreted in light of the study framework. Therefore, the literature review can help locate a framework for the proposed study.

Another purpose of the review of the literature is to help plan the study methodology. Appropriate research methods and research tools for the study may be selected after reading the accounts of other studies. The researcher may be able to capitalize on the successes as well as the mistakes of other investigators.

While the researcher generally begins the literature review with a topic in mind, many published studies contain recommendations for future research; therefore, the idea for a study may actually be formed when reading about a research study.

Literature Sources

Types of Information Sources

There are different types of information sources, and it will be helpful to understand a little about them before beginning a literature search. The question you are researching will influence the sources you use. Finding tools (also called *resources* or *search tools*) will be used to locate literature sources.

Primary and Secondary Sources

Literature sources may be classified as primary or secondary sources. A **primary source** in the research literature is an account of a research study written by the original investigator(s). Primary sources for research studies are frequently found in journal articles. *Nursing Research, Advances in Nursing Science, Applied Nursing Research, Biological Research for Nursing, Clinical Nursing Research, Nursing Science Quarterly, Research in Gerontological Nursing, Research in Nursing and Health,* and *Western Journal of Nursing Research* are examples of journals that publish primary research articles. Clinical journals, such as *Heart & Lung, Journal of Acute and Critical Care,* and *Pediatric Nursing* also contain primary research articles. A **secondary source** is a summary or description of a research study written by someone other than the study investigator(s). A secondary source may review or compare more than one research study. The beginning researcher may be tempted to rely on secondary sources because summaries of studies or theories are easier to read and understand than the original works or primary source. The original or primary source should be read whenever possible. Secondary sources may provide valuable insights into the material, but there is always a risk that the author of a secondary source might interpret information differently from the original researcher, or focus on specific areas of the research and leave out important information that might be valuable to the reader.

Try to begin your search with the most recent primary sources. Read the abstract or summary of the study to determine if the source should be read in depth. These primary sources will frequently contain reference citations for earlier research reports that may be relevant to your proposed study.

Table 7-1 Literature Sources and Search Tools

Literature Sources	Uses and Locations	Suggested Finding Tools
Reference materials (print and electronic) Examples: dictionaries, encyclopedias, yearbooks, biographies, directories, and atlases	Background information, facts, figures, speeches, statistics, definitions, and dates	Library catalogs Discovery catalogs Search engines
Books (print and ebooks)	In-depth coverage of a subject Citations and bibliographies that can be used to identify other sources	Library catalogs Discovery catalogs
Scholarly journals	Primary and secondary research articles Citations and bibliographies that can be used to identify other sources.	Databases Discovery catalogs Search engines
Magazines	Public opinion articles	Multidisciplinary databases Discovery catalogs Search engines
News sources	Current events and developments Firsthand reports of developing situations	News databases Discovery catalogs Search engines
Statistics	Statistical information	Search engines General catalogs Discovery catalogs Databases
Reports, research studies, and conference papers	Examples: government reports and conference papers from print and online depositories. Some materials may not be openly available.	Search engines Repositories Databases
Theses and dissertations	Master's and doctoral dissertations (unpublished)	Databases Repositories
Social media	Source of information available directly from current researchers in the medical and science communities	Internet

Grey Literature

Grey literature, also called gray literature, was defined at the 1999 Fourth International Conference on Grey Literature as "that which is produced on all levels of government, academics, business and industry in print, and electronic formats, but which is not controlled by commercial publishers" (Academy Health, 2006). Reports, conference proceedings, standards, technical documentation, government documents, technical documents, fact sheets, and policy briefs are all examples of grey literature. Grey literature has emerged from being considered simply interesting or supporting information to being recognized as an essential part of research data. Grey literature should be reviewed for inclusion in a comprehensive literature review.

Many research reports never get published because there were no significant findings. Researchers are reluctant to submit a manuscript for this type of study because journal reviewers are unlikely to recommend publication of these manuscripts. Journal editors may be less likely to publish nonsignificant findings than significant findings. This publication bias is one reason grey literature has become increasingly more important, particularly in systematic reviews and meta-analysis studies.

According to the *Health Services Research and Health Policy Grey Literature Project: Summary Report*, much of the grey literature is designed to make technical material or research findings more easily understood by a lay audience. For example, fact sheets are often produced to provide context and to summarize reports, working papers, and other formats of research or technical materials. Research institutes such as the Leonard Davis Institute, the Sheps Center, and the Urban Institute produce working papers and issue briefs. Organizations such as the Alliance for Health Reform write policy briefs that summarize the findings of a number of individual research studies (Health Services Research and Health Policy Grey Literature Project, 2006). The Joanna Briggs Research Library, dissertation abstracts, and many health-related databases such as CINAHL and the Scopus Index often provide access to grey literature along with published research articles.

Search Strategies

Develop a Search Strategy

Searching for information is easier, faster, and often yields better results when you take the time to do a little planning. This pre-search exercise will only take a few minutes, but trust us, it works. It will save you time and help you get a set of results that closely match your topic.

DECIDE ON YOUR SEARCH QUESTION The research question provides the framework for the literature review. It should provide a clear focus and indication of what information is needed to address your question. If the question is too broad, it may lead you in many directions and your search will result in too many sources without a manageable focus.

Example: Is it better to have a baby on a weekday or a weekend?

QUESTION WHETHER THE TOPIC NEEDS TO BE MORE SPECIFIC What do you mean when you ask *is it better*? Are you interested in the health of the mother, the child, or both? What other factors might be important in this study (length of hospital stay, adequate staffing, staff error)? You will make additional changes to your topic as you discover what has already been studied and have seen the results of those existing studies.

How is weekend birth and higher neonatal mortality associated with quality of care?

CREATE A SET OF SEARCH TERMS OR PHRASES Your literature review should include information about how your search terms were selected, modified, and combined to ensure a comprehensive and thorough search:

- Use nouns, noun phrases, and other keywords.
- *Induce, labor, morning, evening*
- Expand your search words with synonyms, antonyms, and other relevant words.
- *Pregnancy, birth, labor, childbirth, delivery, daytime, night, day, time factors*
- Limit your catalog search to specific materials by adding terms such as reference or encyclopedia.
- In databases, add terms such as study, research, measurement, statistics, randomized, validity, and narrative to retrieve research studies.
- Include Medical Subject Headings (MeSH).

DECIDE IF CURRENCY IS IMPORTANT Depending on your topic, you may want to limit your search to the past five or ten years. Remember that currency is important but research studies often cover a significant time period. It may also be important to include historical information for some topics.

USE OPTIONS AND LIMITERS A variety of options and limiters can help you focus your search. Most finding tools offer a set of options and limiters to help you construct a search that will return relevant hits.

> **Combining the terms** *childbirth* and *research* and *weekend* **with the phrase** *time factors*; **limiting to** a 2010–2015 **date range, and limiting to** academic journals **with** references available, resulted in the following citation: Hamilton, P, and E. Restrepo. "Sociodemographic Factors Associated With Weekend Birth and Increased Risk of Neonatal Mortality." *JOGNN: Journal of Obstetric, Gynecologic & Neonatal Nursing* 35.2 (2006): 208-214. *CINAHL Complete*. Web. 20 May 2015. *This is a primary source for a research study and includes the objective, design, samples, main outcome measures, results, conclusions, and keywords.*
>
> **Combining birth and weekend (all of the words) with neonatal mortality (as a phrase) 2000-2015.**
> Hamilton, P. & Restrepo, E. (2003). Weekend Birth and Higher Neonatal Mortality: A Problem of Patient Acuity or Quality of Care? *Journal of Obstetric, Gynecologic, & Neonatal Nursing*, 32: 724–733. doi: 10.1177/0884217503258306

Figure 7–1 Examples of searchers using limiters and other advanced search options

These vary according to the specific resource you are searching. In many cases, the basic or simple search provides a few choices and the advanced search offers additional choices. We recommend you always use the "advanced search" when it is available. A variety of options and limiters can help you focus your search and will result in a more manageable set of results, many of which will be relevant to your topic. A few examples of advanced search options and limiters are: and/or/not/, as a phrase, without the word, date range, language, includes references, audience, URL, research type, age, and peer reviewed.

Ask a Librarian

Searching for information can be overwhelming. Libraries contain a wealth of information and their resources and services are tailored to meet your needs. You can use the library physically or virtually. Most of the services and many of the resources are available in person or online. If you are unfamiliar with a particular library to which you have access, acquaint yourself with that library's facilities and holdings. Tour the library and consult the staff. Librarians have the skills and expertise to assist students with a literature review.

Before beginning your research project, we advise you to make an appointment with a librarian, who will walk you through the organization of information, types of research studies, selection and use of databases and other literature sources, and citation styles and management systems.

Work with your librarian to develop the skills to:

- Identify appropriate search terms (controlled vocabulary, natural language, subject headings, MARC records, metadata, tags, etc.).
- Devise search strategies using limits and modifiers with the specificity to optimize results.
- Gain expertise in the operation of complex search systems.
- Locate and access difficult-to-find resources.
- Assess sources for currency, relevance, authority and accuracy and purpose.

Lisa Federer (2013) has advised that the NIH and the National Science Foundation's current grant funding policies are reinforcing the need for librarians as "research informationists." Research informationists are prepared to work with research teams from project inception and grant-seeking to final publication. Specifically, they may provide "guidance on data management and preservation, bibliometric analysis, expert searching, compliance with grant funder policies regarding data management and open access, and other information-related areas" (Federer, 2013, p. 298).

Librarians love research. Literature reviews are their idea of fun. You will find them knowledgeable and helpful throughout your research process.

Evaluate your result list. Before you print your search results, check to see if all or most of your search terms are included in the title, abstract, description, or keywords. Is the information source authoritative? Is the publication date in line with your topic? Review the record for additional words or phrases to add to your search terms.

Don't forget to note the title, source, and other important information about the source; you will need it for your references. Some records include a citation feature. In order to cite your sources correctly, you must follow the instructions for reference citations in the citation style assigned to you. The American Psychological Association (APA) format has become quite popular in the nursing literature and many nursing education programs use APA style. The APA website offers additional citation information. A great deal of frustration will be avoided if complete reference details are recorded for each literature source at the time you consult it. It is frustrating to have to return to the library or go back to the internet search to find missing items (such as volume numbers). You may discover that some part of the reference citation is missing as you are hurrying to complete your paper at 2 a.m. on the morning before the paper is due. The motto is "Record references accurately" (RRA). One well-respected strategy for relocating a published article is to include the digital object identifier (DOI) within the citation of the article in the reference list. A DOI is the unique number assigned to each article to provide a persistent link to its location on the internet. The American Psychological Association (APA) recommends that DOIs be included for both print and electronic sources when they are available. The DOI is usually located on the first page of the electronic journal article, near the copyright notice. It can also be found on the landing page for the article.

Review the bibliography. Many scholarly literature sources include bibliographies that lead the researcher to additional resources.

Finding Tools

Now we will review the **finding tools** that help you find actual literature sources. Other terms for finding tools are *indices* and *resources*. This section will help you understand how to use finding tools to locate and access the literature sources pertinent to your research topic. Catalogs and databases are examples of finding tools. Some databases that are especially helpful to nursing researchers are CINAHL, MEDLINE, Cochrane, Ovid Nursing, Joanna Briggs EBP, PsychINFO, ProQuest Dissertations and Thesis databases, Science Direct, and Scopus.

CATALOGS Catalogs index the print and electronic holdings of libraries or organizations. Most catalogs are available online. Catalogs contain alphabetical listings of books, multimedia, journals, and other library holdings under several different categories such as title, author, subject heading, and keyword. Catalogs give information on how or where to access these sources. You may find a link that leads you to an online book, journal article, or movie; or you may be given a call number or library location that leads you to print materials. In the past few years, a large number of nursing books have been made available online. *Encyclopedia of Nursing Research, Gale Encyclopedia of Children's Health Infancy through Adolescence, Encyclopedia of Medical Anthropology Health and Illness in the World's Cultures*, and *Gale Encyclopedia of Children's Health Infancy through Adolescence* are examples of excellent nursing reference books. Many of these are offered as full-text online books and they can provide excellent background information for your research topic.

For some time, libraries have been aware that they cannot function as independent units. No one library can afford all the holdings that might be desired. A listing of library collections throughout the world can be found online at WorldCat, a nonprofit, membership-based computer library service and research organization. You can use WorldCat to search many libraries simultaneously for an item, then locate it in a library nearby or request a copy through your library's interlibrary loan or document delivery services.

Discovery catalogs, also called discovery systems, are a recent development in the evolution of the traditional catalog. A traditional catalog is a great finding tool for books but you will find a limited number of links to journal articles. Many libraries now offer a discovery system that includes records and links to some database holdings. These are great finding tools if you only need an article or two on a specific subject, but you must use the databases to do a comprehensive literature review.

DATABASES Databases index journal articles, dissertations, research reviews, and many other literature sources both published and unpublished. Some databases only address specific topics while others are multidisciplinary. Most of the databases are electronic but a few can still be found as print indexes or microforms. There are several databases that index and provide abstracts of articles from nursing, medicine, and other health sciences topics. Nursing researchers will have access to many databases through their campus library (institution-based subscriptions). Other databases such as PubMed and Cochrane are available via the internet at no cost. Some databases are available via the internet through a pay-per-view or other individual access service. Many databases will link directly to full-text sources. If you find a source that does not link to the full-text article, you might locate it on your library shelves, or you can ask a librarian to request it from another library through a document delivery system. Always check the catalog or contact your librarian before you pay for journal articles. This step may save you a significant amount of money.

Selected Databases for Nursing Students

This section is composed from information that was gleaned from vendor and publisher websites as well as through hands-on searching in May, 2015.

CINAHL DATABASES **CINAHL (Cumulative Index to Nursing and Allied Health Literature)** provides indexing of the top nursing and allied health literature available, including nursing journals and publications from the National League for Nursing and the American Nurses Association. It covers a wide range of topics including nursing, biomedicine, health sciences librarianship, alternative/complementary medicine, consumer health, and allied health disciplines. CINAHL also provides access to healthcare books, nursing dissertations, selected conference proceedings, standards of practice, audiovisuals and book chapters, legal cases, clinical innovations, critical paths, research instruments, and clinical trials. It has an easy-to-use interface with basic and advanced search features and searchable cited references. CINAHL Subject Headings follow the structure of the Medical Subject Headings (MeSH) used by the National Library of Medicine and it helps users to effectively search and retrieve information. Coverage is from 1982 to the present. CINAHL is available as an institutional based subscription only.

MEDLINE DATABASES **MEDLINE**, available through the National Library of Medicine (NLM), provides access to journals in the life sciences, with a concentration on biomedicine. It also includes information from nursing, dentistry, veterinary medicine, and pharmacy.

Additional versions of MEDLINE are:

- *MEDLINE with Full Text*, which includes full-text articles for a number of medical journals indexed in *MEDLINE*. Coverage dates back to 1949, with full-text material back to 1965. Institutional subscription only.
- *Medline® Plus*, NLM's free website for consumer health information, covers topics of interest to healthcare consumers and is written in plain language for the general population.
- *PubMed*, the official Database of the NIH, provides free access to the MEDLINE database of references and abstracts on life sciences and biomedical topics. Links to full text are available for some articles.

COCHRANE DATABASE OF SYSTEMATIC REVIEW Cochrane is a global independent network of health practitioners, researchers, patient advocates, and others, who work to identify, appraise, and synthesize individual research findings to produce the best available evidence on what can work, what might harm, and where more research is needed. The **Cochrane Library** is a collection of six databases that contain different types of high-quality, independent evidence to inform healthcare decision making, and a seventh database that provides information about groups in the Cochrane Collaboration. Databases include: Cochrane Database of Systematic Reviews (leading resource for systematic reviews in healthcare), Cochrane Central Register of Controlled Trials, Cochrane Methodology Register, Database of Abstracts of Reviews of Effects, Health Technology Assessment Database, and NHS Economic Evaluation Database. The Cochrane Library is available as an online subscription database; however, much of the information is available at no cost online. The Cochrane Library is working toward achieving universal open access to new and updated Cochrane reviews by the end of 2016. Currently all new reviews become free to access for all readers 12 months after publication.

OVID NURSING DATABASE The **Ovid Nursing Database**, is an institutional subscription database, includes full-text content from current journals through Lippincott Williams & Wilkins, combined with a nursing subset of MEDLINE. The Ovid Nursing Database also provides access to these sources:

> **The Joanna Briggs Institute EBP Database of Evidence Based Recommended Practices** is a comprehensive range of resources including records across seven publication types including literature reviews, recommended practices and procedures, information guideline sheets, comprehensive systematic reviews and protocols, consumer information sheets and technical reports.
>
> **Joanna Briggs Institute (JBI) Library website**, a free internet resource, is a repository for publications and information for policy makers, health professionals, health scientists, and others with a practical or academic interest in evidence-based healthcare. It provides access to the online journal *JBI Database of Systematic Reviews and Implementation Reports*, the JBI PIS (Practice Information Sheets), and many open-access information resources.

PSYCHINFO PsychINFO, prepared by the American Psychological Association, covers literature from psychology and related disciplines, such as nursing. PsychINFO provides abstracting and indexing for journals, book chapters, and books and dissertations. PsychINFO indexes many nursing journals such as *International Journal of Nursing Studies, Advances in Nursing Science, Clinical Nursing Research, Journal of Nursing Measurement, Journal of Nursing Scholarship, Research in Nursing and Health,* and *Journal of Nursing Research*. It is available as an institutional subscription, and by individual pay-per-use access.

PROQUEST DISSERTATIONS & THESES DATABASE (PQDT) **ProQuest Dissertations & Theses Database (PQDT)** is a comprehensive collection of dissertations and theses. Degree-granting institutions submit copies of dissertations and theses to University Microfilms International (UMI) and citations for these dissertations and theses are included in the online database. For works published from 1997 and in some cases before 1997, a full-text PDF will usually be available for free download. The ProQuest Dissertations & Theses Database is available as an institutional-based subscription and also offers an individual search with options for purchase. The ProQuest Nursing & Allied Health database includes abstracting and indexing for nursing journals, videos, dissertations, ebooks, conference papers and other sources in nursing, allied health, alternative and complementary medicine, and other health sciences. Many of the records link to full-text sources. ProQuest Nursing & Allied Health is available as an institutional-based subscription only.

SCIENCE DIRECT **Science Direct**, an Elsevier product, provides abstracting and indexing for scientific, technical, and medical peer-reviewed journals and books. It is a multidisciplinary database that includes nursing, allied health, and other health science sources. Science Direct is available as an institutional subscription. The amount of full-text sources is determined by subscription agreements. Guest User access is also available with several options for obtaining full-text articles.

SCOPUS **Scopus**, another Elsevier product, is an abstract and citation database of scientific journals, books, and conference proceedings. Its objective is to deliver a comprehensive overview of the world's research output in the fields of science, technology, medicine, social sciences, and arts and humanities. Scopus features smart tools to track, analyze, and visualize research. Scopus is available as an institutional-based subscription.

SEARCH ENGINES Search engines are finding tools to help you find literature sources via the internet. Today, libraries are as close as your fingers, with an ever increasing amount of information easily available through your computer and other mobile devices. The biggest challenge for today's student is sorting through this plethora of information to find reputable literature sources that are relevant to your research interest. Google Scholar is this author's choice for locating scholarly sources. For a more focused search remember to use the advanced search feature. Don't pay for articles that your library already owns; use the settings tab to link the Google Scholar search to your library's holdings.

A word of caution is offered here. The internet is ever changing and sites accessed today may change or even disappear tomorrow. Even writing about reviewing the literature is challenging, as information becomes somewhat outdated almost as soon as it becomes available.

Writing the Literature Review

A literature review must include organized information from sources found through a comprehensive search of the literature. Its purpose is to offer the reader a data-based synthesis of existing research relevant to a research topic. The researcher searches the literature to identify research information that is central to the argument for the selected research topic (the claims, the evidence, and the assumptions) and analyzes the strengths and weaknesses that support and oppose the researcher's argument. After the information sources are analyzed the researcher will use a predefined methodology to combine that information and summarize what was discovered.

Analyze: Determine what evidence or information is given in each source to support the points, inferences, or arguments about your topic.

Synthesize: Combine the points, inferences, or arguments from the different sources to provide readers with information about the existing research on your topic.

Extracting Information from Literature Sources

After literature sources are located, pertinent material must be extracted from these sources. Each literature source must be analyzed and interpreted and the findings and conclusions of those deemed pertinent to your topic will be used to write the literature review. This can be a formidable undertaking. Some people try to avoid this task as long as possible by printing every article on a certain topic. However, the researcher must finally read the literature sources and decide what material is appropriate for the study under consideration and determine which literature makes a significant contribution to the understanding of the topic. When taking notes, be as brief as possible, but do not omit important information. It is better to have too much information from a source rather than not enough. For relevant research articles, you will want to record information on the problem of the study, hypotheses, methodology, sample type, findings, and conclusions.

Critiquing the Literature Review in a Research Article

The literature review section of a research article can provide you with a great deal of information about that study as well as past studies of a similar topic. It can be difficult to evaluate the literature review section of a research article if you are not familiar with the literature and previous research for that topic. If all sources appear to be older than 5 years, you might wonder if some recent references may have been omitted. If the topic is one that you know has been studied for many years, such as the effectiveness of mammograms, you would expect to see older studies cited as well as recent studies. Determine if the researcher is citing primary sources or secondary sources when reporting results of studies conducted in the past. An examination of the reference list at the end of the article will provide some clues. If most of the references are from research journals, you will be more confident that the sources are primary ones. If the reference list contains book chapters and literature reviews on a certain topic, it is likely that some secondary sources are being cited. Some of the sources listed in the references may be important for your literature review. If a theorist has been cited, the reference list should contain that theorist's name as the author of the cited material. If, for example, Maslow's theory is being discussed in the article you are critiquing, expect to see a reference that shows Maslow as the author.

Carefully review the citations from the reference list or bibliography. You will likely find additional sources you should include in your own literature review. This is sometimes called parallel searching.

Components of a Literature Review

After you have located your literature sources, you can begin writing the literature review. It should be a structured analysis of the evidence you found to answer your question. Use the list in Box 7–1 to critique your review.

Most literature reviews include an introduction, a body, a section on suggestions for further research, and a closing summary. The introduction includes an overview of the topic, objectives of the review, the research question and thesis statement, a description of the methods used to locate sources, the justification used for inclusion and exclusion of sources, and an explanation of how sources were evaluated and categorized. The body of the literature review is where you document what is known about the research topic. Answer the

---

Box 7–1 Critique Checklist

1. Was the literature search both comprehensive and thorough?
2. Is the literature review comprehensive?
3. Are all sources relevant and focused on evidence pertinent to the topic?
4. Are both primary and secondary sources included?
5. Are both published and grey literature included?
6. Are all sources critically analyzed and synthesized based on your defined methodology?
7. Are both supporting and opposing theory and research discussed?
8. Does the review flow logically from the purposes(s) of the study?
9. Is the literature review concise?
10. Are paraphrases and direct quotes used and appropriately?
11. Does the review include an introduction, analysis, and synthesis of the literature sources; suggestions for further research; and a summary of findings?
12. Are sources cited fully and correctly, offering clear access to the evidence?
13. Will the reader find your literature review interesting and informative?

question, "What is the evidence?" Provide an analysis of how each source supports or opposes a particular position or varies from the other research, and your conclusions about which materials most strongly support your arguments and make the greatest contribution to the understanding and development of their area of research. A section with suggestions for further research is included in most literature reviews. This is based on your questions resulting from what you found or didn't find in the literature. Write about aspects of the topic where further research is needed. Include new research questions. Conclude the literature review with a discussion about the highlights in the body and illustrate how previous research correlates to your thesis statement.

Summary

The most important reason for reviewing the literature before conducting a research study is to determine what is already known about the topic. A literature review analyzes and synthesizes information from literature sources. There are many sources of information including books, journal articles, conference proceedings, dissertations, social media, and more. Catalogs, databases, and internet search engines are finding tools that will help you search for information sources relevant to your research topic. Each literature source is analyzed and interpreted and the findings and conclusions are used to write the literature review.

Literature sources may be classified as primary or secondary. A primary source in the research literature is a description of a study written by the original researcher(s). A secondary source provides a summary or description of a research study written by someone other than the original study investigator(s). Unpublished materials such as reports, conference proceedings, technical documentation, and government documents are called grey literature. In recent years, grey literature has become as an essential part of research data.

Before you begin your search for information sources, you should compose your research question. You can adapt it as needed during your search. Create a broad list of search terms and phrases based on your topic. Use catalogs, databases, and internet search engines to find information sources. Your librarian is available online or face-to-face, to assist you with your search.

After you have located your literature sources, write the literature review. It should be a structured analysis of the evidence you found to answer your question.

Self-Test

Select the best answer.
1. Which statement is true?
   A. Due to concerns of plagiarism, a research study should never be a replication of another study.
   B. Research is an ongoing process that builds on previous knowledge.
   C. Classic information rarely supports new research projects.
   D. An original research study does not need a literature review.
2. What is the difference between primary and secondary sources?
   A. A primary source is a type of study that was first identified by the finding tool and the secondary sources are identified next.
   B. Primary sources are included in literature reviews but secondary sources are not important.
   C. An article written by the researcher who conducted a study is a primary source and

a secondary source is an article that summarizes and comments on the study.
D. A summary of research done on your study topic is a primary source and the original study is a secondary source.

3. Which is not a part of building a search strategy?
    A. discovering whether the topic has already been researched
    B. writing a research question and thesis statement
    C. determining a set of terms and phrases to use for your search
    D. considering whether your topic should include date parameters

4. Which is considered an inappropriate way to ask a librarian for assistance?
    A. Visit the library and ask to speak to a librarian.
    B. Email a specific librarian or use the online *Ask a Librarian* service.
    C. Make an appointment in advance.
    D. Call the librarian at home before your literature review is due.

5. Most research articles that appear in the journal *Nursing Research* are examples of what?
    A. primary sources
    B. secondary sources
    C. meta-analysis studies
    D. systematic reviews

6. Which database provides the most comprehensive research study results on a particular healthcare intervention?
    A. MEDLINE®
    B. CINAHL® Database
    C. CINAHL® Plus
    D. Cochrane Database

7. Which statement is true about databases?
    A. Online databases are not available to the general public.
    B. All databases are online.
    C. Databases, catalogs, and search engines are categories of finding tools.
    D. Databases only include published articles.

8. Which is not a true statement about grey literature?
    A. Grey literature is also called gray literature.
    B. Dissertations are not examples of grey literature.
    C. Grey literature is included in some databases.
    D. Grey literature is published in scholarly journals.

9. Which questions help critique a literature review? Choose all that apply.
    A. Based on defined methodology, are all sources of the review critically analyzed and synthesized?
    B. Are both supporting and opposing theory and research discussed?
    C. Does the review flow logically from the purposes(s) of the study?
    D. Are sources cited fully and correctly?
    E. All of the above help critique literature review.

10. Which search engine is most helpful for finding scholarly articles?
    A. Bing
    B. Scirus
    C. Google Scholar
    D. Web Crawler

See answers to Self-Test in the Answer Section at the back of the book.

References

Academy Health. (2006). Health Services Research and Health Policy Grey Literature Project: Summary Report. http://www.nlm.nih.gov/nichsr/greylitreport_06.html

Federer, L. (2013). The librarian as research informationist: A case study. *Medical Library Association, 101*(4), 298–302. doi:10.3163/1536-5050.101.4.011

Chapter 8

Theory and Nursing Research

Becky Spencer, PhD, RN, IBCLC

 Objectives

On completion of this chapter, you will be prepared to:

1. Summarize the key terminology for nursing theory.
2. Compare types and distinguish scopes of nursing theories.
3. Describe how theory is integrated into nursing research.
4. Summarize how nursing theory is developed, tested, and critiqued.

Introduction

You stop at a grocery store to purchase food items for a backyard cookout. You notice that the cost per pound of chicken has sharply increased over the last several months. What could be causing the increased cost? You suddenly remember a news report about a recent outbreak of avian flu that severely affected chicken farms in the Western and Midwestern United States. Millions of chickens had to be destroyed to control the outbreak. How does this affect the price of chicken at your grocery store in Texas? Could it be the theory of supply and demand? The demand for chicken across the United States remained constant, but the supply of chickens experienced a steep decline. Therefore, suppliers were able to charge higher prices to moderate their loss of profits.

As you drive down the freeway in the busy afternoon traffic, you notice the discourtesy of the drivers and the continual honking of horns. Many drivers appear tense and impatient. You think about the problems these people may have encountered during the day as well as the added inconvenience of the traffic congestion. Without conscious awareness, you may be considering a stress theory as the explanation for the behaviors that you have observed.

People use theories to explain happenings in their lives and in their environments. Nurses also use theories to explain happenings of significance to nursing. Nursing research and nursing practice should be based on theory. When a theoretical framework guides research, the theory guides the research process from the beginning to the end—that is, from the identification of the research problem to the formulation of the study conclusions. You may ask, where does a researcher find a theory for a study or determine which theory would be most appropriate? This chapter helps answer these questions and, it is hoped, helps you to recognize the value of theory-based nursing research.

Theory Terminology

Many nurses experience confusion when confronted with the terms in this chapter. There is no absolute or correct definition for many of these terms. The lack of agreement in terminology sometimes leaves you wondering which definition to use. It is more important for you to gain a basic understanding of the terminology than to memorize definitions. You will be in a better position to recognize the terms when you encounter them in the research literature. Rather than memorizing one correct definition of the word *theory*, for example, try to gain an understanding of what a theory is and how it is useful in nursing.

Some definitions and explanation of terminology are presented first to help you understand the content of this chapter. These definitions and explanations were generated after reviewing both classic and the latest literature on the use of theory in nursing.

Theory

One of the most commonly quoted definitions of a theory was formulated by Kerlinger (1973): "A theory is a set of interrelated constructs (concepts), definitions, and propositions that present a systematic view of phenomena by specifying relations among variables, with the purpose of explaining and predicting the phenomena" (p. 9). Polit and Beck (2012) have defined a theory as "a systematic, abstract explanation of some aspect of reality" (p. 41). Grove, Burns, and Gray (2013) described a theory as "an integrated set of defined concepts and propositions that present a view of a phenomenon and can be used to describe, explain, predict, or control the phenomenon" (p. 41). A more easily understood (although not as comprehensive) definition used in this book is that a **theory** is a set of related statements that describes or explains phenomena in a systematic way. Theories explain why one event is associated with another event or what causes an event to occur. Theories are composed of concepts and the relationships among these concepts. Relationships among concepts are presented in theoretical statements, called **propositional statements**. These propositional statements are connected in a logical system of thought.

Theory development is the basic aim of science (Kerlinger, 1986). Theories make scientific findings meaningful and generalizable. The facts that are derived from many separate and isolated investigations take on meaning when placed within a theoretical context.

Theory comes from the Greek word *theoria*, which means a beholding, spectacle, or speculation. *Speculation* is an appropriate word to use when discussing theories. Theories are always speculative and never considered to be true or proven. They provide description and explanation of the occurrence of phenomena and are always subject to further development or revision. Theories may even be discarded if not supported by empirical evidence.

Concept

Concepts are the building blocks of theory. A **concept** is a word picture or mental idea of a phenomenon. Concepts are words or terms that symbolize some aspect of reality. The meaning of a concept is conveyed by the use of a definition and examples of instances of the concept. A concept may be very concrete, such as the human heart, or very abstract, such as love. Concrete concepts may be specified and defined more easily than abstract concepts.

Construct

A highly abstract, complex phenomenon (concept) is denoted by a made-up, or constructed, term. **Construct** is the term used to indicate a phenomenon that cannot be directly observed but must be inferred by certain concrete or less abstract indicators of the phenomenon. Examples of constructs are wellness, mental health, self-esteem, and assertiveness. Each of these constructs can be identified only through the presence of certain measurable concepts. Wellness might be inferred through laboratory data or clinical observation. The laboratory data would be very objective indicators of wellness, whereas the clinical observation would be a less objective indicator of wellness.

Propositional Statements

A propositional statement asserts the relationship between concepts. Propositional statements are derived from theories or from generalizations based on empirical data. A propositional statement may indicate the relationships among concepts in several ways. A propositional statement may assert simply that two events or phenomena tend to vary together. For example, "There is a relationship between pulse rates and respiration rates." Propositional statements may also assert that one variable causes another variable. For example, "Bacteria cause disease."

Empirical Generalization

When a similar pattern of events is found in the empirical data of a number of different studies, the pattern is called an **empirical generalization** (Reynolds, 1971). Empirical generalizations summarize the results of several empirical studies. Grove, Burns, and Gray (2013) asserted that empirical generalizations are "statements that have been repeatedly tested and have not been disproved" (p. 693). Many studies have shown that women attend church more often than men. The empirical generalization can, therefore, be made that women are more frequent church attendees than men.

Hypothesis

A hypothesis predicts the relationship between two or more variables. Hypotheses present the researcher's expectations about the outcome of a study. Through hypotheses, theoretical propositions are tested in the real world. The investigator can then advance scientific knowledge by providing results that support or fail to support the tested theory.

Model

The more complex the issues, the greater is the need to "create order out of chaos" by constructing models (Blackwell, 1985, p. 169). A **model** is a symbolic representation of some phenomenon or phenomena. Bush (1979) wrote that a model "represents some aspect of reality, concrete or abstract, by means of a likeness which may be structural, pictorial, diagrammatic, or mathematical" (p. 16). Probably the most common usage of the term model is when discussing structural types of models, such as model trains, model airplanes, and models of the human heart. The types of models that nurses are interested in when conducting nursing research are generally of the structural or diagrammatic form. A diagram or a picture can portray a theory in a fashion that clearly demonstrates the structure and parts of the theory. Whereas a theory focuses on statements or explanations of the relationships among phenomena, a model focuses on the structure or composition of the phenomena.

Conceptual Models

Conceptual models are made up of concepts and propositions that state the relationships among the concepts. These concepts are generally very abstract and not readily observable or easily measureable in the empirical world. Conceptual models in nursing represent broad general concepts of interest to nursing. Early nursing theorists developed conceptual models to define and describe practices specific to nursing. These conceptual models are commonly referred to as grand theories of nursing. Examples include Orem's Self-Care Model, Rogers's Science of Unitary Human Beings, Roy's Adaptation Model, and Neuman's Systems Model (Neuman & Fawcett, 2011; Neuman & Young, 1972; Orem, 1971, 2001; Rogers, 1970, 1990; Roy, 1976, 2009).

Paradigm and Metaparadigm

If we could fit all the nurses in the world under one roof and ask them to describe what makes the practice of nursing unique and different from other health-related disciplines, do you think they could agree upon a distinct set of concepts or constructs? Do you think that all nurses share a similar view of the purpose and goals of the professional discipline and science of nursing? A **paradigm** is a philosophical worldview, or a set of beliefs about nature and reality that shape decisions and practices. A **metaparadigm** is a core set of concepts and constructs that are interdependent and uniquely define a discipline. Fawcett (1978, 1995) identified the core concepts of the discipline of nursing as person, environment, health, and nursing. All nursing theory addresses these four central elements in a unique fashion.

Types and Scope of Theories in Nursing Research

Theory development in nursing has evolved along a continuum. The first nursing theorist was Florence Nightingale, who organized the characteristics, principles, and practices of the discipline of nursing in order to develop a training program for nurses (1859/1946). During the 1950s to the 1970s, nursing scholars and theorists began to focus on conducting research that would lead to broad definitions of nursing and a means of differentiating nursing from other health professions, primarily medicine. This focus on scientific inquiry led nursing scholars and theorists in the 1980s and 1990s to conduct research that began to refine the practice of nursing by focusing on concrete and specific nursing situations and actions which led to theories that were more specific to nursing practice. Nursing scholars and theorists of the 21st century have expanded the focus from research and inquiry that is specific to nursing to include a broader focus on interdisciplinary research, which has resulted in a melding of nursing theory with theory from related health disciplines.

Paradigms and Metaparadigms

All nursing research is rooted in a philosophical worldview, or paradigm. The two main paradigms that have most influenced nursing research and the development of nursing theory include positivism and postpositivism (Weaver & Olson, 2006). **Positivism** is a worldview that truth about phenomena can be discovered through systematic inquiry. Positivists strive to discover explanations through the scientific method of observation, empiricism, and quantitative measurement. **Postpositivism** is a worldview that contrasts positivism by asserting that absolute truth or a universal experience of reality does not exist. Postpositivists believe that human beings have differing perspectives of reality; therefore, all science has a subjective component.

The postpositivist paradigm led to the development of many related paradigms that have had a direct influence on nursing theory including, but not limited to, interpretivism, critical social theory, and constructivism (Weaver & Olson, 2006). Interpretivism is concerned with how individuals interpret their experiences. Critical social theory encourages examination of how individuals or groups of individuals are situated within a social context, and how a particular position in society affects the individual or group of individuals. Constructivism posits that humans construct knowledge from a foundation of current knowledge. There is not one correct paradigm, although people who ascribe to one specific paradigm might argue differently. The important point to take away is that all nursing research and theory is conducted and created from a particular paradigm or worldview lens. Nurse researchers should frame their research within the appropriate paradigm (Houghton, Hunter, & Meskell, 2012). For example, if a nurse researcher wants to determine which type of adhesive for endotracheal tubes causes the least amount of skin damage, the appropriate paradigm might be the positivist paradigm because specific quantitative measurements and comparison will be necessary to discover the best answer. Conversely, if a nurse researcher wants to learn about the experience of living with diabetes, the interpretive paradigm would best frame the exploration of individual experiences.

A metaparadigm is a set of concepts that distinguishes one discipline from another; it represents the worldview of members of the discipline. Fawcett's metaparadigm of nursing includes the concepts of person, health, environment, and nursing (1978). Four proposition statements link the four concepts that illuminate the worldview of nursing:

1. The discipline of nursing is concerned with the principles and laws that govern human processes of living and dying.
2. The discipline of nursing is concerned with the patterning of human health experiences within the context of the environment.
3. The discipline of nursing is concerned with the nursing actions or processes that are beneficial to human beings.
4. The discipline of nursing is concerned with the human processes of living and dying, recognizing that human beings are in a continuous relationship with their environments (Fawcett & Desanto-Madeya, 2013).

The above proposition statements represent the purposes and goals of the discipline of nursing and the domain for nursing inquiry. The nursing metaparadigm and philosophical paradigms serve as the large umbrella under which most nursing research is conducted and nursing theory is constructed.

Nursing Conceptual Models

Early nursing theorists, including Dorothea Orem, Martha Rogers, Callista Roy, and Betty Neuman, developed conceptual models that helped to define the discipline of nursing. These conceptual models are broad in scope and are frequently referred to as grand nursing theories. These theories provided the foundation for Fawcett's development of the nursing metaparadigm (1978). While conceptual models, or grand theories, were some of the first theories specific to the nursing discipline developed in the 1950s to the 1970s, they are still used by nurse researchers today. A brief overview of the models introduced by these four nurse theorists is presented.

Orem's Self-Care Model

Dorothea Orem has been developing her ideas about self-care since the early 1950s. Concepts in her model are self-care, self-care agency, self-care demand, self-care deficit, nursing agency, and nursing system. Three theories have been derived from Orem's self-care model: theory of nursing systems, theory of self-care deficit, and theory of self-care. Modifications of her original ideas are found in the sixth edition of her text *Nursing: Concepts of Practice* (2001).

Orem's model is particularly appropriate today with the general public's increased interest in self-care. An article published in *Nursing Science Quarterly* in April 2000 (Taylor, Geden, Isaramalai, & Wongvatunyu, 2000) identified 66 published research studies that had used components of Orem's theories. Many recent studies have also used her theories.

Orem's Nursing Systems Theory

Orem's Theory of Nursing Systems was the framework for a study that evaluated the usefulness and usability of follow-up telehealth medication counseling among a sample of community-based patients with Parkinson's disease (Fincher, Ward, Dawkins, Magee, & Wilson, 2009). A self-care standardized medication educational session lasting 20 to 30 minutes was conducted, and patients and nurses evaluated the usefulness of this intervention.

Rogers's Science of Unitary Human Beings

Martha Rogers proposed a unique conceptual model in nursing. She first presented her science of unitary human beings in her 1970 book, *An Introduction to the Theoretical Basis of Nursing*. By the time she died in 1994, her ideas had made a great impact on nursing and probably will continue to do so for many years to come. Much of Rogers's work is contained in the book *Martha E. Rogers: Her Life and Her Work* by Malinski and Barrett (1994), which was released shortly after Rogers's death.

Rogers continually refined her model, and when she spoke to groups of nurses, she frequently asked that they discuss her most current ideas rather than those presented in her 1970 book (which she called "the purple book"). Just as she viewed humans as continually evolving, her ideas were continually evolving. She originally used the term *man* in her writings. After 1983, she used the term *unitary human beings*. Her most recent ideas were published in *Nursing Science Quarterly* in the article "Nursing Science and the Space Age" (Rogers, 1992).

Humans and their environment are viewed as two energy fields that are always open to each other. Each human field is unique, and change is always toward increasing complexity and diversity. Aging is viewed as a "creative process directed toward growing diversity of field pattern and organization" (Rogers, 1980, p. 336).

Rogers's model is unique in that the person is viewed as a unified whole. No parts or subsystems are separated out. Although other models propose to present a holistic view of people, this view is often contradicted by the models' examination of the parts or subsystems of people.

Rogers's Science of Unitary Human Beings

Farren (2010) used Rogers's Science of Unitary Human Beings to study the relationships among power, uncertainty, self-transcendence, and quality of life in breast cancer survivors. The researcher concluded that there are "complex and synergistic relations among the cluster of field pattern manifestations that contribute to quality of life in breast cancer survivors" (p. 63).

Roy's Adaptation Model

Roy first published her ideas about adaptation as a framework for nursing in a 1970 article in *Nursing Outlook*. She has continued to publish extensively on her model. A thorough presentation of her ideas is found in the second edition of her text *Introduction to Nursing: An Adaptation Model* (1984). Refinements of her model are found in the second edition of *The Roy Adaptation Model* by Roy and Andrews (1999) and in the third edition published in 2008.

Roy has pointed out that nursing focuses on the person as a total being, whereas medicine focuses on the patient's disease process. Humans are considered to be biopsychosocial beings in constant interaction with the changing environment. People are viewed as adaptive systems with cognator and regulator coping mechanisms that act to maintain adaptation in four response modes: physiological, self-concept, role function, and interdependence.

Roy's Adaptation Model

Roy's Adaptation Model (RAM) was the theoretical framework used to study quality of life (QOL) as perceived by lung transplant candidates and their caregivers (Lefaiver, Keough, Letizia, & Lanuza, 2007). The adaptive modes of the caregiver and lung transplant candidate were measured with the Quality of Life Index (QLI). The researchers pointed out parallels between the RAM adaptive modes and the elements of the QLI.

Neuman's Systems Model

The Neuman model first appeared in a 1972 article in *Nursing Research*. It was also outlined in Riehl and Roy's *Conceptual Models for Nursing Practice* (in both the 1974 and 1980 editions). The first edition of Betty Neuman's book, *The Neuman Systems Model*, was published in 1982, with refinements presented in the 1989, 1995, and 2002 editions. A fifth edition was published in 2010, co-authored with Jacqueline Fawcett. According to Günüsen, Üstün, and Gigiotti (2009), more than 200 studies based on Neuman's system model have been published in articles and book chapters.

Neuman has proposed a model that focuses on the total person. The person or client system (individual, group, community) is subject to environmental stressors that are intrapersonal, interpersonal, and extrapersonal. The client system is composed of physiological, psychological, sociocultural, developmental, and spiritual variables. The client is protected from stressors by a flexible line of defense that is dynamic. The next barrier to stressors is the person's normal line of defense that has been built over time. When this defense is penetrated, the internal lines of resistance are activated to stabilize the client system.

Nursing interventions may occur at the primary, secondary, or tertiary levels of prevention. Primary prevention is appropriate before reaction to a stressor has occurred. Secondary prevention is used when reaction to a stressor has already occurred. Tertiary prevention is used to foster rehabilitation and a return to wellness. The nursing process is divided into three steps: nursing diagnosis, nursing goals, and nursing outcomes.

Neuman's Systems Model

Neuman's Systems Model was used as the conceptual framework to study stress in a group of critical care nurses in South Africa (Moola, Ehlers, & Hattingh, 2008). Study results presented perceptions and experiences about stressful events and factors contributing to stress in the critical care environment, as well as the nurses' needs for support systems.

Middle-range and Practice Theories

While grand nursing theories address a broad range of phenomena in the environment or in the experiences of humans, **middle-range theories** have a much more narrow focus. Grand nursing theories contain constructs that are abstract and difficult to test empirically. Middle-range nursing theories are concerned with smaller, more specific areas of the environment or of human experiences and incorporate a small number of concepts that are easier to measure and test (Fawcett, 2005; Meleis, 1995, Walker & Avant, 2011). One critique of conceptual models, or grand theories, of nursing is that the concepts and constructs are so broad and abstract that implementation of these theories into nursing practice is difficult. The **theory–practice gap** is the belief that many nursing theories are too abstract and removed from the reality of nursing practice (Rolfe, 1992). Middle-range theories, in theory, should help close the theory–practice gap because the concepts and propositions are more concrete and applicable to nursing practice. Mishel's Uncertainty in Illness theory (1981, 1990), Pender's Health Promotion Model (2014), and Watson's Theory of Human Caring (2005) are just a few examples of middle-range nursing theories that nurse researchers use when studying phenomena of interest to nursing practice. The following studies are examples of how these middle-range theories were tested in nursing practice.

Mishel's Uncertainty in Illness Theory

Mishel's Uncertainty in Illness theory was used in a study to evaluate the psychometric properties of a new instrument developed to measure uncertainty in children and adolescents (8–17 years) with cancer (Stewart, Lynn & Mishel, 2010). The instrument is called Uncertainty Scale for Kids (USK). The USK demonstrated strong reliability and preliminary evidence for construct and discriminant validity. The researchers contend that these results show promise for further research on uncertainty in illness in children with cancer.

Pender's Health Promotion Model

A tailored intervention based on Pender's Health Promotion Model (HPM) was compared to a generic intervention in a study that sought to increase physical activity and healthy eating among rural women (Walker et al., 2009). Perceived benefits, barriers, self-efficacy, and interpersonal influences were cognitions selected from the HPM in designing the tailored intervention. Although both groups showed gains in physical activity and healthy eating, a higher proportion of the HPM intervention group met the Healthy People 2010 criteria for moderate or greater intensity activity, fruit and vegetable servings, and percentage of calories from fat at 12 months post intervention.

Watson's Theory of Human Caring

Jean Watson's Theory of Human Caring directed a study by Pipe, Bortz, and Dueck (2009) that evaluated a brief stress management intervention for nurse leaders. Nurse leaders (n = 33) were randomly assigned to a brief mindfulness meditation course (MMC) or a leadership course (control). Mindfulness meditation course participants self-reported the most improvement in stress symptoms. Mindfulness "was conceptualized as a way of caring/nurturing the self so that one's leadership could be more caring and effective by extension. (p. 131).

Practice theories have the most specific and narrow scope of application to nursing practice. Practice theories are also referred to as micro theory (Suppe, 1996) and situation-specific theory (Meleis & Im, 2001). While middle-range theories are more specific and applicable to nursing practice, their scope may not include directives for specific nursing interventions. Practice theories produce specific nursing practice guidance for specific patient care situations. The Theory of Heart Failure Self-Care (Riegel & Dickson, 2008) and the Prescriptive Theory of Acute Pain Management in Infants and Children (Huth & Moore, 1998) are two examples of prescriptive theory that postulate specific nursing actions or interventions for a specific population.

The Prescriptive Theory of Acute Pain Management in Infants and Children

Huth and Moore (1998) identified a lack of clinical guidance on alleviating acute pain experienced by infants and children. They acknowledged that several theories of pain explaining the physiological mechanisms of pain in children were present in the literature, but no theories that provided nursing care practice guidelines specific to alleviating children's acute pain. The authors examined existing literature on the physiological mechanisms of children's pain, and national medical guidelines for the prescriptive treatment of acute pain in children. They developed the Prescriptive Theory of Acute Pain Management in Infants and Children as a three-step clinical guideline for assessment and treatment including initial assessment, therapeutic interventions, and reassessment. The goal was satisfactory pain reduction for the child and parent. Important concepts that were expressed as specific nursing actions included assessing verbal report and visual signs of pain, past and current pain history, developmental level, coping strategies, and cultural background. The theory also includes specific guidance on incorporating medications with nonpharmacologic pain therapies and including the child and parent in teaching about adequate pain relief.

Theory of Heart Failure Self-Care

Riegel and Dickson (2008) acknowledged the importance of promoting the concept of self-care to patients. Self-care is a broad concept that does not address the specific needs of patients who have experienced specific illness or injury. The Theory of Heart Failure Self-care was designed to provide guidance to nurses in promoting specific self-care activities for patients who have experienced heart failure. Important concepts that were expressed as specific components of teaching included symptom monitoring, treatment adherence, symptom recognition and evaluation, and treatment implementation and evaluation. Assessing for self-care confidence was also identified as an important nursing action.

The scope of nursing theory ranges from the very broad and abstract worldview lens of paradigms to the very specific and narrowly focused practice theories. The three levels of nursing theory, grand, middle-range, and practice, should stem from the metaparadigm of nursing and draw from the appropriate philosophical paradigm. Figure 8–1 displays the scope of theory in nursing research.

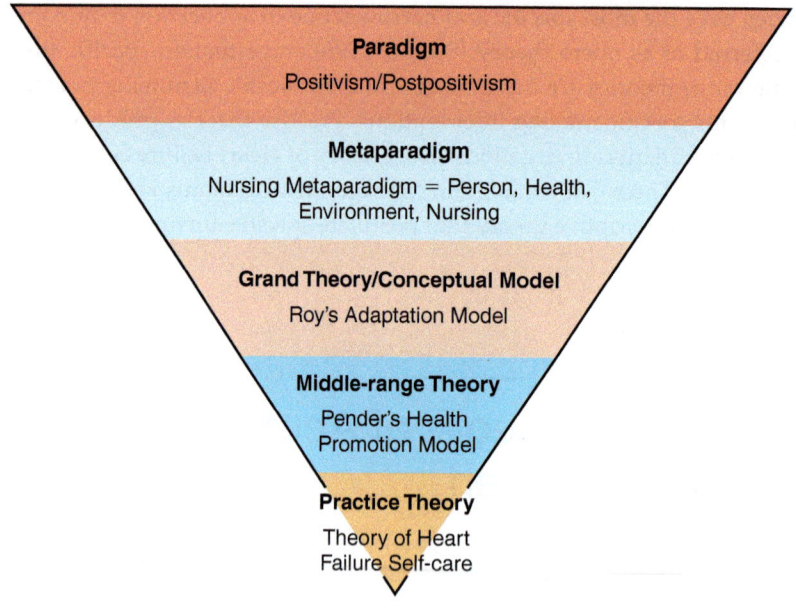

Figure 8–1 Scope of theory in nursing research

Integrating Theory into Nursing Research

Theory should be the foundation of all nursing research, but how do nurse researchers choose a theory for research, and how do nurse researchers apply or integrate a theory into a specific study? Nursing research usually begins with an idea or problem that is relevant to nursing practice. Before designing the study, a nurse researcher should search and examine the literature for research and theories that have been conducted or applied to the problem or idea of interest. A literature search could reveal a theory that has been applied to a similar problem. Once a theory is chosen, the concepts and propositions of the theory will help the nurse researcher identify important variables and ideas that will be explored and measured. The following sections will discuss how nurse researchers choose theories and how they apply them to specific studies.

Theories from Nursing

Do nurse researchers have to use nursing theory for studies that are related to nursing? Can nurse researchers use theories from other disciplines? Nursing scholars have debated this issue. Rosemarie Parse, editor of *Nursing Science Quarterly*, reported on a meeting of doctoral faculty from various schools of nursing around the country (Parse, 2003). Some of the faculty contended that if a nurse conducted a study, it would be considered nursing research. Others disagreed and asserted that for a study to be classified as nursing research, the inquiry must advance nursing knowledge through the use of nursing frameworks and theories. Parse, herself, made a strong plea in 2000 for the use of nursing theories in nursing research. In an editorial in *Nursing Science Quarterly*, Parse (2000) argued that a nursing research study must use a nursing framework or theory. Fawcett (2000) wrote a similar editorial in the *Western Journal of Nursing Research*. The following month Brink (2000) published an editorial in the same journal and disagreed with Fawcett's position. She asserted that any research that has a direct bearing on nursing practice is considered nursing research. She further claimed that nursing is an applied discipline and draws knowledge from many sources. She asserted that if we were to ignore factual data simply because it came from another discipline, we would have to redo a lot of previous research or admit to "culpable ignorance."

Although nurse researchers use theories that were not developed by nurses, the literature has many examples of studies that relied on the theoretical work of nurses. Examples of studies that used the models of Orem, Rogers, Roy, and Neuman were presented earlier in this chapter. Additional theories developed by nurses may be identified in published studies. Some of these include Benner's (1984) model on novice to expert, Cox's (1982) interaction model of client health behavior (IMCHB), King's (1981) theory of goal attainment, and Peplau's interpersonal theory (1988). Nurse researchers need to carefully match theories to the ideas and problems that they want to study. Nursing theorists continually modify their theories based on reasearch findings that support or refute the propositions of the theory. The body of nursing science grows as theories are tested and modified. If a nursing theory exisits that applies to a specific study, it should be used.

Combining Two Nursing Theories

Sometimes nurse researchers combine two nursing theories in their studies. The following example uses Orem's self-care agency, a component of her self-care deficit theory, and Pender's revised health belief model for health promotion.

Combining Two Nursing Theories

Youngkin and Lester (2010) studied the accuracy of a home self-test system for bacterial vaginosis (BV) in women. Orem's self-care agency concept was used to teach women how to understand the disease, assess for BV, and record their findings. The researchers believed that Pender's health promotion model guided the nurses as they helped women to modify their health behaviors through self-care interventions. The goal of secondary prevention in health promotion is health protection, which should decrease the risks of undiagnosed progression of BV.

Theories from Other Disciplines

Nursing is referred to as a practice discipline. It has been said frequently that nursing, as a practice discipline, has borrowed knowledge from other disciplines, such as chemistry, biology, sociology, psychology, and anthropology. Levine (1995) has opposed the use of the term *borrowed*. She said it indicates that something needs to later be "returned." Levine wrote that "knowledge could not be deemed the private domain of one discipline, which needs to be returned like a borrowed cup of sugar to a neighbor" (p. 12).

The use of knowledge from other disciplines is necessary, but frequently this knowledge is not suitable to the needs of the nursing profession. Nurses must find ways to adapt the numerous theories from other disciplines. Once these theories have been adapted, they should be considered as shared knowledge rather than as borrowed theories (Stevens, 1979). Table 8–1 lists theories from other disciplines that are used to explain phenomena in nursing. These theories concern concepts such as social learning, adult learning, role socialization, stress, helplessness, cognitive dissonance, human development, motivation, crisis, relaxation, pain, anxiety, body image, job satisfaction, family interactions, communication, coping, moral reasoning, health behaviors, and change.

The gate control theory of pain by Melzack and Wall (1983) served as the framework for Hatfield's (2008) study of sucrose use to decrease infant biobehavioral responses to immunizations. Sheenan (2009) used Prochaska and DiClemente's (1983) transtheoretical model (TTM) in her study of knowledge of prostate cancer and prostate cancer screening among a group of men at average risk of developing cancer. Bandura's (1985)

Table 8–1 Theories From Other Disciplines

Adult learning theory: Knowles (1990)
Anxiety: Spielberger (1972)
Body image: Schilder (1952)
Change theory: Lewin (1951)
Cognitive dissonance: Festinger (1957)
Coping: Lazarus and Folkman (1984)
Crisis: Caplan (1964)
Developmental theory: Piaget (1926); Freud (1938); Erikson (1950); Havighurst (1952)
Family communication theory: Satir (1967)
Family theory: Minuchin (1974); Duvall (1977)
Health behaviors: Becker (1985)
Helplessness: Seligman (1975)
Job satisfaction: Herzberg (1966)
Moral reasoning: Kohlberg (1978)
Motivation: Maslow (1970)
Pain: Melzack and Wall (1983)
Relaxation: Benson (1975)
Role theory: Mead (1934); Biddle (1986)
Social learning theory: Bandura (1985); Rotter (1954)
Stress: Selye (1976)
Transtheoretical model of behavior change: Prochaska & DiClemente (1983)

self-efficacy theory was used in a simulation study as a teaching–learning method to increase self-efficacy of nursing students during their first clinical course (Bambini, Washburn, & Perkins, 2009). Lazarus and Folkman's (1984) theory of stress, appraisal, and coping was used in a study by Song and Nam (2010) to examine coping strategies, physical function, and social adjustment in people with spinal cord injury. The adult learning theory of Malcom Knowles (1990) was used by Schneiderman, Corbridge, and Zerwic (2009) in a study of the effectiveness of a self-directed online learning module for arterial blood gas interpretation.

Combining Theories from Nursing and Other Disciplines

In some studies, nurse researchers have determined that a combination of theories from nursing and other disciplines would guide their research more appropriately than a theory from only one discipline.

Combining Nursing and Non-nursing Theories

Hoffman et al. (2009) combined the middle-range nursing theory of unpleasant symptoms (TOUS) by Lentz et al. (1997) with Bandura's (1985) self-efficacy theory. The researchers contended that the TOUS helps to understand the multidimensional nature and impact of symptoms, whereas Bandura's theory demonstrates how a persons' belief in his or her ability to self-manage symptoms actually influences that person's performance of corresponding behaviors.

Theoretical and Conceptual Frameworks

A framework for a research study helps organize the study and provides a context for the interpretation of the study findings. Nurses use theoretical and conceptual frameworks to integrate theory into resaerch. Either a theoretical or a conceptual framework should be used in all nursing studies. Theoretical and conceptual frameworks are often used interchangeably in the literature. The two types frameworks are similar in that both provide a background or foundation for a study. However, there are differences in these two types of frameworks.

A **theoretical framework** presents a broad, general explanation of the relationships between the concepts of interest in a research study; it is based on *one* existing theory. When using a theoretical framework, each main study concept is related back to a concept from an existing theory. A proposition from the selected theory will be tested in any study based on that particular theory.

Suppose a teacher wanted to know if contracting for grades would motivate students to earn higher grades. After exploring different theories, she might decide to test a proposition from Carl Rogers's (1969) theory of learning. One of Rogers's propositions is that learning is facilitated when the student participates responsibly in the learning process. The two theory concepts are *learning* and *participates responsibly in the learning process*. The two study concepts that can be matched up with these two theory concepts are *earn higher grades* (which would match up with *learning*) and *contracting for grades* (which would match up with *participates responsibly in the learning process*). Thus, based on the stated proposition from Rogers's theory, the researcher would be able to predict that students who contract for grades would earn higher grades than students who do not contract for grades.

If there is no existing theory that fits the concepts to be studied, the researcher may construct a conceptual framework to be used in the proposed research study. A **conceptual framework** helps explain the relationship between concepts, but rather than being based on one theory, this type of framework links concepts selected from several theories from previous research results or from the researcher's own experiences. The researcher relates the concepts in a logical manner. A conceptual framework is a less well-developed structure than a theoretical framework but may serve as the impetus for the formulation of a theory.

A graduate nursing student decided to examine nurses' job satisfaction levels and their levels of empathy in their interactions with patients. After searching the literature, she was able to find an empathy theory and a job satisfaction theory. However, she could locate no theory that combined these two concepts. Therefore, she constructed a conceptual framework using these two theories. Based on the empathy theory, she reasoned that being empathetic requires being satisfied with self. She further reasoned that if people are happy in their jobs, they will be satisfied with themselves. Therefore, she proposed that job satisfaction and empathy are positively related.

The findings of a study should be related back to the study framework. Otherwise, numerous isolated findings would exist for each study. The concrete findings are linked to the abstract ideas of the theory or to the propositions proposed by the researcher in the conceptual framework. Thus, an explanation for the study findings is presented, and the body of knowledge on the study topic is increased.

Theoretical Development, Testing, and Critique

You have learned about different types of nursing theories and how theory is chosen and applied to research. This section of the chapter will explain how theory is developed and tested. You will also learn how to critique the theoretical framework of a study or how well theory has been integrated and applied in research.

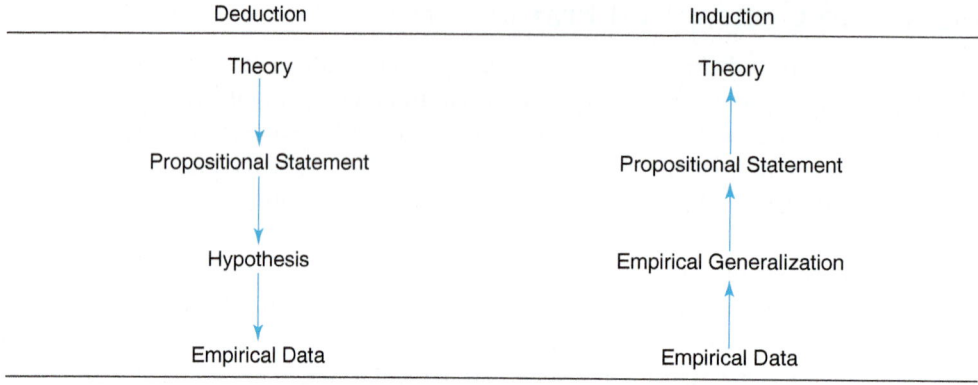

Figure 8–2 Deductive and inductive processes in theory generation and development

Theory Generation and Development

Nurse researchers are concerned with both theory generation and the development of theories. The two activities go hand in hand. Figure 8–2 shows the processes of theory generation and the development of theories through testing. As you can see, theory generation and development involve both inductive and deductive reasoning processes. **Deductive reasoning** proceeds from the general (theory) to the specific (empirical data). **Inductive reasoning**, in contrast, proceeds from the specific (empirical data) to the general (theory).

The deductive process moves from a general abstract explanation to a specific event in the real world. A hypothesis is deduced from a theory, and the hypothesis is empirically tested in a real-life situation. The researcher asks the question, "If this theory is valid, what kind of behavior or event would I expect to find in my study?" For example, you might test a propositional statement from Maslow's (1970) theory of motivation that states "If a person's safety needs are not met, safety needs will take precedence over self-esteem needs." If this statement is valid, you would expect to find that people are more concerned about receiving the correct medications than they are about being told they are "good" patients.

When an inductive process is used, data are gathered from a real-life situation and the researcher tries to derive a general explanation of this behavior or event. The question is asked, "How can I explain what I have been observing?" For example, you might observe that patients who are occupied in some activity, such as watching television, seem to be less anxious than patients who are not involved in a specific activity. You continue to observe many patients and find that this pattern seems to hold true for most of the patients on the unit where you work. Your explanation for this phenomenon would involve an inductive reasoning process. An existing anxiety theory might provide an explanation for the phenomenon just discussed. If no existing theory can be located that explains this phenomenon, the researcher may start the process of generating a new theory. After empirical data are gathered on a number of occasions, empirical generalizations are made. The next step is to develop propositional statements. Finally, the propositional statements are logically related to form a theory.

Theory Testing in Nursing Research

If nursing is to build a scientific knowledge base, nursing studies should be based on a theoretical or conceptual framework so that the findings may be placed within the existing knowledge base for the profession. The most efficient way to obtain a body of knowledge for nursing is to build on the work of other researchers who have used the same theoretical base. Even a small research project becomes quite important when the findings of the study can be added to those of others who have used the same theoretical frame of reference.

Testing theory begins when researchers choose a theory as the foundation for a research study. The chosen theory should be considered throughout the research process. A step-by-step use of the chosen theory requires that the researcher:

1. Review various theories that may be appropriate to examine the identified problem.
2. Select a theory to be tested in the study.
3. Review the literature on this theory.
4. Develop study hypothesis(es) or research questions based on a propositional statement or statements from the theory.
5. Define study variables, using the selected theory as the basis of the theoretical definitions.
6. Choose study instruments that are congruent with the theory.
7. Describe study findings in light of the explanations provided by the theory.
8. Relate study conclusions to the theory.
9. Determine support for the theory based on study findings.
10. Determine implications for nursing based on the explanatory power of the theory.
11. Make recommendations for future research concerning the designated theory.

Theory generation and building through research are essential to the development of scientific knowledge. Because the nursing profession is very concerned at present with the need for nursing knowledge, it can be seen that an understanding and use of theory are critical for all nurses.

Critiquing the Theoretical Framework of a Study

Many nursing studies that are published today contain a clearly identified theoretical or conceptual framework for the study. Other studies do not. Therefore, the first determination to make is whether or not the researcher identified a framework for the study. Sometimes, the research report contains a heading for this section of the study. Other times, the discussion of the theoretical or conceptual framework is included in the introductory section or the review of literature section. The important point is to determine if a framework is clearly identified by the researcher.

If a theoretical or conceptual framework has been clearly identified in the report, the next evaluation step concerns the basis for the framework. Is it based on a nursing theory or a theory from another discipline? At the present time, many nursing studies are based on concepts and theories from other disciplines.

The reader then evaluates the appropriateness of the framework for the study. The entire research report must be read before the evaluation of the framework is made. Then, the reader might ask this question: "Would another theory have been more appropriate to guide the study?" There may be several theories that might have been used in any given study. Imagine that, after reading the research report, it appears to you the researcher was interested in helping subjects alter an unhealthy behavior—smoking. The researcher used a learning theory and taught subjects about the dangers of cigarette smoking. Considering the great amount of publicity about the dangers of cigarette smoking, you might wonder if another theory might have been more useful in helping predict a change in an unhealthy behavior. It is possible that the subjects already had knowledge of the dangers of cigarette smoking, but did not perceive themselves as vulnerable: "Cancer won't happen to me." A theory, such as the health belief model, might have been used. The researcher might focus on the concept of perceived susceptibility of the disease when presenting material about the dangers of smoking to the subjects.

You may be thinking, "I don't know that many theories. How can I evaluate this part of a study and decide whether the most appropriate theory was used?" This is a difficult task, but my guess is that you know more theories than you think you do. You may not know the name of the theorist, but you are familiar with the ideas in the theory. If you have some nagging doubt when you read the framework section of an article, ask other nurses what they think about the framework. If you think that the framework seems appropriate for the study, determine if there is a thorough explanation of the concepts and their relationship to each other.

An entire theory is rarely tested in one study. Thus, is a specific propositional statement from the theory identified that will guide the hypothesis(es) or research question(s)? Are operational definitions provided for the concepts that will be measured in the study? Box 8–1 presents guidelines for critiquing the theoretical or conceptual framework of a study.

Box 8–1 Guidelines for Critiquing the Study Framework

1. Is the framework clearly identified?
2. Is the framework based on a nursing theory or a theory from another discipline?
3. Does the framework appear to be appropriate for the study?
4. Are the concepts clearly defined?
5. Are the relationships among the concepts clearly presented?
6. Is(Are) the propositional statement(s) identified that will guide the research question(s) or hypothesis(es)?
7. Are operational definitions provided for the theoretical concepts that will be tested?
8. Does the researcher relate the study findings back to the study framework?
9. Do the study findings provide support for the study framework?

Summary

An understanding of theory in nursing and the use of theory in research requires familiarity with terms such as *theory, concept, construct, propositional statements, empirical generalization, paradigm, metapdigm, model, conceptual models, theoretical frameworks,* and *conceptual frameworks.*

A theory is a set of statements that describes or explains phenomena in a systematic way. Theories are composed of concepts and the relationship between these concepts. These relationships are presented in propositional statements that are connected in a logical way.

Concepts are the building blocks of theory. A concept is a word picture or mental idea of a phenomenon. Concepts may be concrete or abstract.

A construct is a phenomenon (concept) that cannot be directly observed, but must be inferred by certain concrete or less abstract indicators of the phenomenon. Examples of constructs are wellness and mental health.

Propositional statements present the relationship between concepts in a theory. All theories contain propositional statements.

An empirical generalization is a summary statement of the findings of a number of different studies concerning the same phenomenon.

A paradigm is a philosophical worldview or a set of beliefs about nature and reality that shape decisions and practices.

A metaparadigm is a core set of concepts and constructs that are interdependent and uniquely define a discipline.

A model is a symbolic representation of phenomena. A model can be structural, pictorial, diagrammatic, or mathematical. Models focus on the structure of phenomena rather than on the relationships among phenomena, as is the case with theories.

Conceptual models are made up of concepts and propositions. The concepts are usually abstract. Conceptual models in nursing identify concepts of interest to nursing such as person, environment, health, and nursing.

A theoretical framework differs from a conceptual framework. A theoretical framework is based on propositional statements from one theory, whereas a conceptual framework links concepts from several theories, from previous research results, or from the researcher's own experience. In developing a conceptual framework, the researcher relates concepts in a logical manner to form propositional statements.

Nurse researchers are concerned with the generation and development of theories through testing. Both inductive and deductive reasoning processes are used in theory generation and development. Deductive reasoning proceeds from the general (theory) to the specific (empirical data). Inductive reasoning flows from the specific (empirical data) to the general (theory).

Three types of theories are grand theories (also called conceptual models), middle-range theories, and practice theories. **Grand theories** are concerned with a broad range of phenomena in the environment or in the experiences of humans. Middle-range theories are concerned with only a small area of the environment or human experiences. **Practice theories** have the most narrow focus and produce specific nursing practice guidance for specific patient care situations.

Nurses have used theories from nursing and from other disciplines when conducting nursing research. These theories from other disciplines concern concepts such as social learning, adult learning, role socialization, stress, helplessness, cognitive dissonance, human development, motivation, crisis, relaxation, pain, anxiety, body image, job satisfaction, family interactions, communication, coping, moral reasoning, change, and health behaviors.

A theoretical or conceptual framework should be used in all nursing research. The framework guides the steps in the research process and is the mechanism through which a generalizable body of knowledge is developed.

Self-Test

1. Broad representations of the relationships of concepts and propositions of interest to nursing are called
    A. theoretical frameworks.
    B. conceptual models.
    C. conceptual frameworks.
    D. practice models.
2. A philosophical worldview or a set of beliefs about nature and reality that shape decisions and practices is called a
    A. framework.
    B. theory.
    C. paradigm.
    D. metaparadigm.
3. Statements that have been repeatedly tested and have not been disproved are called
    A. critical social theory.
    B. propositions.
    C. concepts.
    D. empirical generalizations.
4. Which of the following is *not* one of the common concepts that are included in nearly all of the nursing conceptual models?
    A. person
    B. environment
    C. death
    D. health

5. You are trying to help a patient stop consuming foods that are high in complex carbohydrates. Which model/theory would probably be *most* appropriate?
   A. anxiety theory
   B. adult learning theory
   C. health belief model
   D. healthcare system model
6. Which theory was developed by a nurse?
   A. social cognitive theory
   B. uncertainty in illness theory
   C. hierarchy of needs theory
   D. job satisfaction theory
7. Grand theories
   A. are complex and broad in scope.
   B. look at a piece of reality and contain clearly defined variables.
   C. produce specific directions or guidelines for practice.
   D. formulate nursing protocols on specific units.
8. An example of a middle-range theory is
   A. Orem's Self-Care Deficit Theory.
   B. Parse's Human Becoming Theory.
   C. Pender's Health Promotion Model.
   D. Roy's Adaptation Model.
9. Nursing research has used which reasoning process?
   A. inductive
   B. deductive
   C. both inductive and deductive
   D. neither inductive nor deductive
10. Which statement regarding theory is *false*?
    A. It proves the relationship between variables.
    B. It describes the relationship between variables.
    C. It explains the relationship between variables.
    D. It contains propositional statements.

See answers to Self-Test in the Answer Section at the back of the book.

References

Bambini, D., Washburn, J., & Perkins, R. (2009). Outcomes of clinical simulation for novice nursing students: Communication, confidence, clinical judgment. *Nursing Education Perspectives, 30*, 79–82. http://www.nln.org/newsroom/newsletters-and-journal/nursing-education-perspectives-journal

Bandura, A. (1977). *Self-efficacy: The exercise of control.* New York: W. H. Freeman.

Bandura, A. (1985). *Social Foundations of Thought and Action: A Social Cognitive Theory.* Englewood Cliffs, NJ: Prentice-Hall.

Becker, M. H. (1985). Patient adherence to prescribed therapies. *Medical Care, 23*, 539–555.

Benner, P. (1984). *From Novice to Expert: Excellence and Power in Clinical Nursing Practice.* Menlo Park, CA: Addison-Wesley.

Benson, H. (1975). *The relaxation response.* New York: William Morrow.

Biddle, B. J., (1986). Recent developments in role theory. *Annual Review of Sociology, 12*, 67–92. http://www.annualreviews.org/journal/soc

Blackwell, B. (1985). Models: Their virtues and vices. *Cardiac Rehabilitation, 5*, 169–171.

Brink, P. J. (2000). A response to Fawcett. *Western Journal of Nursing Research, 22*, 653–655. http://journals.sagepub.com/home/wjn

Bush, H. (1979). Models for nursing. *Advances in Nursing Science, 1*(2), 13–21. http://journals.lww.com/advancesinnursingscience/Pages/default.aspx

Caplan, G. (1964). *Principles of Preventive Psychiatry.* New York: Basic Books.

Cox, C. (1982). An interaction model of client health behavior: Theoretical prescription for nursing. *Advances in Nursing Science, 5*(1), 41–56. http://journals.lww.com/advancesinnursingscience/Pages/default.aspx

Duvall, E. (1977). *Marriage and Family Development* (5th ed.). Philadelphia: Lippincott.

Erikson, E. (1950). *Childhood and Society.* New York: W. W. Norton.

Farren, A. T. (2010). Power, uncertainty, self-transcendence, and quality of life in breast cancer survivors. *Nursing Science Quarterly, 23,* 63–71. doi:10.1177/0894318409353793

Fawcett, J. (1978). The "what" of theory development. In *Theory development: What, why, how?* (pp. 17–33). New York: National League for Nursing.

Fawcett, J. (1995). *Analysis and Evaluation of Conceptual Models of Nursing* (3rd ed.). Philadelphia: F. A. Davis.

Fawcett, J. (2000). But is it *nursing* research? *Western Journal of Nursing Research, 22,* 524–525. http://journals.sagepub.com/home/wjn

Fawcett, J. (2005). *Contemporary Nursing Knowledge: Analysis and Evaluation of Nursing Models and Theories* (2nd ed.). Philadelphia: F. A. Davis.

Fawcett, J., & Desanto-Madeya, S. (2013). *Contemporary nursing knowledge: Analysis and evaluation of nursing models and theories* (3rd ed.). Philadelphia: F. A. Davis.

Festinger, L. (1957). *A theory of cognitive dissonance.* Stanford, CA: Stanford University Press.

Fincher, L., Ward, C., Dawkins, V., Magee, V. & Willson, P. (2009). Using telehealth to educate Parkinson's disease patients about complicated medication regimens. *Gerontological Nursing, 35*(2), 16–24. http://www.healio.com/nursing/journals/jgn

Freud, S. (1938). *The basic writings of Sigmund Freud.* New York: Random House.

Grove, S., Burns, N., & Gray, J. (2013). *The practice of nursing research: Appraisal, synthesis, generation of evidence* (7th ed.). St. Louis, MO: Saunders Elsevier.

Günüsen, N. P., Üstün, B., & Gigiotti, E. (2009). Conceptualization of burnout from the perspective of the Neuman systems model. *Nursing Science Quarterly, 22,* 200–204. doi:10.1177/0894318409338685

Hatfield, L. A. (2008). Sucrose decreases infant biobehavioral pain response to immunizations: A randomized controlled trial. *Nursing Scholarship, 40,* 219–225. doi: 10.1111/j.1547-5069.2008.00229.x.

Havighurst, R. (1952). *Developmental tasks and education.* New York: Longmans, Green.

Herzberg, F. (1966). *Work and the nature of man.* Cleveland, OH: World Publishing.

Hoffman, A. J., von Eye, A., Gift, A. G., Given, B. A., Given, C. W., & Rothert, M. (2009). Testing a theoretical model of perceived self-efficacy for cancer-related fatigue self-management and optimal physical functional status. *Nursing Research, 58,* 32–41. doi: 10.1097/NNR.0b013e3181903d7b

Houghton, C., Hunter, A., & Meskell, P. (2012). Linking aims, paradigm and method in nursing research. *Nurse Researcher, 20*(2), 34–39. http://dx.doi.org/10.7748/nr2012.11.20.2.34.c9439

Huth, M. M., & Moore, S. M. (1998). Prescriptive theory of acute pain management in infants and children. *Specialists in Pediatric Nursing, 3*(1), 23–32. doi:10.1111/j.1744-6155.1998.tb00206.x

Kerlinger, F. (1973). *Foundations of behavioral research* (2nd ed.). New York: Holt, Rinehart & Winston.

Kerlinger, F. (1986). *Foundations of behavioral research* (3rd ed.). New York: Holt, Rinehart & Winston.

King, I. M. (1981). *A theory for nursing: Systems, concepts, process.* New York: John Wiley.

Knowles, M. (1990). *The adult learner: A neglected species* (4th ed.). Houston, TX: Gulf Press.

Kohlberg, L. (1978). The cognitive developmental approach to moral education. In P. Scharf (Ed.), *Readings in moral education* (pp. 36–51). Minneapolis, MN: Winston Press.

Lazarus, R. S., & Folkman, S. (1984). *Stress, appraisal, and coping.* New York: Springer.

Lefaiver, C. A., Keough, V., Letizia, M., & Lanuza, D. M. (2007). Using the Roy Adaptation Model to explore the dynamics of quality of life and the relationship between lung transplant candidates and their caregivers. *Advances in Nursing Science, 30,* 266–274. doi:10.1097/01.ANS.0000286624.61892.30

Lentz, E. R., Pugh, L. C., Milligan, R. A., Gift, A., & Suppe, F. (1997). The middle-range theory of unpleasant symptoms: An update. *Advances in Nursing Science, 19*(3), 14–27. http://journals.lww.com/advancesinnursingscience/pages/default.aspx

Levine, M. Y. (1995). The rhetoric of nursing theory. *Image: Journal of Nursing Scholarship, 27,* 11–14. doi: 10.1111/j.1547-5069.1995.tb00807.x

Lewin, K. (1951). *Field theory in social science.* Westport, CT: Greenwood.

Malinski, V. M., & Barrett, E. A. M. (Eds.). (1994). *Martha E. Rogers: Her life and her work.* Philadelphia: F. A. Davis.

Maslow, A. (1970). *Motivation and personality* (2nd ed.). New York: Harper & Row.

Mead, G. (1934). *Mind, self and society.* Chicago: University of Chicago Press.

Meleis, A. I. (1997). *Theoretical nursing: Development and progress* (3rd ed.). Philadelphia: Lippincott-Raven.

Meleis, A. I., & Im, E. (2001). From fragmentation to integration in the discipline of nursing: Situation-specific theories. In N. L. Chaska (Ed.), *The nursing profession: Tomorrow and beyond* (pp. 881–891). Thousand Oaks, CA: Sage.

Melzack, R., & Wall, P. (1983). *The challenge of pain* (rev. ed.). New York: Basic Books.

Minuchin, S. (1974). *Families and family therapy.* Cambridge, MA: Harvard University Press.

Mishel, M. H. (1981). The measurement of uncertainty in illness. *Nursing Research, 30,* 258–263. http://journals.lww.com/nursingresearchonline/Pages/default.aspx

Mishel, M. H. (1990). Reconceptualizatin of the uncertainty in illness theory. *Image: Journal of Nursing Scholarship, 22,* 256–262. doi: 10.1111/j.1547-5069.1990.tb00225.x

Moola, S., Ehlers, V. J., & Hattingh, S P. (2008). Critical care nurses' perceptions of stress and stress-related situations in the workplace. *Curationis, 32,* 77–86. http://www.curationis.org.za

Neuman, B. (1982). *The Neuman systems model.* Norwalk, CT: Appleton-Century-Crofts.

Neuman, B., & Fawcett, J. (2011). *The Neuman systems model* (5th ed.) Upper Saddle River, NJ: Prentice Hall.

Neuman, B. & Young, R.J. (1972). A model for teaching total person approach to patient problems. *Nursing Research, 2,* 264–269. http://journals.lww.com/nursingresearchonline/

Nightingale, F. (1859/1946). *Notes on nursing: What it is, and what it is not.* London: Harrison. [Reprinted 1946. Philadelphia: Lippincott.]

Orem, D.E. (1971). *Nursing: Concepts of Practice.* New York: McGraw-Hill.

Orem, D.E. (2001). *Nursing: Concepts of Practice* (6th ed.). St. Louis, MO: Mosby.

Parse, R. R. (2000). Obfuscating: The persistent practice of misnaming. *Nursing Science Quarterly, 13,* 91. http://journals.sagepub.com/home/nsq

Parse, R. R. (2003). What constitutes nursing research? *Nursing Science Quarterly, 16,* 287. http://journals.sagepub.com/home/nsq

Pender, N. J. (2014). *Health promotion in nursing practice* (7th ed.). Norwalk, CT: Appleton & Lange.

Peplau, H. E. (1988). *Interpersonal relations in nursing.* London: Macmillan Education.

Piaget, J. (1926). *The language and thought of the child.* New York: Harcourt, Brace, and World.

Pipe, T. B., Bortz, J. J., & Dueck, A. (2009). Nurse leader mindfulness meditation program for stress management. *Nursing Administration, 39,* 130–137. doi: 10.1097/NNA.0b013e31819894a0

Polit, D. F., & Beck, C. T. (2012). *Nursing Research: Generating and Assessing Evidence for Nursing Practice* (9th ed.). Philadelphia: Lippincott Williams & Wilkins.

Prochaska, J. O., & DiClemente, C. C. (1983). Stages and processes of self-change of smoking: Toward an integrative model of change. *Journal of Consulting and Clinical Psychology, 52,* 390–395. http://dx.doi.org/10.1037/0022-006X.51.3.390

Reynolds, P. (1971). *A primer in theory construction.* Indianapolis: Bobbs-Merrill.

Riegel, B., & Dickson, V. V. (2008). A situation-specific theory of heart failure self-care. *Cardiovascular Nursing, 23*(3), 190–196. doi: 10.1097/01.JCN.0000305091.35259.85

Rogers, C. (1969). *Freedom to learn.* Columbus, OH: Charles E. Merrill.

Rogers, M. (1970). *An introduction to the theoretical basis of nursing.* Philadelphia: F. A. Davis.

Rogers, M. (1980). Nursing: A science of unitary man. In J. P. Riehl and C. Roy (Eds.), *Conceptual models for nursing practice* (2nd ed., pp. 329–337). New York: Appleton-Century-Crofts.

Rogers, M. E. (1990). Nursing: Science of unitary, irreducible, human beings: Update 1990. In E. A. M. Barrett (Ed.), *Visions of Rogers' science-based nursing* (pp. 5–11). New York: National League for Nursing.

Rogers, M. (1992). Nursing science and the space age. *Nursing Science Quarterly, 5,* 27–34. http://journals.sagepub.com/home/nsq

Rolfe, G. (1996). Closing the theory-practice gap a new paradigm for nursing. *Clinical Nursing, 2,* 173–177. http://dx.doi.org/10.7748/nm.3.7.26.s25

Rotter, J. (1954). *Social learning and clinical psychology.* Englewood Cliffs, NJ: Prentice-Hall.

Roy, C. (1976). *Introduction to nursing: An adaptation model.* Englewood Cliffs, NJ: Prentice-Hall.

Roy, C. (1984). *Introduction to nursing: An adaptation model* (2nd ed.). Englewood Cliffs, NJ: Prentice-Hall.

Roy, C. (2009). *The Roy adaptation model* (3rd ed.). Upper Saddle River, NJ: Pearson.

Roy, C., & Andrews, H. A. (1999). *The Roy adaptation model* (2nd ed.). Stamford, CT: Appleton & Lange.

Roy, C., & Andrews, H. A. (2008). *The Roy adaptation model* (3rd ed.). Upper Saddle River, NJ: Prentice-Hall.

Satir, V. (1967). *Conjoint family therapy* (rev. ed.). Palo Alto, CA: Science & Behavior Books.

Schilder, P. (1952). *The image and appearance of the human body.* New York: International University Press.

Schneiderman, J., Corbridge, S., & Zerwic, J. J. (2009). Demonstrating the effectiveness of an online, computer-based learning module for arterial blood gas analysis. *Clinical Nurse Specialist, 33,* 151–155. doi: 10.1097/NUR.0b013e3181a075bc

Seligman, M. (1975). *Helplessness: On depression, development, and death.* San Francisco: W. H. Freeman.

Selye, H. (1976). *The stress of life* (rev. ed.). New York: McGraw-Hill.

Sheehan, C. A. (2009). A brief educational video about prostate cancer screening: A community intervention. *Urologic Nursing, 29,* 103–111, 117. https://www.suna.org/unj

Song, H.-Y., & Nam, K. A. (2010). Coping strategies, physical function, and social adjustment in people with spinal cord injury. *Rehabilitation Nursing, 35,* 8–15. doi: 10.1002/j.2048-7940.2010.tb00025.x

Spielberger, C. (1972). Anxiety as an emotional state. In C. D. Spielberger (Ed.), *Anxiety: Current trends in theory and research* (Vol. 1, pp. 3–47). New York: Academic Press.

Stevens, B. (1979). *Nursing theory.* Boston: Little, Brown.

Stewart, J. L., Lynn, M. R., & Mishel, M. H. (2010). Psychometric evaluation of a new instrument to measure uncertainty in children and adolescents with cancer. *Nursing Research, 59,* 119–125. doi: 10.1097/NNR.0b013e3181d1a8d5

Suppe, F. (1996). Middle-range theory: Role in nursing theory and knowledge development. Proceedings of the Sixth Rosemary Ellis Scholar's Retreat, Nursing Science Implications for the 21st century. Frances Payne Bolton School of Nursing, Case Western Reserve University, Cleveland, OH.

Taylor, S. G., Geden, E., Isaramalai, S., & Wongvatunyu, S. (2000). *Orem's Self-Care Deficit Nursing Theory: Its Philosophic Foundation and the State of the Science Nursing Science Quarterly, 13,* 104–110. http://journals.sagepub.com/home/nsq

Youngkin, E. Q., & Lester, P. B. (2010). Promoting self-care and secondary prevention in women's health: A study to test the accuracy of a home self-test system for bacterial vaginosis. *Applied Nursing Research, 23,* 2–10. doi: 10.1016/j.apnr.2008.02.002.

Walker, L. O., & Avant, K. C. (2011). *Strategies for theory construction in nursing* (5th ed.). Upper Saddle River, NJ: Pearson/ Prentice Hall.

Walker, S. N., Pullen, C. H, Boeckner, L., Hageman, P. A., Hertzog, M., Oberdorfer, M. K., & Rutledge, M. J. (2009). Clinical trial of tailored activity and eating newsletters with older rural women. *Nursing Research, 58,* 74–85. doi: 10.1097/NNR.0b013e31818fcee1

Watson, J. (2005). *Caring science as sacred science.* Philadelphia: F. A. Davis.

Weaver, K., & Olson, J. K. (2006). Understanding paradigms used for nursing research. *Advanced Nursing, 53*(4), 459–469. doi: 10.1111/j.1365-2648.2006.03740.x

Chapter 9
Hypotheses

Rose Marie Nieswiadomy, PhD, RN, and Becky Spencer, PhD, RN, IBCLC

Objectives

On completion of this chapter, you will be prepared to:

1. Describe the role of hypotheses in research studies.
2. Compare classifications of hypotheses.
3. Describe the considerations when developing hypotheses.

Introduction

You wonder why the traffic is moving so slowly. You start thinking of possible reasons. There may have been an accident up ahead. Or maybe a car has stalled and people must switch lanes to get past the stalled car. Maybe road construction is to blame. The next thought that comes to mind is there may be a police officer parked on the side of the road just waiting for speeders. Suddenly, you see flashing lights and hear an ambulance siren. Then you see two crumpled cars and people standing around them. You are now aware that an accident is the cause of the traffic slowdown. The hunches you had about the reasons for the slow traffic could be considered hypotheses. After the facts were gathered, you find that your first hunch was correct. The accident was the cause of the slow traffic.

Hypotheses Overview

In scientific research, hypotheses are intelligent guesses that assist the researcher in seeking the solution to a problem. Kerlinger (1986) has defined a hypothesis as a "conjectural statement of the relations between two or more variables" (p. 17). Polit and Beck (2012) presented a similar definition by calling a hypothesis a "statement of the researcher's expectations about relationships between study variables" (p. 58). Within this book, we define a hypothesis as a statement of the predicted relationship between two or more variables. The hypothesis of a study is the expected outcome of the proposed research question. Earlier, you learned that the research question is the specific question that the nurse researcher expects to be answered by the study. Both quantitative and qualitative studies have research questions, but only quantitative studies have hypotheses. Quantitative research studies may have one or several hypotheses.

The hypothesis links the independent and the dependent variables. Recall that an independent variable is referred to as the cause, and the dependent variable is referred to as the effect in experimental studies. The researcher manipulates, or controls, the independent variable. In nonexperimental studies, the words *cause* and *effect* are not appropriate because the researcher does not manipulate the independent variable. The researcher, however, may be able to determine which variable might have an influence on the other variable. The direction of influence runs from the independent variable to the dependent variable. For example, a researcher might be trying to examine the relationship between age and the amount of exercise that people perform. The independent variable would be *age*, and the dependent variable *exercise performance*. It would not be appropriate to say that age is the cause of the amount of exercise that one performs, although the direction of influence logically flows from age to exercise performance.

Hypotheses should always be written before the study begins, and not changed after the study results are examined. This is like picking the winning horse after you have already watched the race.

Purposes of Hypotheses

Hypotheses serve several purposes in research studies. They lend objectivity to scientific investigations by pinpointing a specific part of a theory to be tested. Through hypotheses, theoretical propositions can be tested in the real world. The investigator can then advance scientific knowledge by supporting or failing to support the tested theory. Even when the research hypothesis is not supported, scientific knowledge is gained. Negative findings are sometimes as important as positive ones. Hypotheses also guide the research design and dictate the type of statistical analysis to be used with the data. Finally, hypotheses provide the reader with an understanding of the researcher's expectations about the study before data collection begins. Hypothesis testing guides evidence-based nursing practice. Nurses need to know that their practice is based on research studies in which hypothesis testing has supported certain nursing care practices or interventions.

Sources or Rationale for Hypotheses

Hypotheses are not wild guesses or shots in the dark. The researcher should be able to state the source or rationale for each hypothesis. This source or rationale for the hypothesis may come from a theory, literature review of prior studies, or personal experience.

The most important source of a hypothesis is the theoretical or conceptual framework developed for the study. This process of hypothesis development involves deductive reasoning. A propositional statement is isolated from the study framework and empirically tested. For example, using Pender's Health Promotion Model (2014), you might decide to test the proposition that self-efficacy increases participation in a healthy behavior. This proposition could then be transferred into a hypothesis to be tested in a research study. You might ask a group of patients how confident they are that they can start an exercise program, and then compare their level of self-efficacy with actual participation in the exercise program.

Hypotheses for nursing research studies can also be derived from the findings of other studies. The researcher may test the assumptions of another study, or test a hypothesis based on the findings of another study. For example, breastfeeding initiation and duration rates increase when women receive a combination of breastfeeding education, peer support, and lactation consultant support (Britton, McCormick, Renfrew, Wade, & King, 2007). However, only adult mothers were included in the studies, and adolescent mothers were excluded. Wambach et al. (2011) conducted a study that tested the same hypothesis, that education and support increase breastfeeding initiation and duration, with adolescent mothers.

Finally, a nurse may have a hunch that comes from personal experiences or observations. For example, you may have noticed that psychiatric patients seem to become more anxious as the time for their discharge approaches. Observations continue to be made. Patients' charts are examined to determine behaviors reported by other staff members. The behaviors recorded on the charts seem to agree with your observations. Thus, an empirical generalization may be made based on these observations: "As the time for discharge draws near, the anxiety levels of psychiatric patients increase." The following hypothesis might then be tested: "The anxiety levels of psychiatric patients are higher immediately before discharge than they are three days before discharge." Recall the difference between induction and deduction. This hypothesis was derived through induction. It was based on an empirical generalization derived from your observations as a nurse. Even when a study is based on empirical generalizations from the researcher's own experiences, a review of the literature should be conducted in the study area to determine what is already known on the topic. Then an attempt should be made to find a theoretical explanation for the observed phenomenon.

Classifications of Hypotheses

Hypotheses can be categorized as simple hypotheses or complex hypotheses. They can also be classified as research hypotheses or null hypotheses. Research hypotheses can be further divided into nondirectional and directional hypotheses, and causal and associative hypotheses.

Simple and Complex Hypotheses

A **simple hypothesis** concerns the relationship between one independent variable and one dependent variable. Independent and dependent variables were previously discussed. If you recall, in experimental studies the independent variable may be considered as the *cause*, or reason that a phenomenon occurs, and the dependent variable may be considered the *effect*, or occurrence of the phenomenon. Independent and dependent variables can also be identified in many nonexperimental studies by examining the direction of the influence of one variable on the other, or by determining which variable occurred before the other one. The independent variable occurs first in chronological time (but not necessarily first in the hypothesis statement itself).

A **complex hypothesis** concerns a relationship in which two or more independent variables, or two or more dependent variables, or both, are being examined in the same study. A simple hypothesis might be called bivariate, and a complex hypothesis multivariate.

Simple hypotheses contain one independent variable and one dependent variable; complex hypotheses contain multiple independent or dependent variables. As long as there is more than one independent variable, or more than one dependent variable, or both, the hypothesis is considered complex. Table 9–1 gives examples of simple and complex hypotheses.

Caution should be exercised when using complex hypotheses. It may be better to divide a complex hypothesis into two or more simple hypotheses. Although you may read about "partial support" for a hypothesis, this is inaccurate. If only part of the hypothesis is supported, the researcher is in the partial support crisis. In actuality, a hypothesis is either supported totally or it is not supported. It is like being pregnant. A woman is either pregnant or not pregnant. She cannot be a little bit pregnant.

Consider this hypothesis: A positive relationship exists between patients' perception of pain control and (a) complaints of pain and (b) requests for pain medications. Statistically, two hypotheses will be tested: (a) the relationship between perception of pain control and complaints of pain, and (b) the relationship between perception of pain control and requests for pain medications. If a significant relationship is found between perception of pain control and complaints of pain, but not between perception of pain control and requests for pain medication, then a *partial* support crisis has occurred. The researcher cannot decide to divide the original hypothesis at this time, but must admit that the research hypothesis has not

Table 9-1 Examples of Types of Hypotheses

Population	Independent Variable	Dependent Variable	Type of Hypothesis	Hypotheses
1. Infants	Level of alcohol use of mothers	Birth weight	Simple, directional, associative	Birth weight is lower among infants of alcoholic mothers than among infants of nonalcoholic mothers
2. Intensive care unit patients	Care clustering	Sleep deprivation	Simple, directional, causal	Care clustering will increase sleep intervals for intensive care unit patients when compared to pateints who receive no care clustering
3. Adults	a. Type of diet b. Exercise	Weight	Complex, directional, causal	Reduced calorie diet and exercise daily will increase daily weight loss for adults when compared to adults who do not follow a reduced calorie diet and do not exercise daily
4. Nurse practitioners	Type of nurse practitioner	Job mobility	Simple, nondirectional, associative	There is an association between the level of job mobility between psychiatric nurse practitioners and medical-surgical nurse practitioners
5. Women	Method of delivery	a. Postpartum depression b. Feelings of inadequacy	Complex, directional, associative	More postpartum depression and feelings of inadequacy are reported by women who give birth by cesarean delivery than by those who deliver vaginally
6. Postmyocardial infarction patients	a. Education videos b. Follow up phone calls	a. Anxiety b. Medication compliance	Complex, nondirectional, causal	Education videos and follow up phone calls have an impact on patient reported anxiety and medication compliance post hospital discharge when compared to patients who receive written discharge instructions and no follow up phone call.

been supported. This problem could have been solved by writing two simple hypotheses rather than one complex hypothesis.

Sometimes complex hypotheses are necessary. Whenever the researcher wants to examine an interaction effect, a complex hypothesis is called for. An **interaction effect** concerns the action of two variables in conjunction with each other. Consider Hypothesis 3 in Table 9–1. The researcher believes that the combination of diet and exercise is necessary for weight loss.

Nondirectional and Directional Research Hypotheses

Research hypotheses may be described as being nondirectional or directional. In a **nondirectional research hypothesis**, the researcher merely predicts that a relationship exists. The direction of the relationship is not presented. When a study is not based on a theory or the findings of related studies are contradictory, the investigator may decide to use a nondirectional hypothesis.

Nondirectional Research Hypothesis

Im, Chang, Chee, Chee, and Mao (2014) examined the relationship between immigration status and depressive symptoms in 1054 women who had immigrated to the United States. The hypotheses tested was, "There is a relationship between immigration status and depressive symptoms in middle-aged women when controlling for background characteristics, self-reported racial/ethnic identity and immigration status." The authors did not predict prior to conducting the study whether immigraiton status would be positively or negatively associated with depressive symptoms. The authors found that immigration status was a predictor of depressive symptoms.

In the **directional research hypothesis**, the researcher predicts the type of relationship that is expected. Directional hypotheses have several advantages: They make clear the researcher's expectation, allow more precise testing of theoretical propositions, and allow the use of one-tailed statistical tests. Statistical significance is more easily achieved when one-tailed tests are used.

Directional Research Hypothesis

Elfering, Nützi, Koch, and Baur (2014) were interested in the effect that interruptions have on patient safety in the operating room. They hypothesized that workflow interruptions would be positively associated with failure in action regulation (slips and lapses in routine action execution) and with near accidents. The authors assumed that interruptions would result in an increase in mistakes and near accidents. Through statistical analysis of observations of workflow interruptions, the researchers found the hypothesis to be true.

Causal and Associative Research Hypotheses

In addition to being directional or nondirectional, hypotheses can express a causal relationship between variables or an associative relationship between variables. Hypotheses that predict causal relationships between variables require an experimental research design, while hypotheses that predict associative relationships between variables require nonexperimental or correlational research designs.

A **causal research hypothesis** predicts that the independent variable will cause something to occur to the dependent variable; the effect on the dependent variable is a direct result of the independent variable.

Causal Research Hypothesis

Ho, Ho, Leung, So, and Chan (2016) were interested in interventions that could decrease pain perception in preterm infants. The hypothesis they tested was that swaddling preterm infants prior to a heelstick procedure would result in decreased pain when compared to preterm infants who were not swaddled prior to a heelstick procedure. The authors measured the preterm infants pain using the Premature Infant Pain Profile (PIPP) scale, heart rate, and oxygen saturation fluctuations. They found that infants who were swaddled had significantly decreased PIPP scores and fewer fluctuations in heart rate and oxygen saturation when compared to preterm infants who were not swaddled. Swaddling appears to have a direct impact on pain perception for preterm infants.

An **associative research hypothesis** predicts that there will be a relationship between the variables. Nurse researchers are frequently interested in examining how different lifestyles or life situation factors are related to patient outcomes or issues. Sociodemographic factors, such as annual income, education, age, gender, race or ethnicity, and so on, often are related or correlated to health conditions and health outcomes such as hypertension, cancer, diabetes, and infant mortality among many, many others. While we know that a particular race or ethnicity does not *cause* hypertension, we know through statistical correlations that African American and Hispanic populations have much higher rates of hypertension than Caucasian populations. Awareness of an association or correlation between two or more variables can help nurse researchers design interventions that are tailored or targeted to the population of greatest need.

Identifying associative versus causal hypotheses can be a little tricky. One hint is that causal hypotheses are generally testing an intervention (independent variable) and the effect of that intervention

Associative Research Hypothesis

Research conducted over many decades has consistently revealed that maternal smoking is associated with an increased risk of preterm birth, low birth weight, and sudden infant death syndrome. Patrick, Warner, Pordes, and Davis (2016) were interested in examining if increases in cost of cigarettes were associated with a decrease in infant mortality between 1999 and 2010 in the United States. The hypothesis they tested was that changes in cigarette taxes and prices over time in the United States were associated with an overall decrease in infant mortality. They found that for every $1 increase in cigarette tax per pack infant mortality decreased −0.19 per 1000 live births. The impact was greater for African American infants. While increasing cigarette cost did not cause a decrease in infant mortality, a logical deduction is that increased costs of cigarettes may have caused women to smoke less, which resulted in healthier pregnancies, births, and infants.

on a specific outcome (dependent variable). A hint for identifying associative hypotheses is that the words *association*, *related to*, or *relationship* will sometimes be found in the hypothesis statement. Take another look at Table 9–1. Cover the middle three columns with a piece of paper and see if you can identify the independent and dependent variables from the hypothesis, and whether the hypotheses are simple or complex, directional or nondirectional, and associative or causal.

Null and Research Hypotheses

Null and research hypotheses are statistical terms for how a relationship between variables is tested. Those of you who have had a course in statistics will recall that a **null hypothesis** (H_0) predicts that no relationship exists between variables, and it is the null hypothesis that is subjected to statistical analysis. A **research hypothesis** or alternative hypothesis (H_1) states the expected relationship between variables. For those of you who have repressed statistics into your unconscious, and for those who have not yet taken a statistics course, you need to know that the null hypothesis is tested even when the research hypothesis is stated in the study. Other names for the research hypothesis are *scientific*, *substantive*, and *theoretical*.

Statistical logic requires that a testable hypothesis state the expectation of no correlation between the variables or no difference between groups or sets of data on the variable being measured. If the research hypothesis proposes that a correlation exists between two variables, the null hypothesis states that no correlation exists. If the research hypothesis states that a difference exists between two groups or sets of data, the null hypothesis states that no difference exists.

Although some research studies express hypotheses in the null form, it is generally more desirable to state the researcher's expectations, according to Batey (1977) and Kerlinger (1986). Polit and Beck (2012) have written that they prefer research hypotheses when there is a reasonable basis for them because these hypotheses "clarify the study's framework and demonstrate that researchers have thought critically about the phenomena under study" (p. 88). A review of the current nursing research journals shows that the research hypothesis has replaced the statistical null hypothesis as the preferred way of expressing the predictions for studies. The use of theoretical frameworks in nursing research has brought about this change. Study predictions should be based on the study framework.

The level of significance for rejecting the statistical null hypothesis should always be stated before data are collected. In nursing, as in many other disciplines, the level of significance is usually set at .05. A significance level of .05 means that the researcher is willing to risk being wrong 5% of the time, or 5 times out of 100, when rejecting the null hypothesis. Generally, the aim of the researcher is to reject the null hypothesis because this provides support for the research hypothesis. Sir Ronald Fisher (1951) stated, "Every experiment may be said to exist only in order to give the facts a chance of disproving the null hypothesis" (p. 16).

Occasionally, the null hypothesis and the research hypothesis are the same. The researcher actually expects no correlation between variables, or no difference between groups being compared on a certain variable. For example, an in-service educator at a hospital might believe that a certain inexpensive teaching program is as effective as an expensive teaching program for patients with diabetes. The educator might predict that there would be no difference in patients' knowledge of the subject matter when the two different teaching programs are used. Usually, the researcher *does* expect to find a difference or a correlation; otherwise, the study would not have been conducted.

As you can see, the null hypothesis was *not* rejected in the study by Harrison et al., but *was* rejected in the Polit and Beck study. Female participants were more numerous than male participants, which is rather surprising. In the past, many research studies were conducted only on men.

Null Hypotheses

A null hypothesis was tested in a study (Harrison, Speroni, Dugan, & Daniel, 2010) that compared the quality of blood specimens drawn on one group of patients (n = 200) by Emergency Medical Services (EMS) staff versus specimens obtained on another group (n = 200) by Emergency Department (ED) staff when the patients reached the emergency department. One aspect of the study examined redraw rates. Study results showed no statistically significant differences in redraw rates between the two groups. The null hypothesis was not rejected.

Polit and Beck (2009) studied gender bias in nursing research. They tested the null hypothesis that males and females are represented equally as participants in nursing research studies. The null hypothesis was rejected. In 834 studies published in eight English-language nursing research journals in 2005–2006, approximately 71% of participants were females. This bias was strong in the United States and Canada; many female participants were also found in studies conducted in Europe, Asia, and Australia.

Developing Hypotheses

A hypothesis should:

1. be written in a declarative sentence.
2. be written in the present tense.
3. contain the population.
4. contain the variables.
5. reflect the problem statement, purpose statement, or research question.
6. be empirically testable.

WRITTEN IN A DECLARATIVE SENTENCE Hypotheses should always be written in declarative sentences. Whereas the research question inquires about some phenomenon or phenomena of interest in the study, the hypothesis presents an answer to the question in the form of a declarative statement.

WRITTEN IN THE PRESENT TENSE Hypotheses found in the published research reports may be written in the future tense. However, hypotheses are tested in the present and should be written in the present tense.

- Future tense: There *will* be a positive relationship between the number of times children have been hospitalized and their fear of hospitalization (incorrect format).
- Present tense: There *is* a positive relationship between the number of times children have been hospitalized and their fear of hospitalization (correct format).

CONTAIN THE POPULATION   The population needs to be specifically identified in the hypothesis, just as it is in the problem statement, purpose statement, or research question. If the research question identifies the population as "middle-aged (40–55 years old) women who are about to undergo a hysterectomy," these same terms should be contained in the hypothesis. It would not be correct to identify the population in the hypothesis only as "hysterectomy patients".

CONTAIN THE VARIABLES   Notice the word *variable* is written as a plural noun in the heading for this paragraph. In the problem statement or research question, you might have only one variable. A univariate research problem statement or research question is acceptable. Remember, however, a scientific hypothesis contains at least two variables, one independent and one dependent, which are linked in the hypothesis.

Frequently, the hypothesis contains the instrument or tool that will be used to measure the dependent variable. This instrument links the hypothesis more closely to the actual data-gathering procedure and helps operationalize the dependent variable. Here is an example of two ways to write the same hypothesis:

- Anxiety levels are lower for preoperative hysterectomy patients who have practiced relaxation exercises than for preoperative hysterectomy patients who have not practiced relaxation exercises.
- Anxiety levels, as measured by the state anxiety scale of Spielberger's State-Trait Anxiety Inventory, are lower for preoperative hysterectomy patients who have practiced relaxation exercises than for preoperative hysterectomy patients who have not practiced relaxation exercises.

As you can see, the second example contains the instrument that will be used to measure the dependent variable. The hypothesis will still need further clarification, however, before it is ready to be tested. For example, relaxation exercises would have to be operationally defined before the study could actually be conducted.

REFLECT THE PROBLEM STATEMENT, PURPOSE STATEMENT, OR RESEARCH QUESTION   To reemphasize the point, the hypothesis should contain essentially the same material as the problem statement, purpose statement, or research question. Occasionally, you read a research report in which it appears that one person wrote the purpose statement, and another person wrote the hypothesis without ever reading the purpose statement. For example, the purpose statement might indicate "depression" as the dependent variable, whereas the hypothesis contains "sadness" as the dependent variable. Congruency is a must.

EMPIRICALLY TESTABLE   The ability to obtain empirical data should have been determined as the research problem was formalized. If there is no possibility of obtaining empirical data, it will not be possible to conduct a quantitative study. A hypothesis that cannot be empirically tested has no scientific merit. Ethical and value issues are two areas that are inappropriate for hypothesis testing because data cannot be obtained that can be empirically verified. Consider the following hypothesis: "Nurse practitioners are better healthcare providers than physicians." This hypothesis is not empirically testable because *better* is a value word. You could, in fact, change the wording of this hypothesis to make it empirically testable: "Nurse practitioners spend more time teaching their clients about preventative healthcare practices than do physicians." The term *time* could be measured empirically.

Hypothesis Format

Research questions that examine more than one variable are usually written in the form of a correlational statement or comparative statement. The same holds true for hypotheses. The issue of correlations and comparisons becomes very important when the data are submitted for statistical analysis. Statistical tests are basically designed to examine correlations between variables or comparisons among sets of data. One study might compare the average pulse rates of *two* different groups, whereas another study might examine the correlation between pulse rates and respirations in *one* group of subjects. A different statistical test would be needed to analyze the data from these two studies.

A directional research hypothesis should contain a predictive term like *less, greater, decrease in*, or *negative correlation*. Let us examine some examples of research questions and corresponding hypotheses. The predictive terms in the two hypotheses are in italics.

- **Research Question:** Is there a correlation between anxiety levels and midterm examination scores of baccalaureate nursing students?
- **Hypothesis:** There is a *negative correlation* between anxiety levels and midterm examination scores of baccalaureate nursing students.
- **Research Question:** Is there a difference in readiness to learn about preoperative teaching between preoperative patients who have high anxiety levels compared with preoperative patients who do not have high anxiety levels?
- **Hypothesis:** Readiness to learn about preoperative teaching is *less* among preoperative patients who have high anxiety levels compared with preoperative patients who do not have high anxiety levels.

Hypotheses and Theory Testing

Though the statistical testing of a hypothesis will be discussed later, it is important at this point to mention hypothesis testing and its relation to theory. A hypothesis usually tests only one proposition from a theory, not an entire theory.

Hypotheses are never proved or disproved. Novice researchers can be spotted easily if they discuss trying to prove their hypotheses. Remember, neither theories nor hypotheses are proved. In my research classes, a student has to bring cookies to the next class if he or she says the word *prove* out loud in a class discussion. (Even I have to bring cookies if I slip and say the "p" word myself.)

If the null hypothesis is rejected, the research hypothesis is supported. If the research hypothesis is supported, the theory from which the hypothesis was derived will also be supported. Likewise, if the research hypothesis is not supported, the theory is also not supported. When the data fail to support the theory, a critical reexamination of the theory is needed. Beginning researchers frequently have difficulty in explaining their findings when these findings fail to support the tested theory. In some cases, the researcher points out all of the limitations of the study and intimates that the theory is probably valid. The researcher then points out that the study results failed to support the theory because of design or methodology problems that are the fault of the researcher. It is possible that study limitations may have, in fact, influenced the results of the study, but it is also possible that the theory is not valid. In some studies where hypotheses are tested, questions may also be posed. These questions may relate to the hypotheses. For example, suppose a researcher is testing a new intervention for weight loss. The hypothesis might be "People who are overweight and allowed to eat a candy bar each day as part of their diet lose more weight over a 6-week period than those who are not allowed to eat a candy bar." (Note: This is my kind of diet.) The researcher might also ask such questions as "Which type of candy bars do people choose?", "How many calories are in the candy bars that are chosen?", and "What percentage of their daily calories is consumed in the candy bars?" My father worked for a candy factory for 50 years before he retired. Although we did not have many material possessions when I was growing up, we always had candy. The neighborhood children were jealous. I must acknowledge that my mother allowed only small amounts of candy in our house, and only on special occasions.

Critiquing Hypotheses

First, the evaluator of a research report determines if the report contains a hypothesis or hypotheses. Optimally, a section heading clearly labels the hypotheses. If the study contains no hypotheses, a determination should be made as to whether or not the study is appropriate for hypothesis testing.

Box 9–1 Guidelines for Critiquing Hypotheses and Research Questions

1. Does the study contain a hypothesis or hypotheses?
2. Is each hypothesis clearly worded and concise?
3. Is the hypothesis written in a declarative sentence?
4. Is each hypothesis directly tied to the study problem?
5. If there is a clearly identified study framework, is each hypothesis derived from this framework?
6. Does each hypothesis contain the population and at least two variables?
7. Is each hypothesis stated as a directional research hypothesis? If not, is the rationale given for the type of hypothesis that is stated?
8. Is it apparent that each hypothesis can be empirically tested?
9. Does each hypothesis contain only one prediction?

If the study report contains a hypothesis or hypotheses, a number of factors must be considered. Box 9–1 presents the criteria for evaluating study hypotheses.

Hypotheses should be clear and concise declarative sentences and written in the present tense. Hypotheses should reflect the problem statement, purpose statement, or research question, and be derived from the study framework if there is a clearly identified study framework. If there is no identified study framework, the source or rationale for each hypothesis should be apparent to the person critiquing the research report. For example, a hypothesis might be based on previous research findings. The preferred type of hypothesis is a directional research hypothesis. It is easy to determine that the hypothesis is directional if it contains a word or phrase such as "greater than," "increase in," or "negative correlation." The hypothesis should contain the population and study variables. Each hypothesis should be empirically testable and contain only one prediction. The hypothesis may contain the name of the specific research instrument(s) that will be used to measure the study variables. If not, the research report should contain an operational definition of each of the study variables.

It is not uncommon for a study to have tested many more hypotheses than are stated. This fact may be discovered when examining the statistical results. For every statistical test result and accompanying probability value (p), the researcher has tested a hypothesis, whether or not the hypothesis was actually stated. Frequently, after eyeballing the data, the researcher may decide to make some additional statistical analyses. For example, suppose a determination was being made about the effectiveness of preoperative relaxation exercises in controlling postoperative anxiety. The study results indicate that the postoperative anxiety levels of subjects are not significantly different between those who practiced relaxation preoperatively, and those who did not. However, when the researcher looked over the data, it appeared that the relaxation exercises might have been effective for women, but not for men. An additional statistical comparison might be made between the women who practiced relaxation and those who did not. This type of statistical analysis is labeled a post hoc (after the fact) comparison.

Summary

A hypothesis is a statement of the predicted relationship between two or more variables. Hypotheses allow theoretical propositions to be tested in the real world, guide the research design, dictate the type of statistical analysis for the data, and provide the reader with an understanding of the researcher's expectations about the study before data collection begins.

The rationale or sources of hypotheses can come from theories, previous research studies, or the researcher's own personal experiences. Nursing research involves both inductive and deductive means of formulating hypotheses.

Hypotheses can be categorized as simple or complex. Simple hypotheses contain one independent and one dependent variable; complex hypotheses contain two or more independent variables, or two or more dependent variables, or both. An interaction effect concerns the action of two variables in conjunction with each other. The nondirectional research hypothesis indicates that a difference or correlation exists, but does not predict the type. The directional research hypothesis states the type of correlation or difference that the researcher expects to find. The directional research hypothesis is the preferred type for nursing research studies, unless the study is not based on theory or if previous studies in the area have demonstrated contradictory findings.

Hypotheses are also classified as causal or associative. A causal research hypothesis predicts that the independent variable will cause something to occur to the dependent variable. An associative research hypothesis predicts that there will be a relationship between the variables.

Hypotheses may also be classified as statistical null hypotheses or research hypotheses. The null hypothesis states that no difference exists between groups or sets of data or that there is no correlation between variables. The research hypothesis states that a difference or correlation does exist.

A hypothesis should (a) be written in a declarative sentence; (b) be written in the present tense; (c) include the population; (d) include the variables; (e) reflect the problem statement, purpose statement, or research question; and (f) be empirically testable.

The results of statistical analysis will either support or fail to support the hypothesis. Hypotheses are never proved or disproved. If the null hypothesis is rejected, then the research hypothesis is supported. Thus, if a theoretical proposition is being tested and support is found for the research hypothesis, the theory is also supported.

Self-Test

1. The main purpose of a hypothesis in a research study is to
   A. predict the expected results or outcome of a study.
   B. define the theoretical framework for the study.
   C. identify the source of the problem under study.
   D. clarify the concepts used in the study.
2. Which of the following is true about the relationship between the hypotheses and the theoretical framework of a study?
   A. If the hypotheses are stated, the researcher does not need to have a framework.
   B. The framework is tested, not the hypothesis.
   C. The framework and hypotheses must be congruent with each other.
   D. Hypotheses are inductively identified within the stated framework.
3. What is the relationship between the research question and the hypothesis of a study?
   A. There is no relationship between the research question and the hypothesis.

B. The hypothesis is the expected outcome of the research question.
C. The research question is empirically tested while the hypothesis is theoretically tested.
D. The research question and the hypothesis are exactly the same.

4. "Gel pillows will reduce bilateral head flattening in preterm infants." This hypothesis is which of the following:
   A. causal, directional, simple
   B. causal, nondirectional, simple
   C. associative, directional, complex
   D. associative, nondirectional, complex

5. "There is a relationship between the use of formula and the incidence of necrotizing enterocolitis in preterm infants." This hypothesis is which of the following:
   A. causal, directional
   B. causal, nondirectional
   C. associative, directional
   D. associative, nondirectional

6. Which of the following hypotheses is complex and demonstrates an associative, directional relationship between variables?
   A. Older adults demonstrate a lower self-image after retirement than before retirement.
   B. The job turnover rate and job dissatisfaction levels of graduate nurses who have worked less than 2 years is higher than for those who have worked 2 or more years.
   C. New mothers who participate in support groups report less postpartum depression and higher self-confidence than new mothers who do not attend support groups.
   D. There is a higher incidence of marijuana usage among first-year high school students than among high school seniors.

7. Which of the following hypotheses is simple and demonstrates a causal, nondirectional relationship between variables?
   A. Cancer patients who receive music therapy complain less frequently of pain and require less pain medication than cancer patients not receiving music therapy.
   B. Normal saline flush with heparin is more effective than normal saline flush alone in maintaining patency of an intermittent intravenous site.
   C. Low-fat diet is related to lower total cholesterol and higher HDL (high-density lipoprotein).
   D. Delaying the first bath of newborns until 12 hours after birth affects the number of breastfeeding attempts in the first 48 hours of life when compared to not delaying the first bath of newborns.

8. "Preoperative pain medication education is more effective in reducing surgical patients' perception of pain and anxiety postoperatively than no preoperative pain medication education." What type of variable is "anxiety"?
   A. independent
   B. extraneous
   C. dependent
   D. confounding

9. Which of the following are requirements in the structure of a hypothesis? (Select all that apply.)
   A. written in present tense
   B. written as a question
   C. contains the population of interest
   D. contains the independent and dependent variables
   E. contains the statistical test to be applied

10. If a nurse researcher wanted to examine if there is decrease in the number of medication errors in a pediatric clinic when nurses use prefilled syringes for vaccines, which would be the best hypothesis statement?
    A. The use of prefilled syringes will have an effect on medication errors for pediatric clinic patients when compared to the use of nurse-prepared syringes.
    B. Will the use of prefilled syringes have an effect on medication errors for pediatric clinic patients when compared to the use of nurse-prepared syringes?
    C. The use of prefilled syringes will result in decreased medication errors for pediatric clinic patients when compared to the use of nurse-prepared syringes.
    D. Will the use of prefilled syringes result in decreased medication errors for pediatric clinic patients when compared to the use of nurse-prepared syringes?

See answers to Self-Test in the Answer Section at the back of the book.

References

Batey, M. (1977). Conceptualization: Knowledge and logic guiding empirical research. *Nursing Research, 26*, 324–329. http://journals.lww.com/nursingresearchonline/Pages/default.aspx

Britton, C., McCormick, F. M., Renfrew, M. J., Wade, A., & King, S. E. (2007). Support for breastfeeding mothers (Review). *Cochrane Database Syst Rev, 1*, CD001141. doi:10.1002/14651858.CD001141.pub3

Elfering, A., Nützi, M., Koch, P., & Baur, H. (2014). Workflow interruptions and failed action regulation in surgery personnel. *Safety and Health at Work, 5*(1), 1–6. http://dx.doi.org/10.1016/j.shaw.2013.11.001

Fisher, R. (1951). *The design of experiments* (6th ed.). New York: Hafner.

Harrison, G., Speroni, K. G., Dugan, L., & Daniel, M. G. (2010). A comparison of the quality of blood specimens drawn in the field by EMS versus specimens obtained in the emergency department. *Emergency Nursing, 36*, 16–20. doi:10.1016/j.jen.2008.11.001

Ho, L. P., Ho, S. S., Leung, D. Y., So, W. K., & Chan, C. W. (2016). A feasibility and efficacy randomized controlled trial of swaddling for controlling procedural pain in perterm infants. *Clinical Nursing, 25*, 472–482. doi:10.1111/jocn.13075.

Im, E. O., Chang, S. J., Chee, W., Chee, E., & Mao, J. J. (2015). Immigration transition and depressive symptoms: Four major ethnic groups of midlife women in the United States. *Health Care for Women International, 36*(4), 439–456. doi:10.1080/07399332.2014.924518

Kerlinger, F. (1986). *Foundations of behavioral research* (3rd ed.). New York: Holt, Rinehart & Winston.

Patrick, S. W., Warner, K. E., Pordes, E., & Davis, M. M. (2016). Cigarette Tax Increase and Infant Mortality. *Pediatrics, 137*, 1–8. doi:10.1542/peds.2015-2901

Pender, N. J. (2014). *Health promotion in nursing practice* (7th ed.). Norwalk, CT: Appleton & Lange.

Polit, D. F., & Beck. C. T. (2012). *Nursing research: Principles and methods* (9th ed.). Philadelphia: Lippincott Williams & Wilkins.

Polit, D. F., & Beck, C. T. (2009). International gender bias in nursing research, 2005–2006: A quantitative content analysis. *International Journal of Nursing Studies, 46*, 1102–1110. doi:10.1016/j.ijnurstu.2009.02.002

Wambach, K. A., Aaronson, L., Breedlove, G., Domian, E. W., Rojjanasrirat, W., & Yeh, H. W. (2011). A randomized controlled trial of breastfeeding support and education for adolescent mothers. *Western Journal of Nursing Research, 33*, 486–505. doi:10.1177/0193945910380408

PART III Research Designs

Chapter 10
Quantitative Research Designs

Rose Marie Nieswiadomy, PhD, RN, and Sharon Souter, RN, PhD, CNE

Objectives

On completion of this chapter, you will be prepared to:

1. Summarize criteria for exploratory, descriptive, and explanatory research studies.
2. Distinguish between the types of internal and external validity and threats to each seen in experimental designs.
3. Distinguish among true, quasi-, and pre-experimental designs.
4. Compare and contrast five types of nonexperimental designs.

Introduction

Do you travel? Do you cook? If so, you probably use plans and recipes. These plans and recipes provide guidelines that help you have a great travel outcome visiting the places you wanted to see, or cook a delicious meal with all the ingredients included in their correct amounts.

This chapter introduces the concept of research design, which is the outline or plan for a research study. The choice of a research design concerns the overall intended plan and outcome for the study. It is concerned with the type of data that will be collected, and the means used to obtain the needed data. For example, the researcher must decide if the study will try to determine causative factors, explore relationships, or examine historical data. The design is not concerned with the specific data-collection methods, such as questionnaires or interviews, but with the overall plan for data gathering and analyzing the data obtained. The design must be appropriate to test the study hypothesis(es) or answer the research question(s). General guidelines for critiquing a quantitative design are presented at the end of this chapter.

Exploratory, Descriptive, and Explanatory Studies

The amount of existing knowledge about the variable(s) can be used as the criterion for classifying research as exploratory, descriptive, or explanatory. Although there can be an overlap between the first two categories, it is helpful to examine them separately.

Exploratory studies are conducted when little is known about the phenomenon of interest. For instance, you might decide to examine the needs of family members of a patient who will be receiving IV antibiotics at home with treatments and interventions managed by family members. To determine what questions need to be asked, you would conduct a review of the literature. It is likely that you may find little data on this topic. An exploratory research study would, therefore, be appropriate and findings would add to the body of knowledge.

A flexible approach rather than a structured approach to data collection would be used. In exploratory studies, there is interest in examining the qualitative aspects of the data as well as the quantitative aspects. Hypotheses are generally not appropriate for these types of studies. Although there is interest in the qualitative data, this type of study would not be classified as a qualitative study because the researcher would be interested in gathering data that could be grouped, categorized, and eventually generalized to other groups of patients and their caregivers.

In **descriptive studies**, phenomena are described or the relationships between variables are examined. A descriptive study is similar to an exploratory study. However, the two categories can be distinguished by considering the amount of information that is available about the variable(s) under investigation. As previously stated, exploratory studies are appropriate when little is known about the area of interest. When enough information exists to examine relationships between variables, descriptive studies may be conducted in which hypotheses are tested.

Explanatory studies search for causal explanations and are much more rigorous than exploratory or descriptive studies. This type of research is usually experimental. Enough knowledge exists about the variables and their relationships that the investigator is able to exercise some degree of control over the research conditions and manipulate one or more of the variables. Returning to the example about IV therapy at home, the researcher may have enough information to design an explanatory study. An intervention might be designed to help families reduce the incidence of complications in intravenous therapy.

To summarize, exploratory and descriptive studies describe phenomena and examine relationships among phenomena, whereas explanatory studies help provide explanations for the relationships among phenomena. Many nursing studies have been exploratory or descriptive in nature. A large number of explanatory studies have also been reported in the nursing literature.

Research Designs

Although the terms *exploratory*, *descriptive*, and *explanatory research* can be used to determine the type of study being conducted, these terms do not clearly indicate the study plan or specific design. There are several ways to classify research designs. This text presents designs under the two broad categories of quantitative and qualitative designs. As mentioned earlier in this textbook, some studies combine aspects of quantitative and qualitative research in the same study, and are referred to as mixed methods studies.

Quantitative designs are discussed in this chapter, and qualitative designs will be presented in another chapter of this book. Quantitative designs are divided into experimental and nonexperimental designs. Table 10–1 presents some of the various experimental and nonexperimental designs.

Table 10-1 Quantitative Research Designs

Experimental Designs	Nonexperimental Designs
True experimental designs	Action studies
Pretest-posttest control group	Comparative studies
Posttest-only control group	Correlational studies
Solomon four-group	Evaluation studies
Quasi-experimental designs	Meta-analysis studies
Nonequivalent control group	Metasynthesis studies
Time-series	Methodological studies
Pre-experimental designs	Secondary analysis studies
One-shot case study	Survey studies
One-group pretest-posttest	

Experimental Research

Experimental research is concerned with cause-and-effect relationships. A **cause-and-effect relationship** occurs when one object or event makes some other object or event happen. For example, weight gain could be considered an effect (object) as a side effect of taking certain medications (cause).

All experimental studies involve manipulation or control of the independent variable (cause) and measurement of the dependent variable (effect). Although experimental research designs are highly respected in the scientific world, causal relations are difficult to establish, and, as discussed elsewhere in this book, researchers should avoid using the word *prove* when discussing research results. Controls are difficult to apply when experimental research is conducted with human beings. This is one of the reasons that many nursing studies have employed nonexperimental designs.

Validity of Experimental Designs

In experimental studies, as well as in other types of research, the researcher is interested in controlling extraneous variables that can influence study results. **Extraneous variables** are those variables the researcher is unable to control, or does not choose to control, and which can influence the results of a study. Other names for extraneous variables are *confounding* and *intervening*. These variables are also called **study limitations**. The researcher acknowledges these study limitations in the discussion section of a research report. In experimental studies, the extraneous variables, or competing explanations for the results, are labeled threats to internal and external validity (Campbell & Stanley, 1963).

In an experimental study, the researcher is trying to establish a cause-and-effect relationship. The **internal validity** of an experimental design concerns the degree to which changes in the dependent variable (effect) can be attributed to the independent variable (cause). Threats to internal validity are factors other than the independent variable that influence the dependent variable. These factors constitute rival explanations or competing hypotheses that might explain the study results.

External validity concerns the degree to which study results can be generalized to other people and other settings. These kinds of questions should be answered about external validity: With what degree of confidence can the study findings be transferred from the sample to the entire population? Will these study findings hold true with other groups in other times and places?

Internal and external validity are related in that as the researcher attempts to control for internal validity, external validity is usually decreased. Conversely, when the researcher is concerned with external validity or the generalizability of the findings to other settings and other people, the strict control necessary for high internal validity may be affected. Therefore, the researcher must decide how to balance internal and external validity.

Threats to internal and external validity are addressed before the discussion of the types of experimental designs so you can better determine the strengths and weaknesses of the various designs as you read about them in this chapter.

Threats to Internal Validity

Campbell and Stanley (1963) and Cook and Campbell (1979) have identified threats to the internal validity of a study. Six of these threats are discussed in this chapter: selection bias, history, maturation, testing, instrumentation change, and mortality.

SELECTION BIAS The **selection bias** threat occurs when study results are attributed to the experimental treatment or the researcher's manipulation of the independent variable when, in fact, the results are related to subject differences before the independent variable was manipulated. This selection threat should be considered in experimental studies when subjects are not randomly assigned to experimental and comparison groups. For example, suppose the researcher decides to offer a seminar to help people stop cigarette smoking. Fifteen volunteers are obtained who indicate they would like to stop smoking. This group is designated as the experimental group. Fifteen other people are recruited who have not shown a desire to stop smoking. This group becomes the control group. The 15 subjects in the experimental group may have been more motivated to stop smoking before the treatment than the 15 subjects in the control group. The selection process for the groups may, therefore, have biased the eventual results of the study.

HISTORY The threat of history (**history threat**) occurs when some event besides the experimental treatment occurs during the course of a study, and this event influences the dependent variable. A researcher might be interested in determining the incidence of breast self-examination (BSE) among women after they attended a three-week teaching program on BSE. During the time the study is being conducted, an article is published in the newspaper concerning the rise in the number of women with breast cancer. This history event could result in an increase in the incidence of BSE behaviors. At the conclusion of the study, the researcher would not be able to determine if the teaching program (independent variable) was the reason for the increase in the incidence of BSE (dependent variable), or if the newspaper article was the impetus for an increase in BSE among the study subjects.

History is controlled by the inclusion of at least one simultaneous control or comparison group in a study. Additionally, random assignment of subjects to groups helps control the threat of history. Environmental events (history) would, therefore, be as likely to occur for subjects in one group as in another. If a difference is found between the groups at the conclusion of the study, the researcher is much more confident that the manipulation of the independent variable is the cause of this difference.

MATURATION Maturation becomes a threat when changes that occur within the subjects during an experimental study influence the study results. People may become older, taller, or sleepier from the time of the pretest to the posttest. If a school nurse were interested in the weight gain of children who receive a hot breakfast at school each day, she would have to keep in mind that changes may occur in these children during the course of the study that are not related to the experimental treatment. The children will probably gain some weight as they eat more and grow older, regardless of whether they eat a hot breakfast at school or not. Again, a comparison group of similar children helps control for this threat. Maturation processes are then as likely to occur in one group as in another.

TESTING The testing threat may occur in studies where a pretest is given or where subjects have knowledge of baseline data. **Testing** refers to the influence of the pretest or knowledge of baseline data on the posttest scores. Subjects may remember the answers they put on the pretest and put the same answers on the posttest. Also, subjects' scores may be altered on the posttest as a result of their knowledge of baseline data. For example, if subjects were weighed and told their weight before an experimental weight reduction program, these subjects might make some effort on their own to lose weight because they have discovered they are overweight. This knowledge of baseline data could be considered a pretest (Hudson & Llosa, 2015).

Testing Threats

Hudson and Llosa (2015) identified one of the threats to validity in evaluating relationships is testing. Using experimental second language (L2) research, the authors desired to discover causal relationships among manipulated variables and to answer questions, including: To what extent does the presence/absence/amount of X (independent variable) cause Y (the dependent variable) to change? They suggested that in a true experiment, a researcher would manipulate the presence/absence/amount of X and measure the effects on Y. Subjects would be randomly selected from the target population and randomly assigned to differing conditions representing categories of X. The subjects would then be measured on a reliable and valid measure of Y and appropriate analyses would be carried out. These measures included testing. The authors suggested that taking a pretest affects performance on subsequent testing observations. These effects may be in motivation of the subjects or in areas such as strategy development. They cautioned that a pretest might predispose the subjects to appreciate some particular aspects of the treatment that they might not have been attracted to in other circumstances. Such concerns may lead the researcher to move to a random assignment as identified in the study to ensure that experimental and control groups begin the intervention with the same level playing field.

INSTRUMENTATION CHANGE When mechanical instruments or judges are used in the pretest and posttest phases of a study, the threat of instrumentation must be considered. **Instrumentation change** involves the difference between the pretest and posttest measurement caused by a change in the accuracy of the instrument or the judges' ratings, rather than as a result of the experimental treatment. Judges may become more adept at the ratings or, on the contrary, become tired and make less exact observations. Training sessions for judges and trial runs to check for fatigue factors may help control for instrumentation changes. Also, if mechanical instruments are used, such as sphygmomanometers, these instruments should be checked for their accuracy throughout the study.

MORTALITY The **mortality threat** occurs when the subjects do not complete a study. **Attrition** or dropout may occur in any research study. However, the term mortality is reserved for experimental studies in which the dropout rate is different between the experimental and the comparison groups. The observed effects may occur because the subjects who dropped out of a particular group are different from those who remained in the study. For example, if a large number of experimental group subjects who scored very high on an anxiety pretest dropped out of the study, the average anxiety scores on the posttest for the experimental group might be deceivingly low. The researcher might falsely conclude that the treatment really worked well. There is no research design that will control for mortality because, for ethical reasons, participants can never be forced to remain in a study.

The longer a study lasts, the more likely that subject dropout will occur. Hudson and Llosa (2015) suggested that subjects drop out of studies due to lack of interest and motivation. This may be of particular concern in randomization where subjects drop out of one group at a rate higher than another group.

For example, if the dependent variable was depression, it is possible that people with the highest or lowest levels of depression would be the ones to drop out of the study.

Subject mortality is a problem that plagues nurse researchers in nearly all clinical studies, even animal-based studies (Holman et al., 2016). To control for this threat, the researcher should try to establish a relationship with the study participants and help them recognize the importance of their continued participation in a particular study.

Threats to External Validity

Campbell and Stanley (1963) have identified four threats to external validity, and Bracht and Glass (1968) delineated 10 threats to the external validity of a study. Three threats are discussed in this chapter: the Hawthorne effect, the experimenter effect, and the reactive effects of the pretest.

HAWTHORNE EFFECT The **Hawthorne effect** occurs when study participants respond in a certain manner because they are aware that they are being observed. This term came about as the result of the studies on worker productivity at the Hawthorne plant of the Western Electric Company. Working conditions, such as changing the length of the working day, were varied. Worker productivity was found to increase no matter what changes were made. The increase in productivity was finally determined to be the result of the subjects' knowledge that they were involved in a research study, and that someone was interested in them.

Hawthorne Effect

Hagel et al. (2015) wanted to quantify the Hawthorne effect on performance of hand hygiene through an observational approach. Their experiment included direct observations of hand hygiene and electronically recorded observations of hand hygiene. What do you suppose they found? At an almost three-to-one ratio, more healthcare workers under direct supervision performed hand hygiene.

The Hawthorne effect may also be considered a threat to internal validity. It might be possible to control this threat by using a double-blind experiment. In a **double-blind experiment**, neither the researcher nor the research participants are aware of which participants are in the experimental group and which participants are in the control group.

EXPERIMENTER EFFECT The **experimenter effect** is a threat to study results that occurs when researcher characteristics or behaviors influence subject behaviors. Examples of researcher characteristics or behaviors that may be influential are facial expressions, clothing, age, gender, and body build. Although the term experimenter effect is appropriate to use only when discussing experimental research, a term with a similar meaning is used in nonexperimental research. The **Rosenthal effect**, named after the person who identified this phenomenon, is used to indicate the influence of an interviewer on respondents' answers. It has been shown that researcher characteristics such as gender, dress, and type of jewelry may influence study participants' answers to questions in nonexperimental studies.

REACTIVE EFFECTS OF THE PRETEST When a pretest and a posttest are used in an experimental study, the researcher must be aware not only of the internal validity threat that may occur, but also of the external validity threat that may exist. The **reactive effects of the pretest** occur when subjects have been sensitized to the treatment because they took the pretest. This sensitization may affect the posttest results. People might not respond to the treatment in the same manner if they had not received a pretest. The pretest does not have to be from a questionnaire-like test. As mentioned previously, if study participants were told their weight prior to a weight-reduction study, this knowledge of baseline data would be considered a pretest.

Symbolic Presentation of Research Designs

Research designs are often easier to understand when seen in a symbolic form. The symbols used to depict the designs in this chapter are based on the notation scheme of Campbell and Stanley (1963).

R = random assignment of subjects to groups

X = experimental treatment or intervention

O = observation or measurement of dependent variable

The Xs and Os on one line apply to a specific group. The time sequence of events is read from left to right. If an X appears first and then an O, this means the intervention occurred first then an observation was made. If a subscript appears after an X or O (X_1; X_2; O_1; O_2), the numbers indicate the first treatment, second treatment, first observation, second observation, and so forth.

$R\ O_1\ X\ O_2$ (Experimental group)

$R\ O_1\ O_2$ (Comparison group)

This example has two groups, both of which were formed through random assignment (R) of subjects to groups. **Random assignment** is a procedure that ensures that each subject has an equal chance of being assigned or placed in any of the groups in an experimental study. Both groups in the example were measured or given a pretest (O_1) on the phenomenon of interest (dependent variable). The experimental group was exposed to an experimental treatment (independent variable); the comparison group was not exposed to this treatment. Then, both groups were again measured or given the posttest (O_2) on the phenomenon of interest (dependent variable).

There are a number of ways of carrying out random assignment. Today, it is often done through a computer-generated process.

Types of Experimental Designs

The three broad categories of experimental research designs are true experimental, quasi-experimental, and pre-experimental. The distinctions among these designs are determined by the amount of control the researcher is able to exercise over the research conditions.

True Experimental Designs

The **true experimental designs** are those in which the researcher has a great deal of control over the research situation. Threats to the internal validity of the study are minimized. Only with the use of true experimental designs may causality be inferred with any degree of confidence. With these types of designs, the researcher has some confidence that the independent variable was the cause of the change in the dependent variable. A true experimental design has three criteria:

1. The researcher manipulates the experimental variable(s).
2. At least one experimental and one comparison group are included in the study.
3. Subjects are randomly assigned to either the experimental or the comparison group.

The first criterion for a true experimental design is manipulation of the independent variable. Sometimes, there is a misunderstanding of the term *manipulation* as it is used in experimental studies. The concept of manipulation might bring to mind the picture of puppets on a string; however, in research, the term **manipulation** means that the independent, or experimental, variable is controlled by the researcher. The researcher has control over the type of experimental treatment administered and who will receive the treatment.

The experimental treatment in nursing research usually concerns some type of nursing intervention. The researcher manipulates the independent variable, or nursing intervention, by administering it to some subjects and withholding it from others. The dependent variable, or the effect(s) of the nursing intervention, is then observed. For example, a nurse researcher might implement a new, structured, preoperative teaching program with a group of preoperative patients and use the routine teaching program with another group of preoperative patients. The anxiety levels of both groups of patients might be the dependent variable that is observed.

The second criterion for a true experimental design is the use of a comparison or control group. The term *control group* is seen more frequently in the literature than the term *comparison group*. A **control group** usually indicates a group in an experimental study that does not receive the experimental treatment. In nursing research, the withholding of a treatment may be unethical. In the previous example concerning preoperative patients, the withholding of preoperative teaching would not be considered ethical. In many nursing studies, therefore, a comparison group is used rather than a control group that receives no intervention. The comparison group usually receives the "normal" or routine intervention. The term **comparison group** is used in this text to indicate any group in an experimental study that either receives no treatment, or a treatment that is not thought to be as effective as the experimental treatment.

Finally, the third criterion for true experimental studies is the random assignment of subjects to groups. As previously mentioned, random assignment ensures that each subject has an equal chance of being placed into any of the groups in an experimental study. Keep in mind that random sampling and random assignment are two entirely different concepts. These concepts will be discussed more extensively in another chapter of this book. At this point, be aware that random assignment concerns the equality of groups in experimental studies. The random assignment of subjects to groups eliminates selection bias as a threat to the internal validity of the study.

The following sections discuss three types of true experimental designs: pretest-posttest control group design, posttest-only control group design, and Solomon four-group design.

PRETEST-POSTTEST CONTROL GROUP DESIGN The **pretest-posttest control group design** is probably the most frequently used experimental design. In this design, (a) the subjects are randomly assigned to groups, (b) a pretest is given to both groups, (c) the experimental group receives the experimental treatment and the comparison group receives the routine treatment or no treatment, and (d) a posttest is given to both groups.

$$R\ O_1\ X\ O_2\ \text{(Experimental group)}$$

$$R\ O_1\ \ O_2\ \text{(Comparison group)}$$

The researcher is able to determine if the groups were equal before the treatment was administered. If the groups were not equivalent, the posttest scores may be adjusted statistically to control for the initial differences between the two groups that were reflected in the pretest scores.

A nurse researcher might be interested in the usefulness of a diabetic teaching film. A group of clients with diabetes are randomly assigned to the experimental or comparison group. Both groups are then pretested on their knowledge of diabetes. Members of the experimental group watch the diabetic teaching film. Members of the comparison group are asked to read printed material that is similar to the information covered in the teaching film. Both groups are then posttested on their knowledge of diabetes. Finally, the difference between the posttest scores of the two groups is compared.

The pretest-posttest control group design controls for all threats to internal validity. The disadvantage of this design concerns the external threat of the reactive effects of the pretest. The results of the study can be generalized only to situations in which a pretest would be administered before the treatment.

Pretest-Posttest Control Group Design

Fitzgerald, Rorie, and Salem (2015) studied the acceptability of a mobile health (mHealth) application among nursing students for health promotion education and secondary prevention health recommendations for hospitalized patients. A pretest-posttest design was used with a convenience sample of 169 prelicensure master's entry clinical nursing students in a large urban public university. The students were assessed on many areas regarding the application including: their intention to use, perceived usefulness of, perceived ease of use, clinical area relevance and output quality, and resultant demonstrability of the U.S. Preventive Services Task Force (USPSTF) evidence-based practice guidelines using the mHealth application. Pre- and posttest scores demonstrated statistically significant differences ($p < 0.1$) between intention to use, perceived usefulness, clinical relevance, and resultant demonstrability. The pre- and posttest scores for ease of use were not significantly different.

POSTTEST-ONLY CONTROL GROUP DESIGN In the **posttest-only control group design**, (a) subjects are randomly assigned to groups, (b) the experimental group receives the experimental treatment and the comparison group receives the routine treatment or no treatment, and (c) a posttest is given to both groups.

$$R \; X \; O_1 \text{ (Experimental group)}$$
$$R \quad\;\; O_1 \text{ (Comparison group)}$$

The posttest-only control group design is easier to carry out and superior to the pretest-posttest design. The researcher does not have to be concerned with the reactive effects of the pretest on the posttest. The generalizability of the results would be more extensive. A study similar to the example described regarding the pretest-posttest control group design could be developed. The only difference would be that the two groups would not receive a pretest on their knowledge of diabetes.

Random assignment of subjects into groups in the posttest-only control group design helps ensure equality of the groups. The use of a large sample size will increase the effectiveness of random assignment. Although random assignment should ensure equality of groups, researchers seem to be fearful that the groups may not, in fact, be similar. Therefore, they sometimes choose to administer a pretest.

The posttest-only control group design should be used when it is not possible to administer a pretest or when it would not make sense to administer a pretest.

Posttest-Only Control Group Design

Schlegel, Bonvin, Rethan, and van der Vleuten (2015) examined the impact of video recording for standardized patients (SP) in the training on SPs' role accuracy, investigating how the use of different types of video during SP training improves the accuracy of SP portrayal. In a randomized posttest-only control group design, three groups of 12 SPs each with different types of video training, and one control group of 12 SPs without video use in SP training, were compared. The three training intervention groups used a role-modeling video, a performance-feedback video, or a combination of both. Each SP from each group had four student encounters. Two blinded faculty members rated the 192 video-recorded encounters, using a case-specific rating instrument to assess SPs' role accuracy. Researchers reported that SPs trained by video showed statistically significant ($p < 0.001$) better role accuracy than SPs trained without video over the four sequential portrayals. There was no difference between the other three types of video training.

SOLOMON FOUR-GROUP DESIGN In the **Solomon four-group design**, (a) subjects are randomly assigned to one of the four groups; (b) two of the groups, experimental group 1 and comparison group 1, are pretested; (c) two of the groups, experimental group 1 and experimental group 2, receive the experimental treatment, whereas two of the groups, comparison group 1 and comparison group 2, receive the routine treatment or no treatment; and (d) a posttest is given to all four groups.

$$R\ O_1\ X\ O_2\ \text{(Experimental group 1)}$$
$$R\ O_1\ \ O_2\ \text{(Comparison group 1)}$$
$$R\ \ X\ O_2\ \text{(Experimental group 2)}$$
$$R\ \ O_2\ \text{(Comparison group 2)}$$

The Solomon four-group design is considered to be the most prestigious experimental design (Campbell & Stanley, 1963) because it minimizes threats to internal and external validity. This design not only controls for all of the threats to internal validity, but also controls for the reactive effects of the pretest. Any differences between the experimental and the comparison groups can be more confidently associated with the experimental treatment. Unfortunately, this design requires a large sample, and statistical analysis of the data is complicated. Only one Solomon four-group design could be located in the nursing literature of the past 5 years.

Solomon Four-Group Design

A Solomon four-group design was used to determine if introducing acceptance and commitment to therapy in the prevention of mother-to-infant HIV transmission with the use of weekly telephone messaging would result in improved health status in HIV-positive women (Ishola & Chips, 2015). The study participants were randomly assigned to two intervention groups and two control groups. The intervention groups received weekly messages by mobile phone for three months during their pregnancy. The messages contained information with value-based health messages. The control group received only post-HIV test counseling. On the pretest, the groups did not differ. On the posttest, the intervention group received significantly higher acceptance scores.

Quasi-Experimental Designs

Sometimes researchers are not able to randomly assign subjects to groups, or for various reasons, no comparison group is available for an experimental study. **Quasi-experimental designs** are those in which there is either no comparison group or subjects are not randomly assigned to groups. The researcher uses existing, or intact, groups for the experimental and comparison groups. Although the researcher does not have as much control in a quasi-experimental study as in a true experiment, there are some advantages to the use of quasi-experimental designs. By conducting experiments with naturally occurring groups, the real world is more closely approximated than when subjects are randomly assigned to groups.

Many different designs fall into the category of quasi-experimental designs. Two of these are discussed next: nonequivalent control group design and time-series design.

NONEQUIVALENT CONTROL GROUP DESIGN The **nonequivalent control group design** is similar to the pretest-posttest control group design except there is no random assignment of subjects to the experimental and comparison groups.

$$O_1\ X\ O_2\ \text{(Experimental group)}$$
$$O_1\ \ O_2\ \text{(Comparison group)}$$

A researcher might choose a group of patients with diabetes on one hospital floor for the experimental group and a group of patients with diabetes on another floor for the comparison group. The experimental treatment would be administered to the experimental group; the comparison group would receive the routine treatment or some alternative treatment.

Threats to internal validity controlled by the nonequivalent control group design are history, testing, maturation, and instrumentation change. The biggest threat to internal validity is selection bias. As the two groups may not be similar at the beginning of the study, it is possible to test statistically for differences in the groups. For example, it could be determined if the ages and educational backgrounds of the subjects in both groups were similar. If the groups were similar at the beginning of the study, more confidence could be placed in a cause-and-effect relationship between variables. A statistical test called analysis of covariance (ANCOVA) can be used to help control for differences that might have existed, through chance, between the experimental and control groups at the beginning of the study.

TIME-SERIES DESIGN In a **time-series design**, the researcher periodically observes or measures the subjects. The experimental treatment is administered between two of the observations.

$$O_1 \; O_2 \; O_3 \; X \; O_4 \; O_5 \; O_6$$

A researcher might assess the pain levels of a group of clients with low back pain. After three weeks of pain assessment (O_1, O_2, O_3), subjects could be taught a special exercise to alleviate low back pain. During the next three weeks, pain levels would again be measured (O_4, O_5, O_6). The results of this study would help the researcher determine if low back pain persists, if a specific exercise is effective in reducing low back pain, and if the effectiveness of the exercise persists.

The time-series design with its numerous observations or measurements of the dependent variable helps strengthen the validity of the design. The greatest threats to validity are history and testing.

Pre-Experimental Designs

Pre-experimental designs is the name applied by Campbell and Stanley (1963) to experimental designs that are considered very weak and in which the researcher has little control over the research. Sometimes these types of designs are discussed to provide examples of how not to do research. The two pre-experimental designs discussed here are the one-shot case study and the one-group pretest-posttest design.

ONE-SHOT CASE STUDY In a **one-shot case study**, a single group is exposed to an experimental treatment and observed after the treatment.

$$X \; O$$

A group of patients with diabetes might attend a diabetic education class (X) and be tested on their knowledge of diabetes (O) after the class is completed. This design does not call for any comparisons to be made. There is no way to determine if the level of knowledge about diabetes was the result of the class. The patients could have already possessed this knowledge before the class.

Threats to internal validity are history, maturation, and selection bias. The threats of testing and instrumentation change would not be applicable in this design. Selection bias would be a very serious threat in this particular design. The one-shot case study is the weakest of all the experimental designs because it controls for no threats to internal validity. No example of this type of study was found in the recent nursing literature.

ONE-GROUP PRETEST-POSTTEST DESIGN The **one-group pretest-posttest design** provides a comparison between a group of subjects before and after the experimental treatment.

$$O_1 \; X \; O_2$$

A group of patients with diabetes could be given a pretest of their diabetes knowledge (O_1). This group would then attend a diabetic education class (X) and be posttested (O_2) at the end of the class.

Threats to internal validity would be history, maturation, testing, and instrumentation change. Note this design has two threats that were not applicable in the last design. Because of the existence of a pretest and posttest, testing and instrumentation change now become threats to internal validity.

One-Group Pretest-Posttest Design

A one-group pretest-posttest design was used to study students' knowledge of empowering discourse to determine how students understand the structure of discourse as it relates to practice and supporting patient empowerment as an essential part of patient education. The researchers found that students lacked a holistic perspective of the knowledge of empowering discourse (Virtanen, Leino-Kilpi, & Salantera, 2015).

Nonexperimental Research

Nurse researchers have made great use of the nonexperimental research designs. Many times, experimental research cannot be conducted with human beings because of ethical reasons. At other times, nonexperimental research is the most proper type of research to obtain the needed data. In trying to determine clients' perceptions of pain, the only way to obtain this information would be to ask these clients about their pain. An experimental study would not be appropriate. All nonexperimental research is descriptive because there is no manipulation or control of variables, and the researcher can describe the phenomenon only as it exists. Although the researcher cannot talk about a cause-and-effect relationship in nonexperimental research, it is important to obtain valid study results in this type of research. The researcher must attempt to control for extraneous variables through such means as careful selection of the study sample. Threats to internal validity and external validity are terms that are reserved for use in discussing experimental studies. However, in nonexperimental research, extraneous variables or study limitations must also be considered.

Types of Nonexperimental Designs

Table 10–1 lists nine types of nonexperimental research; five of these designs will be discussed in the following sections: survey, correlational, comparative, methodological, and secondary analysis studies.

Survey Studies

Survey studies are investigations in which self-report data are collected from samples with the purpose of describing populations on some variable(s) of interest. Surveys have probably been conducted as long as humankind has been in existence. Accounts of surveys are recorded in the Bible and in other historical books. Probably everyone who is reading this material has been involved in some type of survey. Two of the more common public opinion surveys conducted in the United States are the Gallup and Harris polls. These national polls use scientific sampling techniques to obtain information about large groups of people through the sampling of a small percentage of the total groups.

The control exercised by the researcher in survey research lies in the sampling technique. The ability to generalize sample results to the population of interest depends on the sampling method. Probability sampling techniques and adequate sample sizes, which are discussed in another chapter are very important in survey research.

Many disciplines, especially the social sciences, have used survey research. Surveys generally ask subjects to report their attitudes, opinions, perceptions, or behaviors. A nurse researcher might use a survey to gather data on the health needs of clients, their sleep patterns, or their perceptions of the nursing care they have received.

Surveys may be conducted by phone, mail, the Internet, or through personal contact with the subjects. The most common data-collection techniques used in survey research are questionnaires and interviews. In surveys, participants may be studied using a cross-sectional or a longitudinal approach. In a cross-sectional survey, subjects are studied at one point in time. Longitudinal surveys follow subjects over an extended period of time.

One of the chief virtues of survey research is its ability to provide accurate information on populations while using relatively small samples. Another advantage of survey research concerns the large amount of data that can be obtained rather quickly and with minimal cost. However, self-report responses may be unreliable because people may provide socially acceptable responses.

Correlational Studies

In **correlational studies**, the researcher examines the strength of relationships between variables by determining how changes in one variable are associated with changes in another variable. A correlation indicates the extent to which one variable (X) is related to another variable (Y). As X increases, does Y increase or decrease? In a simple correlational study, one group of subjects is measured on two variables (X and Y) to determine if there is a relationship between these variables. Other correlational studies may examine the relationship among more than two variables.

The magnitude and direction of the relationship between two variables is indicated by a **correlation coefficient**. Correlation coefficients may be positive (+) or negative (−) and range from −1.00 (perfect negative correlation) to 1.00 (perfect positive correlation). If the correlation coefficient has no sign in front of it (e.g., .80), a positive relationship is indicated. A negative correlation coefficient is preceded by a negative sign (e.g., −.80). A correlation coefficient of .00 indicates there is no relationship between variables. Correlation coefficients are reported through various statistics such as the Pearson's product-moment correlation (more commonly called the Pearson r) and the Spearman rho.

A **positive relationship**, or direct relationship, means that as the value of one variable increases, the value of the other variable increases. A **negative relationship**, or inverse relationship, means that as the value of one variable increases, the value of the other variable decreases. Suppose data are gathered on age and assertiveness levels of registered nurses. A correlation coefficient of .80 would indicate a fairly strong positive relationship between age and assertiveness levels of registered nurses. The older the nurse, the more assertive she or he is. Conversely, a correlation coefficient of −.80 would indicate a strong negative relationship. The older the nurse, the less assertive she or he is.

The identification of an independent and a dependent variable may not be appropriate in some correlational studies. Generally, however, the independent variable is that variable that comes first in chronological order and that influences the other variable. For example, if you were trying to determine if there is a correlation between age and assertiveness levels, the independent variable would be age, and the dependent variable would be assertiveness levels. The subject's age is a nonmanipulated, inherent variable that exists in time, or chronological order, before the variable of assertiveness. Even if a strong correlation were found between these two variables, the researcher should not conclude that age *causes* assertiveness. There may be some other variable(s) that bring about the assertiveness levels of people. For example, you would probably find a strong positive relationship between the number of churches in a city and the number of people who dine out each week. Do you think the number of churches would be the *cause* of the large number of people who dine out in a week? No, the probable causative factor is the number of people who live in that city. A large city will probably have more people and more churches than a small city. Therefore, if a city has a large population, there is probably going to be a large number of people who dine out each week.

Correlational Study

Chen, Chen, and Chu (2015) conducted a correlational study in Taiwan to examine the relationships among caregiver burden on, health status of, and learned resourcefulness of older caregivers who managed the care of disabled older adults. The results indicated that the caregiver burden negatively correlated with physical health, mental health, and learned resourcefulness ($p < .001$) and that physical and mental health were positively correlated with learned resourcefulness ($r = .40, p < .001$).

Comparative Studies

Comparative studies examine the differences between intact groups on some dependent variable of interest. This description may sound like the aim of many experimental studies. The difference between comparative studies and experimental studies lies in the researcher's ability to manipulate the independent variable. In comparative studies, there is no manipulation of the independent variable. Frequently, the independent variable is some inherent characteristic of the subjects, such as personality type, educational level, or medical condition.

There are many reasons for the choice of a comparative research design. One reason involves the ethics of research. When human subjects are studied, the manipulation of the independent variable may not be possible. A researcher could not examine child abuse as an independent variable in an experimental study. It would not be ethical to select one group of children who would receive abusive treatment and another group of children who would not receive abusive treatment. However, the researcher could choose a group of children who had experienced abuse during their life and compare them with a group of children who had not been abused. The dependent variable might be self-esteem.

Comparative studies are frequently classified as retrospective or prospective. In **retrospective studies**, the dependent variable (effect) is identified in the present (a disease condition, for example), and an attempt is made to determine the independent variable (cause of the disease) that occurred in the past. In **prospective studies**, the independent variable or presumed cause (high cholesterol blood levels, for example) is identified at the present time, then subjects are followed in the future to observe the dependent variable (incidence of coronary artery disease, for example).

Retrospective studies are frequently called *ex post facto*. In **ex post facto studies**, data are collected after the fact. Variations in the independent variable are studied after the variations have occurred, rather than at the time of the occurrence. For example, a researcher might be interested in the fear responses of children during physical examinations. A study might be conducted to examine previous unpleasant experiences during physical exams that might have influenced the children's present behaviors. These previous experiences might be considered the "cause", and the present fear responses might be the "effect."

A retrospective study starts by examining an effect and then looks back in time to determine the cause; a prospective study starts with the determination of a cause and then looks forward in time to determine

Comparative Study

A comparative study by Alfes (2015) focused on the preparation of students for patient interactions in a psychiatric setting after exposure to a simulated patient compared to role-playing in a similar scenario. The study compared pre-licensure nursing students' knowledge, attitudes, and self-efficacy after exposure to both experiences. The results suggested that the order of teaching strategies (role-play first versus simulated patient interaction first) did not significantly impact the students' perceptions of knowledge, attitude, or self-efficacy.

the effect on subjects. An example of prospective research is the well-publicized study concerning Agent Orange and Vietnam veterans. During the war in Vietnam, many American servicemen were exposed to the chemical defoliant Agent Orange. After years of examining the effects of this chemical on veterans and their offspring, the Air Force finally issued a report in 1984 that revealed some of the problems linked with exposure to the herbicide Agent Orange, which was named after the color-coded bands on storage drums. Among the problems found were high rates of benign skin lesions, liver disorders, leg pulses that could indicate hardening of the arteries, and minor birth defects in their children ("Agent Orange Study," 1984). Prospective studies may use an experimental approach, whereas retrospective studies would never use this type of design. In prospective studies, the researcher might manipulate the independent variable, or the cause, then observe study participants in the future for the dependent variable, or the effect. Prospective studies are costly, and subject dropout may occur. These types of studies are less common than retrospective studies.

Methodological Studies

Nurse researchers must be sure to use instruments in research projects that are valid and reliable measures of the variables of interest. **Methodological studies** are concerned with the development, testing, and evaluation of research instruments and methods. Nurses frequently use tools developed by researchers in other disciplines. If these tools are appropriate for nursing research, they definitely should be used. Frequently, however, tools are used because of their availability rather than for their appropriateness to measure the variables of the study.

Secondary Analysis Studies

In the process of implementing a study, researchers gather a lot of data. It may not be possible or feasible to analyze all of the data that were gathered. In secondary analysis studies, data from a previous study may be analyzed in light of new research questions or new hypotheses. This type of study is efficient and economical, because data collection is the most time-consuming part of most studies. Trinkoff et al. (2015) suggest that secondary analysis can also aid in further understanding of how treatments work and for whom. Secondary analysis studies have become very popular among investigators, especially as they relate to the existence of national databases that provide data from large cohorts of patients. However, it should be noted that the use of secondary analysis is controversial due to the possible misrepresentation

Secondary Analysis Study

Trinkoff et al. (2015) used cross-sectional secondary analysis to examine associations between education and certification among Nursing Home Administrators (NHAs) and Directors of Nurses (DONs) with resident outcomes with a focus on levels of pain. Resident outcomes were measured using facility-level nursing home quality indicator rates selected from the Minimum Data Set (MDS). (According to the Centers for Medicare and Medicaid Services website, the MDS is a standardized screening and assessment tool of health status that forms the foundation of the comprehensive assessment for all residents in a Medicare- and/or Medicaid-certified long-term care facility. The MDS helps nursing home staff identify health problems and each resident's functional capabilities). Facility-level quality indicators were regressed onto leadership variables in models that also held constant facility size and ownership status. The researchers found that patients in nursing homes led by NHAs with both master's degrees or higher and certifications, and by DONs with bachelor's degrees or higher plus certifications, had significantly better pain management outcomes than those from nursing homes led by administrators with less educational preparation and no certification.

of study results. Thus, researchers should carefully examine the inclusion and exclusion sampling criteria used by the original reseachers and make certain that certain population groups are not under- or overrepresented.

Settings for Research

Research may be classified as laboratory or field studies, according to the setting in which the study is conducted. In **laboratory studies**, subjects are studied in a special environment created by the researcher. Although laboratory studies are not always highly standardized, the investigator usually attempts to control the research environment as much as possible. **Field studies** are conducted in a real-life situation, what is called "in the field," where not as much control can be maintained.

Simulation studies are considered to be laboratory studies. In a simulation study, the researcher might measure subjects' responses to descriptions of case studies that are intended to represent real-life situations. The control of the environment in this situation is through the researcher's descriptions of the events in the case studies.

Simulation Study

Two groups of nursing students in Pennsylvania were taught about the care of patients with acute coronary syndrome and acute ischemic stroke (Howard, Ross, Mitchell, & Nelson, 2010). Some participants were taught using a human patient simulator, and others using interactive case studies. Students in the human patient simulator group scored higher on the posttest than students in the interactive case studies group. The researchers concluded that students responded favorably to human patient simulators as a teaching method.

A research study receives the classification of *field* study when conducted in a real-life setting. Phenomena are studied in the natural environments in which they occur. Most nursing research has been conducted in the field. The field approach is particularly appropriate for the nurse researcher because nursing is a practice discipline.

Critiquing Quantitative Research Designs

It may be very difficult for the reader to determine if an appropriate design has been used in a study. As said previously, critiquing is not easy. Advanced research knowledge may be necessary to make an accurate determination of the appropriateness of a study design. However, the beginning researcher or critic can make some overall evaluations of the design section of a research report. Box 10–1 presents criteria for evaluating quantitative research designs.

The entire research report must be read before a determination can be made of whether the research design is appropriate for the study. The major consideration when critiquing a study design concerns the ability of the study design to test the hypothesis(es) or answer the research question(s). Is the researcher trying to determine a cause-and-effect relationship, or describe a phenomenon from the point of view of the research subject?

The research design determines how much control the researcher has over the research situation. In some studies, very tight controls are needed; in other studies, tight controls would inhibit the collection of valid data. Therefore, the reader of a research report must determine the purpose of the study and what the researcher hoped to add to the body of knowledge on the selected phenomenon or phenomena.

> **Box 10–1 Guidelines for Critiquing Quantitative Research Designs**
>
> 1. Is the design clearly identified and described in the research report?
> 2. Is the design appropriate to test the study hypothesis(es) or answer the research question(s)?
> 3. If the study used an experimental design, was the most appropriate type of experimental design used?
> 4. If the study used an experimental design, what means were used to control for threats to internal validity? External validity?
> 5. Was assignment of subjects to the experimental and control group clearly described?
> 6. Does the research design allow the researcher to draw a cause-and-effect relationship between the variables?
> 7. If a nonexperimental design was used, would an experimental design have been more appropriate?
> 8. What means were used to control for extraneous variables, such as subject characteristics, if a nonexperimental design was used?

Summary

Exploratory, descriptive, and explanatory studies are classified according to the amount of knowledge about the variable(s) of interest. Exploratory studies are conducted when little is known about the topic of interest. In descriptive studies, the phenomenon of interest may have already been studied in the past, and there is enough information to ask questions about the relationship between variables. Explanatory studies search for causal explanations. The researcher exercises control over the research situation by manipulating one or more of the variables and examining the influence of this manipulation on another variable(s).

Experimental research is concerned with cause-and-effect relationships. All experimental studies involve manipulation of the independent variable (cause) and measurement of the dependent variable (effect).

Extraneous variables, also called *study limitations, confounding variables*, and *intervening variables*, are uncontrolled variables that may influence study results. In experimental studies, these extraneous variables are called threats to internal and external validity. Internal validity concerns the degree to which changes in the dependent variable (effect) can be attributed to the independent variable (cause). External validity concerns the degree to which study results can be generalized to other people and settings.

Six threats to internal validity are selection bias, history, maturation, testing, instrumentation change, and mortality. Selection bias occurs when study results are attributed to the experimental treatment when, in fact, the results occur because of subject differences before the treatment. History occurs when some event other than the experimental treatment occurs during the course of the study, and this event influences the dependent variable. Maturation is a threat to internal validity when changes that occur within the subjects during an experimental study influence the study results. The testing threat involves the influence of the pretest on the posttest scores. Instrumentation change concerns the difference between the pretest and posttest measurements related to a change in the accuracy of the instrument or judges' ratings. The mortality threat occurs when the subject dropout rate is different between the experimental and comparison groups, and this difference influences the posttest results. Attrition, or dropout, may occur in any research study. However, the term mortality is reserved for experimental studies in which the dropout rate is different between the experimental and the comparison groups.

Three threats to external validity are the Hawthorne effect, the experimenter effect, and the reactive effects of the pretest. The Hawthorne effect occurs when study participants respond in a certain manner because they are aware that they are being observed. In a double-blind experiment, neither the researcher nor the research participants know who is in the experimental and control groups. A researcher's behavior that influences subject behavior is called the experimenter effect. In a nonexperimental study, the influence of the interviewer on the respondents is called the Rosenthal effect. The reactive effects of the pretest threat occurs when subjects' responses to the experimental treatment are indirectly influenced by the pretest.

Random assignment is a procedure that ensures that each subject has an equal chance of being assigned or placed into any of the groups in an experimental study.

The three broad categories of experimental research designs are: true experimental, quasi-experimental, and pre-experimental. True experimental designs are determined by three criteria: The researcher manipulates the experimental variable, at least one experimental and one comparison group or control group are included in the study, and subjects are randomly assigned to either the experimental or comparison group. Manipulation means that the independent variable is controlled by the researcher. Three types of true experimental designs are the pretest-posttest control group design, the posttest-only control group design, and the Solomon four-group design.

Quasi-experimental designs have either no comparison group or no random assignment of subjects to groups. Two quasi-experimental designs are the nonequivalent control group design and the time-series design.

Pre-experimental designs are those in which the researcher has little control over the research. Two types of pre-experimental designs are the one-shot case study and the one-group pretest-posttest design. There are many different types of nonexperimental designs. Survey studies obtain data from samples on certain variables to determine the characteristics of populations on those same variables.

Correlational studies examine the strength of relationships between variables. A correlation indicates the extent to which one variable (X) is related to another variable (Y). The magnitude and direction of the relationship between two variables is indicated by a correlation coefficient. These coefficients may be positive (+) or negative (−) and range from −1.00 (perfect negative correlation) to 1.00 (perfect positive correlation). A positive relationship (direct) means that as the value of one variable increases, the value of the other variable increases. A negative relationship (inverse) means that as the value of one variable increases, the value of the other variable decreases.

Comparative studies examine the difference between intact groups on some dependent variable of interest. Many comparative studies are called ex post facto studies because the variation in the independent variable has already occurred, and the researcher tries to determine "after the fact" if the variation that has occurred in the independent variable has any influence on the dependent variable that is being measured in the present. Ex post facto studies may also be called retrospective studies. Prospective studies are comparative studies in which the independent variable is identified in the present and the dependent variable is measured in the future.

Methodological studies are concerned with the development, testing, and evaluation of research instruments and methods. A growing number of instruments have been developed to measure the specific phenomena of interest to nurses.

In secondary analysis studies, a researcher analyzes data gathered in a previous study. The purpose may be to test new hypotheses or answer new research questions.

Research may be conducted in a laboratory or field setting. Laboratory studies are conducted in a special environment created by the researcher. Simulation studies are a type of laboratory study. Field studies are conducted in real-life settings. Most experimental studies in nursing research have been field studies.

Self-Test

1. What threat to internal or external validity does this statement suggest: "It's a good thing that I'm in this new diet study. I couldn't believe it when the researcher told me that I was 10 lbs. overweight."
   A. History
   B. Testing
   C. Selection bias
   D. Hawthorne effect

2. What threat to internal or external validity does this statement suggest: "I'm glad I remembered those questions from the first test."
   A. History
   B. Testing
   C. Selection bias
   D. Hawthorne effect

3. What threat to internal or external validity does this statement suggest: "That researcher scares me. I guess I'd better act like he wants me to act."
   A. History
   B. Testing
   C. Selection bias
   D. Hawthorne effect

4. What threat to internal or external validity does this statement suggest: "I really like the researcher's bracelet. This study should be fun!"
   A. History
   B. Testing
   C. Selection bias
   D. Rosenthal effect

5. What threat to internal or external validity does this statement suggest: "I watched this show about lung cancer. It made me realize that I really should try to stop smoking while I'm in this smoking cessation study."
   A. History
   B. Testing
   C. Selection bias
   D. Rosenthal effect

6. Which item distinguishes true experimental research from quasi-experimental research?
   A. size of sample
   B. use of a nonprobability sample
   C. random assignment of subjects to groups
   D. introduction of an experimental treatment

7. Which design would be most appropriate to use in trying to determine if clients' low back pain changes after they were taught an exercise to help correct back alignment?
   A. one-group pretest-posttest design
   B. posttest-only control group design
   C. one-shot case study
   D. pretest-posttest control group design

8. Which design controls for the sensitization of subjects to a pretest?
   A. pretest-posttest control group design
   B. Solomon four-group design
   C. one-shot case study
   D. time-series design

9. A researcher is studying the use of a new realistic model of the heart to teach people what happens during a heart attack. Two weeks later, she will test their recall of the information taught. Which situation that might occur *during* the study would concern the researcher *most* about the validity of her study?
   A. A television celebrity had a heart attack and later announced on television that it is important for people to understand how their heart functions.
   B. Two of the study participants drop out of the study.

C. The researcher has just learned that the new realistic heart model has increased in price.
D. The CDC released a report that the number of heart attacks has increased slightly in the last 5 years.

10. A researcher wants to use a true experimental design in her study. However, which circumstance would require the use of a quasi-experimental design rather than a true experimental design?

A. The researcher is going to administer a pretest to study participants.
B. It will not be possible for the researcher to use random sampling to obtain study participants.
C. The health care agency will not allow the researcher to assign study participants to groups randomly.
D. The study will use a longitudinal design.

See answers to Self-Test in the Answer Section at the back of the book.

References

Agent orange study finds health problems (1984, February 25). *Dallas Morning News*, pp. 1A, 5A.

Alfes, C. M. (2015) Standardized patient versus role-play strategies: A comparative study measuring patient-centered care and safety in psychiatric mental health nursing. *Nursing Education Perspectives, 36*(6), 403–405. doi:10.5480/14-1535

Bracht, G., & Glass, G. (1968). The external validity of experiments. *American Educational Research Journal, 5,* 437–474. http://www.jstor.org/publisher/aera

Campbell, C., & Stanley, J. (1963). *Experimental and quasi-experimental designs for research.* Chicago: Rand McNally.

Chen, M.-C., Chen, K.-M., and Chu, T.-P. (2015). Caregiver burden, health status and learned resourcefulness of older caregivers. *Western Journal of Nursing Research, 37*(6), 767–780. doi:10.1177/0193945914525280

Cook, C., & Campbell, D. (1979). *Quasi-experimentation: Design and analysis issues for field settings.* Chicago: Rand McNally.

Fitzgerald, L. A., Rorie, A., & Salem, R. E. (2015). Improving secondary prevention screening in clinical encounters using mHealth among prelicensure master's entry clinical nursing students. *Worldviews of Evidence-Based Nursing, 12*(2), 79–87. doi:10.1111/wvn.12081

Hagel, S., Reischke, J., Kesselmeier, M., Winning, J., Gastmeier, P., Brunkhorst, F. M., Scherage, A., & Pletz, M. W. (2015). Quantifying the Hawthorne effect in hand hygiene. Compliance through comparing direct observation with automated hand hygiene monitoring. *Infection Control and Hosptial Epidemiology, 36*(8), 957–862. doi:10.1136/bmjqs-2014-003080

Holman, C., Piper, S. K., Grittner, U., Diamantaras, A. A., Kimmelman, J., Siegerink, B., & Dimagl, U. (2016). Where have all the rodents gone? The effects of attrition in experimental research on cancer and stroke, *PLoS Biol 14*(1). doi:org/10.1371/journal.pbio.1002331

Howard, V. M., Ross, C., Mitchell, A. M., & Nelson, G. M. (2010). Human patient simulator and interactive case studies. *CIN: Computers, Informatics, Nursing, 28,* 42–48. http://journals.lww.com/cinjournal/pages/default.aspx

Hudson, T., & Llosa, L. (2015). Design issues and inference in experimental L2 research. *Language Learning, 65*(S1), 76–96. doi:10.1111/lang.12113

Ishola, A. G., & Chips, J. (2015). The use of mobile phones to deliver acceptance and commitment therapy in the prevention of HIV transmission in Nigeria. *Telemedicine and Telecare, 21*(8), 423–426. doi:10.1177/1357633X15605408.

Schlegel, C., Bonvin, R., Rethans, J. J., & van der Vleuten, C. (2015). The use of video in standardized patient training to improve portrayal accuracy: A randomized post-test control group study. *Medical Teacher, 37*(8), 730–737. doi:10.3109/0142159X.2014.970989

Trinkoff, A. M., Lerner, N. B., Storr, C. L., Han, K., Johantgen, M. E., & Gartrell, K. (2015). Leadership education, certification and resident outcomes in US nursing homes: Cross-sectional secondary analysis. *International Journal of Nursing Studies, 52*(1), 334–344. doi:http://dx.doi.org/10.1016/j.ijnurstu.2014.10.002

Virtanen, H., Leino-Kilpi, H., & Salantera, S. (2015). Nursing students' knowledge about an empowering discourse: Pretest and posttest assessment. *Collegian,* 2015. (In press.) doi:10.1016/j.colegn.2015.06.004

Chapter 11
Qualitative and Mixed Methods Research Designs

Donna Scott Tilley, PhD, RN, CNE, CA SANE

 Objectives

On completion of this chapter, you will be prepared to:

1. Summarize the important features of six common types of qualitative designs.
2. Discuss the main principles and purposes that guide researchers to use more than one method.
3. Describe the strategies a researcher might use in a mixed method study.

Introduction

Qualitative and mixed methods research are increasingly accepted in academe and practice, and sought out as a way for nurses to understand more about human responses to actual or potential illness and disease (Morse, 2015). Qualitative studies are particularly well-suited for questions about which there is little or no research. Qualitative studies can often help answer questions about processes humans use to avoid, cope with, or adjust to illness and disease.

When knowledge gained from qualitative research is used alongside knowledge gained from quantitative research, the result can be powerful and impactful. For example, consider the early days of the HIV epidemic in the early 1980s. While quantitative researchers garnered evidence about the virus itself, how the virus replicated, and how the virus might be eliminated, qualitative researchers were conducting essential ethnographic and case studies to learn more about how the disease was spreading from person to person, and the context in which the disease was spreading. This important qualitative work, combined with the bench science about the virus, helped health officials take measures to slow the spread of HIV disease.

There are many different types of qualitative research. Sometimes people new to qualitative research can feel overwhelmed with the number of different approaches to qualitative research and the different language that is often used in discussing qualitative research. While reading this chapter, don't try to learn everything about each method. Expert qualitative researchers often spend years becoming adept in using their preferred qualitative method. Just try to gain an appreciation of the value of qualitative research to the nursing profession. At some later time, you may be interested in learning more about one or more types of qualitative research. The words *approaches, types*, and *designs* are used interchangeably here in discussing qualitative research.

Qualitative Research Designs

There are many qualitative research designs, and they vary widely in their approach and purpose. The researchers should have a clear sense of the research problem before they select a research design for their study. While there are many different qualitative approaches, we will focus on the six most common qualitative approaches in this chapter. The six most common qualitative designs are phenomenology, ethnography, grounded theory, narrative inquiry, case study, and action research. Excerpts from published nursing studies are presented for each of these six types of qualitative research.

Phenomenology

Phenomenological studies examine human experiences through the descriptions provided by the people involved. These experiences are called *lived experiences.* The goal of phenomenological studies is to describe the meaning that experiences hold for each participant.

In phenomenological research, participants are asked to describe their experiences as they perceive them. They may write about their experiences (for example in diaries) but information is generally obtained through interviews. Bevan (2015) stated that the interview is a very important but often underemphasized part of a phenomenological study. He proposes that the researcher must have an accurate and clear notion of the phenomenon of interest, and use descriptive questions to elicit the most complete responses from participants.

To understand the lived experience from the perspective of the participant, the researcher must take into account the researcher's own beliefs and feelings. The researcher must first identify what she or he expects to discover and deliberately put aside these ideas; this process is called **bracketing**. Some researchers believe that only when the researcher puts aside her or his own ideas about the phenomenon will it be possible to see the experience from the eyes of the person who has lived the experience. Other researchers believe that our experiences and beliefs are a part of who we are and can't be put aside (Bevan, 2015). These researchers would say that instead of bracketing, the researcher should attempt to clearly identify their values and beliefs as they relate to the topic and how they may influence the research. This process of self-reflection is also called **reflexivity**, reflectivity, or critical reflection. Researchers who are reflexive are able to focus on self-knowledge and carefully monitor how their beliefs, biases, and experiences may affect their research (Berger, 2015).

Phenomenological research would begin with a question such as, "What is the lived experience of a mother with a teenage child who is dying of cancer?" The researcher might perceive that she, herself, would feel very hopeless and frightened. These feelings would need to be identified and acknowledged or put aside, or bracketed, to listen to what the mother is saying about how she is living through this experience.

Phenomenological research methods are very different from the methods used in quantitative research and can be difficult to understand, particularly if a person has had a limited background in philosophy. The beginning phenomenological researcher should seek a mentor with experience in phenomenological research.

Phenomenological Study

Loaring, Larkin, Shaw, and Flowers (2015) used the phenomenologic approach to study how breast cancer diagnosis and treatments may affect the relational context of women's coping and the impact upon their intimate partners. Their study focused on couples' experiences of breast cancer surgery, and its impact on body image and sexual intimacy. Using interpretative phenomenological analysis, the researchers conducted an in-depth analysis of the personal meaning of experiences. The researchers concluded that gendered coping styles and normative sexual scripts are an important part of the experience and that management of expectations regarding breast reconstruction may be helpful.

Ethnographic Studies

Ethnographic studies involve the collection and analysis of data about cultural groups. According to Leininger (1985), ethnography can be defined as "the systematic process of observing, detailing, describing, documenting, and analyzing the lifeways or particular patterns of a culture (or subculture) in order to grasp the lifeways or patterns of the people in their familiar environment" (p. 35). Ethnography is a form of qualitative research that focuses on social relationships and the context in which they occur (Mannay & Morgan, 2015). There are several types of ethnography: classical, natural, interpretive, critical, digital, autoethnography, and subjective evidence-based ethnography (Lahlou, Bellu, & Boesen-Mariani, 2015; Mannay & Morgan, 2015; Pink, S., 2015). These variations of ethnography share some common characteristics which include establishing trust, extended periods of time with the culture, the need for the researcher to practice reflexivity, and careful analysis of the various sources of data (Lahlou et al., 2015; Mannay & Morgan, 2015; Pink, 2015).

In ethnographic research, the researcher frequently spends extended periods of time with the group and becomes a part of their culture. The researcher explores with the group their rituals and customs. An entire cultural group or just a subgroup may be studied. The term *culture* may be used in the broad sense to mean an ethnic community, for example, or in a more narrow sense to mean one nursing care unit or one group of nurses. Sources of data may include but are not limited to interviews, images, observations, or interactions between researcher and participants (Lahlou et al., 2015; Mannay & Morgan, 2015; Pink, 2015).

Protecting participant confidentiality is important in all qualitative research, but perhaps more so in ethnographic research. Because of the extended periods of time the researcher spends in the field and the level of trust that is necessary for ethnographic research, researchers must produce work that is transparent and subject to outside scrutiny for rigor, but that also protects the participants. The difficulties in maintaining this balance made national headlines when a researcher did an ethnography of young black men caught up in the criminal justice system (Parry, 2015). The researcher, who became immersed in the community, had firsthand knowledge of many illegal activities committed by participants in her study. There is no agreement as to the correct way to deal with this difficult ethical issue, but it does point out the need to have a clearly defined research plan to avoid ethical dilemmas such as this (Parry, 2015).

The following example of an ethnography is an excellent example of studying a specific group within the context of a healthcare setting who have cultural rules and rituals of interest to a researcher.

Although ethnography is relatively new to nurse researchers, the method has been used in anthropological research for a long time. Margaret Mead (1929) used it to study the Samoans. Ethnography has been the principal method used by anthropologists to study people all over the world. Ethnographers study how people live and how they communicate with each other.

Ethnographic Study

Saleem et al. (2015) conducted an ethnographic study of clinical end-users interacting with electronic medical records systems in Veterans Affairs Medical Centers. They analyzed data and identified barriers to effective adoption and optimization of electronic medical records systems. Identifying the barriers explained some of the challenges with the optimization of the electronic medical records systems across the Veterans Affairs Medical system. They were then able to make recommendations about how to improve adoption of systems for more effective use by Veterans Affairs healthcare providers.

Grounded Theory

Grounded theory is a qualitative research approach developed by two sociologists, Glaser and Strauss (1967). Although the grounded theory approach was developed by sociologists, the approach is very appropriate for use by nurse researchers. When a researcher is interested in an area in which little research has been done or in which existing theories are not sufficient, grounded theory studies are a good choice. The outcome of a grounded theory study is a theory that is grounded in data from the study.

Rather than using probability sampling procedures, purposeful (sometimes called purposive) sampling is used. The researcher looks for certain participants who will be able to shed new light on the phenomenon being studied. As hypotheses and theories begin to emerge, the researcher may deliberately choose participants to fill in missing information or who might be able to disprove emerging theory. Diversity rather than similarity is sought in the people who are sampled.

Data are gathered in natural settings (field settings). Data collection primarily consists of participant interviews, and data are recorded through audio recordings and handwritten notes, called field notes. However, many grounded theorists use a variety of data sources including quantitative instruments alongside qualitative data. Data collection and data analysis occur simultaneously. Data analysis is done using the **constant comparison method**, where data are constantly compared to data that have already been gathered. Pertinent concepts are identified and assigned codes. These codes are constantly reviewed as new interpretations are made of the data. The researcher keeps an open mind and uses an intuitive process in interpreting data. Once concepts have been identified and their relationships specified, the researcher consults the literature to determine if any similar associations have already been uncovered. Despite the great diversity of the data that are gathered, the grounded theory approach presumes it is possible to discover fundamental patterns in all social life. These patterns are called *basic social processes*.

Grounded theory is more concerned with the generation of new theory rather than the testing of hypotheses. The theory that is generated is self-correcting, which means that as data are gathered, adjustments are made to the theory to allow for the interpretation of new data that are obtained.

Grounded Theory

Fritz (2015) used grounded theory method to examine the process by which low-income (mostly minority) women develop the skills to integrate diabetes self-management into daily life and the conditions that affect the process. The researcher used semistructured interviews, photo elicitation, time geographic diaries, and a standardized assessment to collect data from ten low-income women with type 2 diabetes. The resulting theory, the Transactional Model of Diabetes Self-Management (DSM) Integration, depicts the theorized process whereby low-income women accept aspects of diabetes education and training as a part of their circumstances, act on them, and practice with them until they become integrated into daily life.

Narrative Inquiry

Narrative inquiry is a method that seeks to explore experiences of participants through the stories told by participants. The researcher elicits stories of experiences from the participants and enters into the experience through the hearing of the stories and the relationship with the participant that develops during the study. The researcher attends to the story through attention to verbal elements of the story and nonverbal elements of the story (Clandinin, 2013). Nonverbal elements may include pauses, rhythm and pacing, sighs or smiles, and other expressions. Elements such as environment, time, location, and social elements of the story are all important. The researcher transcribes the story into written form and notes their perceptions of nonverbal elements in field notes. Photos, drawings, or recordings provided by the participants about the story may all be used to shape understanding of the story. These layers of information provide an in-depth understanding of experience from the participant's point of view (Wang & Geale, 2015) Together, the participant and researcher begin to assign meaning to the stories shared by participants.

Narrative Inquiry

Elliott (2015) used narrative inquiry to describe ten military nurses' experiences and their meaning with returning to personal and professional roles post-deployment. Description of the experience had five themes: 'learning to manage changes in the environment'; 'facing the reality of multiple losses'; 'feeling like it's all so trivial now'; 'figuring out where I 'fit' in all the chaos'; and 'working through the guilt to move forward'. Description of the meaning of the experience had two themes: 'serving a greater purpose' and 'looking at life through a new lens'. Elliott concluded that it is important for nurses who work alongside military nurses to understand these experiences and be able to provide support to nurses in the post-deployment phase.

Case Studies

Case studies are in-depth examinations of people or groups of people. A case study could also examine an institution, such as hospice care for the dying. The case method has its roots in sociology and has also been used a great deal in anthropology, law, and medicine. In medicine, case studies have frequently been concerned with a particular disease. In nursing, the case study approach might be used to answer a question such as "How do nurse practitioners handle pre-exposure prophylaxis for HIV prevention in high risk groups?" (Rowniak, 2015). This topic is a good example of the utility of the case study method since the topic is important and has clinical relevance, but may not occur often enough to lend itself well to other qualitative research methods.

A case study may be considered as quantitative, qualitative, or mixed methods research, depending on the purpose of the study and the design chosen by the researcher. As is true of other types of qualitative studies, for a case study to be considered as a qualitative study, the researcher must be interested in the meaning of experiences to the participants themselves, rather than in generalizing results to other groups of people. The objective of the case study is to help us understand the details of a case from several perspectives; thus, multiple data sources and the context of a case are important (Abma & Stake, 2014).

Patricia Benner is a qualitative researcher who is widely recognized as an expert in understanding how a nurse moves from novice to expert. She has used the case study approach extensively. She contends that case studies help us formalize experiential knowledge and, thus, promote quality nursing care (Benner, 1983).

Data may be collected in case studies through various means such as questionnaires, interviews, observations, or written accounts by the participants. A nurse researcher might be interested in how people with diabetes respond to an insulin pump. One person or a group of people with diabetes could be studied for a time to determine their responses to the use of an insulin pump. Diaries might be used for the day-to-day recording of information. The nurse researcher would then analyze these diaries and try to interpret the written comments.

When participants are chosen for case studies, care must be taken in the selection process. In the previously discussed example, the researcher should avoid choosing only those clients who are expected to respond favorably or unfavorably to the insulin pump. The concept of purposive sampling also applies here; the researcher should select participants who can fill in missing information.

Case Study

Kobler (2014) presented a case study of one unit's response to the unexpected death of a long-term patient, which caused caregivers to lean in to support each other. Using a case study approach, the author identified strategies to guide teams caring for patients who die unexpectedly and provides ideas for co-creating ritual to honor relationship in the midst of tragedy.

Action Research Studies

Action research is a type of qualitative research that actively engages the community of interest in solving a problem. Unlike other qualitative research designs, action research is not intended to increase theoretical knowledge. Rather, solutions are sought to practice problems in one particular hospital or healthcare setting. In action research, the implementation of solutions occurs as an actual part of the research process. There is no delay in implementation of the solutions.

Action research became popular in the 1940s. Kurt Lewin (1946) was influential in spreading action research, which he used to help social workers improve their practice.

Participatory action research (PAR) is a special kind of community-based action research in which there is collaboration between the study participants and the researcher in all steps of the study: determining the problem, the research methods to use, the analysis of data, and how the study results will be used. This kind of research may also be called community-engaged research. The participants and the researcher are co-researchers throughout the entire research study. Researchers used community-engaged research very effectively to develop interventions to improve rates of human papilloma virus vaccination among adolescents in a high risk community (Katz & Paskett, 2015).

Action Research

Purpose: VanDevanter, Gennaro, Budin, Calalang-Javiera, and Minh (2014) conducted an action research study to evaluate the implementation of a United Nations Children's Fund (UNICEF)/WHO Baby-Friendly Hospital Initiative (BFHI) in a large urban hospital in New York City. Evaluation of the program included focus groups, key informant interviews, and observations of the clinical environment using a community-based participatory research approach with healthcare providers. Strengths and challenges of the system were identified and strategies for enhancing program implementation and outcomes were devised. The researchers concluded that evaluation of program implementation at multiple levels of the organization in collaboration with providers is critical to understanding program outcomes.

Mixed Methods Research

Because healthcare is complex, mixed methods research is increasingly popular as a way to explore complex problems that influence health and health outcomes (Shneerson & Gale, 2015). Though increasingly popular, mixed methods research is not new. The first mixed methods study was published by Cora DuBois, an anthropologist, in 1938 (Pelto, 2015).

Mixed methods research was defined by a working group commissioned by the National Institutes of Health as "a research approach or methodology focusing on research questions that call for real-lfe contextual understandings, multi-level perspectives, and cultural influences; employing rigorous quantitative research assessing magnitude and frequency of constructs and rigorous qualitative research exploring the meaning and understanding of constructs; utilizing multiple methods; intentionally integrating or combining these methods to draw on the strengths of each; and framing the investigation within philosophical and theoretical positions" (Creswell, Klassen, Plano Clark, & Clegg Smith, n.d., page 4).

Mixed methods research is a very practical approach to solving complex problems of interest to nurse researchers because it allows researchers to use all of the qualitative and quantitative data-gathering and analyzing methods available (Pelto, 2015), overcome the weaknesses of a single design, or complement the strengths of a single design (Biddix, n.d.; Creswell et al., n.d.; Shneerson & Gale, 2015).

The research methods selected for any study should be chosen because they are the best method to answer the research question or problem. Mixed methods research is complex; it is far more than adding an open-ended question to the end of a survey or simply mixing qualitative and quantitative data sources. When designing a mixed methods study, the researcher should consider the underlying philosophical and theoretical framework, the resources available to conduct the work, and the research question or problem. The researcher should always consider the needs of human subjects, and plan for data-collection methods that adequately answer the research question or address the research problem.

Strategies for Mixed Methods Research

Creswell (2003) identified six strategies for mixed methods research:

1. sequential explanatory
2. sequential exploratory
3. sequential transformative
4. concurrent triangulation
5. concurrent nested
6. concurrent transformative

As the names imply, these strategies vary by the order of data collection, the intent of the research, and the presence or absence of a theoretical framework.

The sequential explanatory strategy involves collecting qualitative data after analyzing quantitative data to explain quantitative findings. For instance, results of a quantitative study may be unexpected, and the researcher might choose to follow up with interviews to help understand these quantitative results. In sequential explanatory research, data are integrated during the interpretation of data. In the example of the follow-up interviews, the results from both phases would be discussed to make clearer the meaning of the results of both phases of data collection and analysis.

The sequential exploratory strategy involves an initial period of qualitative data collection and analysis followed by a quantative data collection and analysis. This strategy may be used when a phenomenon is poorly understood, to test elements of a theory, to explore possible generalization of qualitative data to a specific population, or for instrument development and testing.

The sequential transformative strategy is used when a specific theoretical perspective, such as feminism, is the guiding framework for the study. Using the sequential transformative strategy, the researcher has two distinct phases of data collection, and either type of data can be collected first. A researcher might choose the sequential transformative strategy to give voice to varying perspectives, or to understand a phenomenon that might change as a result of being studied (Cresswell, 2003).

When using the concurrent triangulation strategy, both types of data are collected concurrently to confirm or corroborate findings within the study. This strategy allows the researcher to compensate for the weaknesses of one method.

With the concurrent nested strategy, the researcher collects data using one primary approach with the secondary approach nested within. For example, the primary approach might be semistructured interview with a brief quantitative element to obtain a different perspective or additional information.

In the concurrent transformative strategy, data are collected concurrently with equal priority given to each type of data collection. As with the sequential transformative strategy, the defining feature of this strategy that the research is guided by a specific theoretical perspective.

Each of these strategies has value when used appropriately. All require that the researcher have a firm grasp of the phenomenon being studied and expertise in both qualitative and quantitative methodologies. It is a rare researcher who can truly claim expertise in both qualitative and quantitative methods, which points to the need to researchers to work in teams where team members can provide needed expertise in both methods (Hesse-Biber, 2015). The concurrent strategies require less time than other strategies, since data are being collected at once, but require a good deal of organization and planning. Researchers who plan to use the sequential strategies should plan for the additional time required to collect and analyze data before moving to the second data collection and analysis phase.

Multiple approaches to studying a phenomenon can provide a broad perspective, but should be approached with the same care, deliberate planning, attention to detail, and valuing of methodological thinking (Greene, 2015) expected in single-method studies. As with all studies, the method should be chosen that is the best fit to answer the research question or problem.

Summary

Qualitative studies are particularly well-suited for questions about which there is little or no research. Mixed methods studies can be powerful and impactful. There are many qualitative research designs, but the six most common approaches are phenomenology, ethnography, grounded theory, narrative inquiry, case study, and action research. Phenomenological studies are interested in experiences and meanings of experiences as described by those who experienced them; this is called lived experience. Ethnographic studies are helpful in understanding groups of people, particularly social norms and the context in which they occur.

Though there are several types of ethnography, each requires the researcher to spend time in the culture, establish trust, practice reflective thinking, and examine all data sources carefully. Grounded theory studies are helpful for studying an area in which explanatory theory is inadequate or absent. As the name implies, grounded theory studies seek to ultimately arrive at explanatory theories that are grounded in data. Case studies are in-depth examinations of people, groups of people, or institutions. Case studies are helpful in understanding problems that are important but occur infrequently. Action research is qualitative research that actively engages the community of interest in solving an identified problem. The implementation of solutions becomes part of the research process.

Mixed methods research, though not new, has recently become widely accepted as a research methodology in health sciences research. There are six strategies a researcher can use to conduct a mixed methods study: (1) sequential explanatory, (2) sequential exploratory, (3) sequential transformative, (4) concurrent triangulation, (5) concurrent nested, and (6) concurrent transformative. As the names imply, these strategies vary by the order of data collection, the intent of the research, and the presence or absence of a theoretical framework. Mixed methods research requires the same amount of deliberate planning, attention to detail, and expertise as single-method studies. Most researchers do not possess the expertise required to conduct mixed method studies without consultation from other expert researchers.

Self-Test

Select T (True) or F (False) for the following statements:

____ 1. Phenomenology is concerned with creating a theory that is grounded in research data.

____ 2. The researcher who identifies and sets aside personal beliefs about the subject of the study is engaging in reflexivity or self-reflection.

____ 3. Ethnographic studies involve the collection and analysis of data about cultural groups.

____ 4. When a researcher is interested in an area in which little research has been done or in which existing theories are not sufficient, grounded theory studies are a good choice.

____ 5. When data collection and data analysis occur simultaneously, the researcher is using the constant comparison method of data analysis.

____ 6. The number of subjects is generally larger in qualitative research than in quantitative research.

____ 7. Because healthcare is complex, mixed methods research is increasingly popular as a way to explore complex problems that influence health and health outcomes.

8. Which statement is true when describing sequential exploratory mixed methods?
   A. This method involves choosing participants who can fill in gaps in the data.
   B. This method involves collecting qualitative data after analyzing quantitative data to explain quantitative findings.
   C. This method involves collecting qualitative and qualitative data simultaneously.
   D. This method involves an initial period of qualitative data collection and analysis followed by a quantative data collection and analysis.

9. If a researcher were planning a qualitative study, which data-collection methods would most likely be considered? Select all that apply.
   A. closed-ended questions and nonparticipant observations
   B. participant observations and semistructured interviews
   C. structured interviews and physiological measures
   D. closed-ended questions and structured interviews
   E. All of these data collections methods would probably be considered.

10. Consider the study title, "The Lived Experience of Long-Term Complications from a Football-Related Concussion." Which design is most likely for this title?
    A. grounded theory
    B. action research
    C. phenomenology
    D. case study

See answers to Self-Test in the Answer Section at the back of the book.

References

Abma, T., & Stake, R. (2014). Science of the particular: An advocacy of naturalistic case study in health research. *Qualitative Health Research, 24* (8), 1150–1161. doi:10.1177/1049732314543196

Benner, P. (1983). Uncovering the knowledge embedded in clinical practice. *Image: Journal of Nursing Scholarship, 19*, 36–41. doi: 10.1111/j.1547-5069.1983.tb01353.x

Berger, R. (2015). Now I see it, now I don't: Researcher's position and reflexivity in qualitative research. *Qualitative Research, 15*(2), 219–234. doi:10.1177/1468794112468475

Bevan, M. T. (2015). A method of phenomenological interviewing. *Qualitative Health Research, 24*(1), 136–144. doi:10.1177-104973231359710

Biddix, J. P. (n.d.). Ressearch rundowns: Mixed methods research designs. https://researchrundowns.wordpress.com/mixed/mixed-methods-research-designs/

Clandinin, D. J. (2013). Engaging in narrative Inquiry. Walnut Creek, CA: Left Coast Press, Inc.

Creswell, J. (2003). *Research design: Qualitative, quantitative, and mixed method approaches.* Thousand Oaks, CA: Sage.

Creswell, J., Klassen, A.C., Plano Clark, V. L., Clegg Smith, K. (n.d.). Best practices for mixed methods research in the health sciences. Office of Behavioral and Social Sciences Research, National Institutes of Health.

Elliott, B. (2015). Military nurses' experiences returning from war. *Journal Of Advanced Nursing, 71*(5), 1066–1075. doi:10.1111/jan.12588

Fritz, H. A. (2015). Learning to do better: The transactional model of diabetes self-management integration. *Qualitative Health Research, 25*(7), 875–886. doi:10.1177/1049732314552453

Glaser, B. G., & Strauss, A. C. (1967). *The discovery of grounded theory: Strategies for qualitative research.* New York: Aldine.

Greene, J. C. (2015). The emergence of mixing methods in the field of evaluation. *Qualitative Health Research, 25*(6), 746–750. doi:10.1177/1049732315576499

Hesse-Biber, S. (2015). Mixed methods research: The "thing-ness" problem. *Qualitative Health Research, 25*(6), 775–788. doi:10.1177/1049732315580558

Katz, M. L., & Paskett, E. D. (2015). The process of engaging members from two underserved populations in the development of interventions to promote the uptake of the HPV vaccine. *Health Promotion Practice, 16*(3), 443–453. doi:10.1177/1524839914559776

Kobler, K. (2014). Leaning in and holding on: Team support with unexpected death. *MCN: American Journal of Maternal Child Nursing, 39*(3), 148–156. doi:10.1097/NMC.0000000000000028

Lahlou, S., Bellu, A., & Boesen-Mariani, S. (2015). Subjective evidence based ethnography: Method and applications. *Integrative Psychological & Behavioral Science, 49*, 216–238. doi:10.1007/s12124-014-9288-9

Leininger, M. M. (Ed.). (1985). *Qualitative research methods in nursing.* Orlando, FL: Grune & Stratton.

Lewin, K. (1946). Action research and minority problems. *Social Issues, 2*(4), 34–46. doi: 10.1111/j.1540-4560.1946.tb02295.x

Loaring, J. M., Larkin, M., Shaw, R., & Flowers, P. (2015). Renegotiating sexual intimacy in the context of altered embodiment: The experiences of women with breast cancer and their male partners following mastectomy and reconstruction. *Health Psychology, 34*(4), 426–436. doi:10.1037/hea0000195

Mannay, D., & Morgan, M. (2015). Doing ethnography or applying a qualitative technique? Reflections from the "waiting field." *Qualitative Research, 15*(2), 166–182. doi:10.2277/468794113517391

Mead, M. (1929). *Coming of age in Samoa.* New York: New American Library.

Morse, J. (2015). Qualitative health research: One quarter of a century. *Qualitative Health Research, 25*(1), 3–4. doi:10.1177-1049732314561207

Parry, M. (2015, June 12). Conflict over sociologist's narrative puts spotlight on ethnography. *Chronicle of Higher Education.* http://www.chronicle.com/

Pelto, P. (2015). What is so new about mixed methods? *Qualitative Health Research, 25*(6), 734–745. doi:10.1177/1049732315573209

Pink, S. (2015). Going forward through the world: Thinking theoretically about the first person perspective digital ethnography. *Integrative Psychological & Behavioral Science, 49,* 239–252. doi:10.1007/s12124-014-9292-0

Rowniak, S. (2015). PrEP: A case study. *American Association of Nurse Practitioners, 27*(6), 296–299. doi:10.1002/2327-6924.12240

Saleem, J. J., Plew, W. R., Speir, R. C., Herout, J., Wilck, N. R., Ryan, D. M., & ... Phillips, T. (2015). Understanding barriers and facilitators to the use of clinical informationsystems for intensive care units and anesthesia record keeping: A rapid ethnography. *International Journal of Medical Informatics, 84*(7), 500–511. doi:10.1016/j.ijmedinf.2015.03.006

Shneerson, C., & Gale, N. (2015). Using mixed methods to identify and answer clinically relevant research questions. *Qualitative Health Research, 25*(6), 845–856. doi:10.1177/1049732315580107

VanDevanter, N., Gennaro, S., Budin, W., Calalang-Javiera, H., & Minh, N. (2014). Evaluating implementation of a baby friendly hospital initiative. *MCN:American Journal of Maternal Child Nursing, 39*(4), 231–237. doi:10.1097/NMC.0000000000000046

Wang, C. and Geale, S. (2015). The power of story: Narrative inquiry as a methodology in nursing research. *International Journal of Nursing Sciences 2,* 195–198

PART IV Obtaining Study Participants and Collection of Data

Chapter 12
Populations and Samples

Rose Marie Nieswiadomy, PhD, RN, and Renae L. Dougal, MSN, RN, CLNC, CCRP

 Objectives

On completion of this chapter, you will be prepared to:

1. Summarize the concepts related to populations and samples in research design.
2. Differentiate among various types of probability and nonprobability sampling methods.
3. Explain sampling size, sampling error and sampling bias.

Introduction

Did you check out some new blog site today, taste a new food, or turn on a different TV program that you have never watched before? If so, you have been sampling. Sampling is a part of our everyday life. Frequently, decisions in life are made on limited sampling from all of the available options. For instance, if you are thinking about going shopping for new clothes today, would you plan to try on all of the clothes in the store before you purchased one item? Probably not, or the store would close before you made your decision.

Researchers also make decisions based on data from samples. However, the consequences of basing decisions on inadequate samples may be much more serious for the researcher than for the shopper. If you chose the wrong size or changed your mind about the style of shoes you bought, you are usually allowed to exchange the item or return it and receive your money back. However, the researcher is not able to change a decision about the selection of a sample for a study once the sample has been chosen. Of course, the safest choice then would be to study total populations. Just as it is unlikely that you would buy a whole "population" of shoes, researchers rarely study entire populations. Therefore, an understanding of the means of selecting samples for research studies is important for nurse researchers.

Populations

A population is a complete set of persons or objects that possess some common characteristic of interest to the researcher. Quantitative research is very interested in populations. Qualitative research focuses more on individuals themselves. This chapter focuses on obtaining a sample for a quantitative study. The goal of sampling in quantitative research is to be able to make generalizations about the population from which the sample was drawn.

The population for a study is composed of two groups: the target population and the accessible population. The target population is composed of the entire group of people or objects to which the researcher wishes to generalize the findings of a study. The target population consists of people or things that meet the designated set of criteria of interest to the researcher. Examples of target populations might be all people who are institutionalized for psychiatric problems in one state, or all the charts from well-child clinics for the year 2010. Because the likelihood of being able to obtain a list of these populations is quite low, the researcher usually samples from an available group, called the *accessible population* or *study population*. The need to identify the accessible population is quite important for nurse researchers. By clearly identifying the group from which the study sample was chosen, the investigator enables readers of a research report to come to their own conclusions about the generalizability of the study findings. The conclusions of a research study are based on data obtained from the accessible population, and statistical inferences should be made only to the group from which the sample was randomly selected.

Target and Accessible Populations

A study was conducted to explore and compare predictors of hospital length of stay (LOS), acute LOS (ALOS), emergency room (ER) wait times, rate of admission (ROA), and costs of inpatient hospital care for older adults with and without mental illness (MI) diagnoses in Canadian provinces (Adams, Koop, Quan, & Norris, 2015). The target population was identified as people who were 65 years and older and admitted to an acute care hospital. The accessible population was participants who were 65 years of age and older, permanent residents of the province, and admitted to one of the province's acute care hospitals between April 1, 2008 and March 31, 2009. This population consisted of 12,283 eligible participants.

Samples and Sampling

Although researchers are always interested in populations, an entire population is generally not used in a research study. The accuracy gained when all members are included is often not worth the time and money involved, and it is probably not possible to gain access to the whole population. In most nursing research studies, a sample or subset of the population is selected to represent the population. When a sample is chosen properly, the researcher is able to make claims about the population based on data from the sample alone. The method of selection and the sample size determine how representative a sample is of the population.

A single member of a population is called an **element**. The terms *population member* and *population element* are often used interchangeably. Elements, or members of a population, are selected from a **sampling frame**, which is a listing of all elements of a population. Sometimes listings of populations such as membership lists, hospital patient census sheets, and vital statistics listings are readily available. However, it may be necessary for the researcher to prepare the sampling frame by listing all members of the accessible population. This can be a time-consuming task. For example, you might examine a large group of charts and make a list of all patients who were admitted for their second major surgical procedure within the past two years.

Although examining each member of a population would generally produce more accurate data, occasionally data obtained from a sample are more exact. For example, in large-scale survey studies in which many interviewers have to be trained, the quality of the interviews would be difficult to control. A small number of interviews conducted by a well-trained group of interviewers might produce more accurate data than would be produced by a large group of interviewers. Also, when resources are spread thin, a weak study may result.

Samples are chosen through two types of sampling procedures: probability and nonprobability. The various types of probability and nonprobability sampling methods are discussed next.

Probability Sampling Methods

Probability sampling, or random sampling, involves the use of a random selection process to obtain a sample from members or elements of a population. The goal of probability sampling is to obtain representative elements of populations.

The term *random* can be confusing to the beginning researcher. The dictionary definition of this word suggests that something occurs haphazardly or without direction. However, random sampling is anything but haphazard. It is a very systematic, scientific process. The investigator can specify the chance of any one element of the population being selected for the sample. Each population element has a known chance or probability of being selected for the sample. Selections are independent of each other, and the investigator's bias does not enter into the selection of the sample.

When a random sample is selected, the researcher hopes that the variables of interest in the population will be present in the sample in approximately the same proportions as would be found in the total population. Unfortunately, there is never any guarantee. Probability sampling enables the researcher only to estimate the chance that any given population element will be included in the sample. When probability samples are chosen, inferential statistics may be used with greater confidence. Without the use of random sampling procedures, the ability to generalize the findings of a study is greatly reduced. Four types of random sampling procedures are examined here: simple, stratified, cluster, and systematic.

SIMPLE RANDOM SAMPLING **Simple random sampling** is a type of probability sampling method that ensures each element of the population has an equal and independent chance of being chosen. This method is generally used in at least one phase of the other three types of random sampling procedures and, therefore, is examined first. Table 12–1 lists the advantages and disadvantages of simple random sampling.

The word *simple* does not mean easy or uncomplicated. In fact, simple random sampling can be quite complex and time-consuming, especially if a large sample is desired.

The first step is to identify the accessible population and enumerate or list all the elements of the population. After this sampling frame is developed, a method must be selected to choose the sample. Slips of paper representing each element in the population could be placed in a hat or bowl, and the sample selected by reaching in and drawing out as many slips of paper as the desired size of the sample.

Although random sampling can be achieved in this manner, the most commonly used and accurate procedure for selecting a simple random sample is through the use of a **table of random numbers**. A table of random numbers includes a group of numbers that has been generated in such a manner that there is no order or sequencing of the numbers. Each number has an equal chance of following any other number. Tables of random numbers are still found in some research and statistical textbooks. However, today these tables are usually computer-generated, and there are several websites that enable you to generate your own table of random numbers.

Simple Random Sample

A simple random sample of second-year nursing students attending a selected nursing college of Mangalore Taluk in India was identified by using a lottery method (Pradap, 2015). The author provided no other details associated with the process of selecting participants from the accessible population. A total of 60 students completed a questionnaire regarding knowledge of body mechanics.

STRATIFIED RANDOM SAMPLING In **stratified random sampling**, the population is divided into subgroups, or strata, according to some variable(s) of importance to the research study. After the population is divided into two or more strata, a simple random sample is taken from each of these subgroups.

Many different characteristics of populations may call for the use of stratified sampling. Subject characteristics such as age, gender, and educational background are examples of variables that might be used as criteria for dividing populations into subgroups. For example, a school nurse might be interested in studying marijuana usage among high school students. To determine if marijuana usage is different among freshmen, sophomores, juniors, and seniors, the total high school population could be stratified into four separate sampling units, and a random sample selected from each grade. If a simple random sample technique is used, the four grades might not be represented in large enough numbers to make valid comparisons. Generally, there are more freshmen in a school than there are seniors. Some dropout occurs as students progress through high school. By dividing the total population into the four grades, the school nurse would be more certain that sufficient numbers of students from all four grades will be selected for inclusion in the study.

After dividing the population into subgroups, the researcher must decide how large a sample to obtain from each of these strata. Two approaches may be used. The first is called **proportional stratified sampling** and involves obtaining a sample from each stratum that is in proportion to the size of that stratum in the total population. If there were 400 freshmen, 300 sophomores, 200 juniors, and 100 seniors (highly unlikely) in a total high school population of 1000 students, the size of the sample from each of these groups should be freshmen, 40%; sophomores, 30%; juniors, 20%; and seniors, 10%. If a sample of 100 students was desired, the selection should include 40 freshmen, 30 sophomores, 20 juniors, and 10 seniors.

What if the school nurse decided that 10 seniors was not a large enough sample to get a clear picture of marijuana usage among that group? She might decide to choose 25 subjects from each class. The selection of members from strata in which the number of members chosen from each stratum is not in proportion to the size of the stratum in the total population is called **disproportional stratified sampling**. Whenever disproportional sampling is used, an adjustment process known as *weighting* should be considered. This process involves simple computations that are described in many texts on sampling procedures. These adjustments allow a better estimate of the actual population values.

As previously mentioned, simple random sampling is used to obtain the sample elements from each stratum when a stratified random sampling method is used. Table 12–1 lists the advantages and disadvantages of stratified sampling.

Table 12–1 Probability Sampling Chart

Type of Sampling	Description of Methodology	Advantages	Disadvantages
A. Simple random	Assign a number to each member of the population. Select the sample through a table of random numbers.	1. Little knowledge of population is needed. 2. Most unbiased of probability methods 3. Easy to analyze data and compute errors	1. A complete listing of population is necessary. 2. Time-consuming 3. Expensive
B. Stratified	Divide population into strata. Determine number of cases desired in each stratum. Random sample these subgroups.	1. Increases probability of sample being representative 2. Assures adequate number of cases for subgroups	1. Requires accurate knowledge of population 2. May be costly to prepare stratified lists 3. Statistics are more complicated.
1. Proportionate	Determine sampling fraction for each stratum that is equal to its proportion in the total population.		
2. Disproportionate	Sample is drawn in manner to ensure that each stratum is well represented. Used when strata are very unequal.		
C. Cluster	Groups rather than people are selected from population. Successive steps of selection are done (state, city, county). Then sample is randomly selected from clusters.	1. Saves time and money 2. Arrangements made with small number of sampling units 3. Characteristics of clusters as well as those of population can be estimated.	1. Larger sampling errors than other probability samples 2. Requires assignment of each member of population uniquely to a cluster 3. Statistics are more complicated.
D. Systematic	Obtain listing of population. Determine sample size. Determine sampling interval ($k = N/n$). Select random starting point. Select every kth element.	1. Easy to draw sample 2. Economical 3. Time-saving technique	1. Samples may be biased if ordering of population is not random. 2. After the first sampling element is chosen, population members no longer have equal chance of being chosen.

Stratified Random Sample

Chen and Lo (2015) conducted a nationwide survey to understand the satisfaction of associate of science in nursing (ASN) students with their nursing programs as a whole during 2008 and 2009. Students were recruited from 138 ASN or ADN programs from 46 states; students from 31 states which represented 56 ASN or ADN programs agreed to participate in this study. Stratified random sampling of the agreed upon participants from the nursing programs was done to collect data on student satisfaction with ASN programs in the United States during 2008 and 2009. The study results revealed that the students rated their satisfaction with the nursing program as close to "satisfied." Additionally, the faculty, curriculum, and social interaction significantly and positively demonstrated a predicted overall student satisfaction with a nursing program.

CLUSTER RANDOM SAMPLING In large-scale studies in which the population is geographically spread out, sampling procedures may be very difficult and time-consuming. Also, it may not be possible to get a total listing of some populations. Suppose a researcher wanted to interview 100 nurse administrators in the United States. If the 100 names were chosen through a simple random sampling procedure, it is likely the investigator would be faced with traveling to 100 different cities in the United States to conduct the interviews. This would be a very expensive and time-consuming activity. Another approach that might be used to obtain this sample of nurse administrators is cluster sampling.

In **cluster random sampling**, large groups, or clusters, become the sampling units. To obtain the sample of nurse administrators, the first clusters to be sampled would be acquired by drawing a simple random sample or stratified random sample of states in the United States. Then, cities would be chosen from these states. Next, hospitals from within those cities would be selected, and, finally, the nurse administrators from some of these hospitals would be interviewed. During each phase of sampling from the clusters, simple, stratified, or systematic random sampling may be used. Because the sample is selected from clusters in two or more separate stages, the approach is sometimes called multistage sampling.

Although cluster sampling may be necessary for large-scale survey studies, the likelihood of sampling error increases with each stage of sampling. A simple random sample is subject to a single sampling error, whereas a cluster sample is subject to as many sampling errors as there are stages in the sampling procedure. To compensate for the sampling error when cluster sampling is used, larger samples should be selected than would normally be chosen for a simple or stratified random sample. Table 12–1 lists the advantages and disadvantages of cluster sampling.

Cluster Random Sample

A study to describe how often family carers of nursing home residents who died with dementia were aware that their relative had dementia was conducted in Belgium (Penders, Albers, Deliens, Vander Stichele, & Van den Block, 2015). Another purpose of the study was to identify the care characteristics associated with awareness among the residents, nursing staff, general practitioners and family carers of the deceased nursing home residents. In order to collect data that was representative of the area, a random sample of 134 high-care nursing homes was taken and stratified according to region, type, and size. Then the researcher worked with a contact person from the nursing homes to identify those residents who had died from dementia. Structured questionnaires were completed by each of the participants who met the eligibility criteria.

SYSTEMATIC RANDOM SAMPLING **Systematic random sampling** involves selecting every kth element of the population, such as every fifth, eighth, or twenty-first element. The first step is to obtain a list of the total population (N). Then, the sample size (n) is determined. Next, the sampling interval width (k) is determined by N/n. For instance, if the researcher were seeking a sample of 50 from a population of 500, the sampling interval would be:

$$k = 500/50 = 10$$

Every tenth element of the population list would be selected for the sample. This method may be used to obtain any sample size from a given population.

This sampling method is the most controversial type of random sampling procedure. In fact, systematic sampling may be classified as either a probability or a nonprobability sampling method. Two criteria are necessary for a systematic sampling procedure to be classified as probability sampling: (a) the listing of the population (sampling frame) must be random with respect to the variable of interest, and (b) the first element or member of the sample must be selected randomly. If either of these criteria is not met, the sample becomes a nonprobability sample.

The first criterion for the inclusion of systematic sampling as a probability sampling method is the requirement that the listing of the elements of the population must be in random order. Suppose a researcher was choosing names from an alphabetized list. Certain ethnic groups have large numbers of surnames that begin with the same initial and are grouped together alphabetically. If systematic sampling is used, these ethnic groups may be underrepresented or overrepresented. As another example, the sample to be selected might be patients in hospital rooms. The decision might be made to sample every fifth hospital room. It might happen that every fifth room is a private room. Patients in private rooms may not respond in the same manner that patients in semiprivate rooms might respond.

The second criterion for considering systematic sampling as a type of probability sampling is that a random starting point must be chosen. The best way to obtain this starting point is through a table of random numbers. If the population size is 500 and a sample size of 50 is desired, a number between 1 and 500 is selected as the starting point. Suppose the first number randomly selected is 289. The sampling interval width ($k + 10$) is added to this number ($289 + 10 = 299$), and the next element selected would correspond to number 299. When 500 is reached, the researcher starts back over at the beginning of the list and continues, adding 10 to select each additional element of the sample. An alternate procedure, recommended in most texts, is to select the first element randomly from within the first sampling interval. If the sampling interval width was 10, a number between 1 and 10 would be selected as the random starting point. For example, suppose the number 4 is randomly chosen. The next element selected would correspond to number 14 ($4 + 10 = 14$). Although this latter procedure is technically correct, choosing a random starting point from across the total population of elements is appealing to the authors of this text because every element has a chance to be chosen for the sample during the first selection step.

When careful attention is paid to obtaining an unbiased listing of the population elements, and the first element is randomly selected, systematic random sampling is similar to simple random sampling and much easier. Drawing 50 numbers from a table of random numbers is a much more laborious task than choosing 50 numbers through systematic sampling (see Table 12–1 for the advantages and disadvantages of systematic random sampling). A review of the published nursing research literature suggests that few studies mention systematic random sampling.

Systematic Random Sample

Systematic random sampling was used in a study of nurses who worked in teaching hospitals in Zanjan, Iran (Amini, Negarandeh, Ramezani-Badr, Moosaeifard, & Fallah, 2015). From the accessible population of 1029 nurses, 252 valid questionnaires were completed and entered into the analysis through systematic random sampling. The authors did not provide the details of this process of sampling.

Nonprobability Sampling Methods

In **nonprobability sampling**, the sample elements are chosen from the population by nonrandom methods. Nonrandom methods of sampling are more likely to produce a biased sample than are random methods. The investigator cannot estimate the probability that each element of the population will be included in the sample. In fact, in nonprobability sampling, certain elements of the population may have no chance of being included in the sample. This restricts the generalizations that can be made about the study findings. Despite the limitations of nonprobability sampling, most nursing research studies involve this type of sampling procedure. True random samples are rare in nursing research.

The most frequent reasons for the use of nonprobability samples involve convenience and the desire to use available subjects. Samples may be chosen from available groups of subjects by several different methods, including convenience, quota, and purposive.

CONVENIENCE SAMPLING **Convenience sampling** is also referred to as *accidental* or *incidental*, and involves choosing readily available people or objects for a study. These elements may or may not be typical of the population. There is no accurate way to determine their representativeness. It is easy to see that this may be a very unreliable method of sampling. However, convenience sampling has probably been the most frequently used sampling method in nursing research. A search of the literature confirms that this type of sampling continues to be popular among current researchers.

Convenience samples are chosen because of the savings in time and money. The researcher may choose a convenience sample from familiar people, as when a teacher uses students in her or his class, or from strangers, such as might be encountered when a nurse researcher conducts a survey among family members in an intensive care unit waiting room to determine their attitudes about visiting hours.

Convenience Sample

Poreddi et al. (2016) utilized a convenience sample of 172 nursing students enrolled in the second, third, and fourth year of the nursing program, with 158 students who completed the questionnaires. The intent was to examine nursing students' knowledge and attitudes regarding child abuse and neglect, and the relationships between the research variables.

Another method of obtaining a convenience sample is through **snowball sampling**, also called **network sampling**. This term is used to describe a method of sampling that involves the assistance of study subjects to help obtain other potential subjects. Suppose the researcher wanted to determine how to help people stop cigarette smoking. The researcher might know of someone who has been successful in refraining from cigarette smoking for 10 years. This person is contacted and asked if he or she knows others who have also been successful. This type of networking is particularly helpful in finding people who may be reluctant to make their identity known, such as substance abusers.

Snowball Sample

Gazarian (2014) used a snowball sampling technique to recruit nurses to participate in a study that was focused on the observations of RNs in a milieu of monitor alarms with any correlations to patient deterioration. The 2011 study included continuous monitoring, ECG monitoring, frequency and types of alarms, associated nursing interventions, and impact on the patient's plan of care.

QUOTA SAMPLING Quota sampling is similar to stratified random sampling in that the first step involves dividing the population into homogeneous strata and selecting sample elements from each of these strata. The difference lies in the means of securing potential subjects from these strata. Stratified random sampling involves a random sampling method of obtaining sample members, whereas quota sampling obtains members through convenience samples.

The term *quota* arises from the researcher's establishment of a desired quota or proportion for some population variable of interest. The basis of stratification should be a variable of importance to the study. These variables frequently include subject attributes such as age, gender, and educational background. The number of elements chosen from each stratum is generally in proportion to the size of that stratum in the total population. For example, if the researcher wanted to determine whether more males or females receive yearly physical examinations, an equal proportion of males and females should be approached for the study. If convenience sampling is used, the two genders may not be equally represented in the sample. If a sample of 100 were desired, a quota of 50% males and 50% females would be set. Then, the first 50 males and first 50 females approached by the researcher would be asked to participate in the survey. Of course, because this would not be a probability sample, there is a risk that the sample would not be typical of all males and females. Examples of quota samples are difficult to find in recent studies published by nurses.

Quota Sample

From 2012 to 2013, Petkovšek-Gregorin and Skela-Savic (2015) obtained a quota sample to interview Slovenian nursing employees for their opinions on the importance of nursing documentation. A total of 592 respondents, nurses with at least a college degree, attributed more importance to documentation compared to those with only a secondary education.

PURPOSIVE SAMPLING **Purposive sampling** involves handpicking of subjects. This method is also called **judgmental sampling**. Subjects the researcher or an expert believes represent the accessible population may be recruited to join the study. This type of sampling is based on the assumption that the researcher or chosen expert has enough knowledge about the population of interest to select specific subjects for the study.

An investigator might want to determine some of the problems that are experienced by individuals with cancer who have a Port-a-Cath inserted for the administration of their chemotherapy. The investigator works in an oncology clinic and personally knows several clients who have been experiencing problems with their ports. These potential subjects are viewed as typical cases and asked to participate in the planned research study. It is evident that bias can enter into the selection of samples through purposive sampling procedures. Researchers may believe that errors in judgment will tend to balance out; purposive samples are not uncommon in nursing research. Most qualitative studies use purposive samples.

Purposive Sample

A purposive sample of Russian students from three nursing schools were recruited to respond to questionnaires regarding their knowledge of HIV and Acquired Immuno-Deficiency Syndrome (AIDS) and their attitudes toward caring for people/patients living with HIV or AIDS in 2010 (Suominen et al., 2015). The researchers also explored responses that were suggestive of the subjects' possible homophobic attitudes. The study questionnaires were offered to 107 students; the response rate was 95.3%.

Time Frame for Studying the Sample

The time frame for selecting and studying subjects in a research study is the criterion by which research studies are classified as longitudinal or cross-sectional. A **longitudinal study** follows subjects over a period of time in the future; a **cross-sectional study** examines subjects at one point in time. There is no agreed-upon time period for designating a study as longitudinal. Technically, if the researcher is interested in changes that occur over time, the research should be considered longitudinal, even if the time period is only 1 month or even 1 week.

A special type of longitudinal study is a cohort study. In a **cohort study**, the focus is on a subgroup of the population, frequently persons who are of a similar age group. In 1976, a large cohort of registered nurses became participants in the Nurses' Health Study (NHS), a longitudinal study that was conducted by researchers at Harvard Medical School. The population consisted of married female RNs born between January 1, 1921, and December 31, 1946, and residing in 11 states with the largest number of RNs: New York, California, Pennsylvania, Ohio, Massachusetts, New Jersey, Michigan, Texas, Florida, Connecticut, and Maryland. The original sample for this study was composed of approximately 122,000 nurses. The study was designed to examine some of the health risks that pose a special threat to women. Some of the identified risks were cigarette smoking, the use of hair dyes, and the use of oral contraceptives. Nurses were chosen as the subjects for this study, according to Frank Speizer, the principal investigator, because the study called for "a sophisticated group of individuals who could report exposure and diseases more accurately than the general population" ("Massive Nurses' Health Study," 1983, p. 998). The study was later expanded to examine dietary patterns, stress factors, and the use of prescription drugs. In one of the study's more publicized aspects, 68,000 nurses sent their toenail clippings to be examined for dietary intakes of selenium. The relationship between selenium intake and cancer was being examined.

The Nurses' Health Study was originally intended to last for only 4 years, but additional funding has been received through the years, and the study has continued for approximately 35 years. A similar but younger cohort group of approximately 123,000 nurses began participating in the Nurses' Health Study II (NHS II) in 1989. One of the purposes of this study was to examine the long-term effects of contraceptive use. By 1989, most of those in the original study group no longer had to worry about contraceptives. A third arm of the Nurses' Health Study began in 1996 with approximately 11,000 children of the Nurses Health Study II participants. The main purpose of this study was to explore adolescent weight gain. Hundreds of articles have been published about the results of data gathered in all of these studies. The Nurses' Health Study III (NHS III) was begun in 2008. For more details on these studies and the entire project, visit the Nurse's Health study website.

The data-collection process in a cross-sectional study is quite different from that of a longitudinal study. Data are gathered on subjects at *one* specific point in time, but the data are collected from separate groups of people who represent different ages, time periods, or developmental states. Consider the previous example in which the school nurse was interested in studying marijuana usage among high school students. She wanted to know if changes in usage occur as students progress through high school. A longitudinal study might be conducted in which freshman students would be followed until graduation, and their marijuana usage compared over the 4 years of high school. Because of the time factor and cost involved in such a lengthy study, the nurse researcher might decide to gather all of the data at one time by sampling students in all four grades of high school and comparing the marijuana usage among these groups. Of course, the danger in this type of study is that an assumption must be made that the seniors will reply as the freshmen would have replied at the end of 4 years. This might be a risky assumption. A longitudinal study is a more accurate means of studying changes that occur over time. However, cross-sectional studies are conducted because they are less expensive and easier to conduct than longitudinal studies.

Cross-Sectional Study

Lukewich et al. (2015) studied undergraduate nursing students' self-reported confidence in learning about key patient safety competency areas outlined in the Safety Competency Framework from 2010 to 2013.

The researchers used a nested cohort of students enrolled in a bachelor of nursing science program at one Canadian university.

Sampling Concepts and Factors

Sample Size

One of the most frequent questions posed to statisticians is "How large should my sample be?" Unfortunately, there is no simple answer. An important issue is whether the study will be of a quantitative or qualitative nature. Qualitative studies use much smaller samples than quantitative studies. Qualitative studies may use samples that are quite small, sometimes even smaller than 10. After patterns and themes have been extracted from the participants and no more new ideas are being uncovered, sampling ceases. Generally speaking, quantitative studies seek to obtain sample sizes large enough to talk about the population of interest.

There are no simple rules for determining the desired sample size for a quantitative study. Some factors to be considered are the homogeneity of the population, the degree of precision desired by the researcher, and the type of sampling procedure that will be used. If the population is very homogeneous, or alike, on all variables other than the one being measured, a small sample size may be sufficient. But if the researcher wants to be very precise in generalizing to the population based on sample data, a large sample may be necessary for the sample to represent the population accurately. Finally, when probability sampling methods are used, smaller samples are required than when nonprobability sampling techniques are employed.

According to Roscoe (1975), there are few instances in descriptive behavioral research when a sample size smaller than 30 or larger than 500 can be justified. A sample size of 100 ensures the benefits of the central limit theorem. Sample sizes as small as 30 are generally adequate to ensure that the sampling distribution of the mean will closely approximate the normal curve (Shott, 1990).

Large sample sizes may be needed in the following instances:

1. Many uncontrolled variables are present. The researcher thinks age may influence study results, but is not able to control for this variable.
2. Small differences are expected in members of the population on the variable of interest. Small, but important, differences between members of the population may not be uncovered when small samples are used.
3. The population must be divided into subgroups. Sample sizes must be increased to assure inclusion of members of each of the subgroups.
4. The dropout rate among subjects is expected to be high. This problem is especially likely to occur in longitudinal studies.
5. Statistical tests are used that require minimum sample sizes. Certain statistical tests require minimum numbers of responses in each cell of the data.

Although large samples are desirable, the law of diminishing returns applies. A sample of 100, or 10%, may be necessary to obtain the required precision desired for a population of 1000. A 10% sample of a population of 1 million would require 100,000 elements. This would be a huge sample and would be unnecessary. In fact, samples of 5000 or 6000 are often sufficient to estimate the characteristics of the entire population of the United States. The next time you see a Gallup survey report, make a note of the number of participants who were included in the sample. A more important issue than the size of the sample is the representativeness of the sample. Election results can be predicted with very small percentages of votes counted because the polled voters have been thoroughly examined for representativeness in voting behavior. Does it make you angry when you see the media predict the winner of an election when only 25% of the votes are in?

It is always wise to set the sample size a little bit larger than what is actually desired (to allow for nonresponse or subject dropout). Also, an absolute minimum sample size should be declared at the beginning of a study. Should the study be conducted if only five people agree to participate? The researcher must make the decision about the minimum acceptable sample size before data collection begins.

Power analysis is a procedure that can be used to determine the needed sample size for a research study. Researchers want to ensure that they have enough sample elements to detect a difference or a correlation, if one actually exists between groups or within groups on some variable of interest. This procedure is very important in experimental studies. The power of a statistical test is its ability to detect statistical significance in a study, when it is present. When power is low, the likelihood of making a type II error is high. One factor that influences the power of a test is the sample size that was used in the study. In many studies, researchers erroneously conclude that no significant difference exists between the experimental and the control group when, in fact, a difference would have been detected if the sample had been larger.

Connelly (2008) asserted that a trade-off exists between obtaining the desired sample size and the amount of time and resources available for a study. She also contended that it would be unethical to sample more people than is really needed, especially if the study is invasive.

Power Analysis

A study was conducted to investigate the levels of the implementation of knowledge management and outcomes of nursing performance from a sample of 192 nurses from three large healthcare organizations in South Korea (Lee, Kim, & Kim, 2014). The researchers examined the relationships between core knowledge management factors and nursing performance outcomes, and identified core knowledge management factors that affect these outcomes. The sample size for this study was calculated using G Power 3 analysis software, and it was determined that 191 subjects would be needed to complete the study to avoid the risk of a type II error.

Polit and Sherman (1990) studied 62 articles that were published in *Nursing Research* and *Research in Nursing and Health* during 1989. They concluded that a substantial number of published studies (and they presumed that even more unpublished studies) had insufficient power because of small sample sizes. However, a more recent review of the literature indicates that an increasing number of researchers have discussed the use of power analysis to determine their sample size. Cohen, Jia, and Larson (2009) evaluated the use of power analysis in 152 studies published between September 2005 and August 2007 in five top nursing research journals. They concluded that power analysis was included in about one third (46 of 122) of the studies in which power analysis would have been appropriate.

A review of nursing literature in the past few years revealed many examples of studies in which power analysis was used: Bryer, Cherkis, and Raman (2013); Choi and Staggs (2014); and Gaskin and Happell, (2013; 2014).

The researcher would be wise to perform a power analysis before conducting a study. If this analysis indicates that the needed sample size would be very difficult to obtain, the researcher might decide not to conduct the study. Nearly all external funding sources require that grant proposals present the results of the power analysis conducted to determine the optimum sample size for the proposed study. Although the procedure is not very difficult to perform, it is not discussed in this text. For more information, consult Cohen's (1988) book on power analysis.

Many nursing research studies are limited to small convenience samples. Generalizations to total populations, therefore, are usually difficult to make with any degree of confidence. The use of small sample sizes dictates the need for studies to be replicated. If several investigators find similar results when studying the same topic, generalizations to other populations are more appropriate.

Sampling Error and Sampling Bias

Although sampling error and sampling bias are sometimes discussed interchangeably, these two concepts should be considered separately. **Sampling error** may be defined as the difference between data obtained from a random sample and the data that would be obtained if an entire population were measured. Error may be contained in sample data even when the most careful random sampling procedure was used to obtain the sample. Sampling error is not under the researcher's control; it is caused by the chance variations that may occur when a sample is chosen to represent a population. Table 12–2 demonstrates how random samples vary from the true population values. The table contains pulse measurements on a population of 20 subjects. The mean pulse rate for the population is 71. The mean pulse rate for random sample 3 is also 71. The mean pulse rate for random sample 1 is considerably below the average for the population; the mean pulse rate for random sample 2 is well above the average.

Whereas sampling error occurs by chance, sampling bias is caused by the researcher. **Sampling bias** occurs when samples are not carefully selected. If names are written on slips of paper and placed in a hat, each piece of paper would have to be the same size and thickness or bias could occur. Bias could also occur if the slips of paper stuck together in clumps. The literature is replete with examples of bias in sample selections. One of the most famous examples concerns the U.S. presidential election of 1936. *Literary Digest* magazine conducted a large poll among eligible voters to determine if people planned to vote for Alfred Landon, the Republican candidate, or Franklin Roosevelt, the Democratic candidate. The magazine predicted, on the basis of this poll, that Landon would win by a landslide margin. Roosevelt soundly defeated Landon. It was determined that biased sampling occurred as the result of selecting subjects from the telephone directory and through listings of automobile registrations. Depressed economic conditions were present in 1936, and members of the Republican Party were more likely than members of the Democratic Party to own telephones and automobiles.

All nonprobability sampling methods are subject to sampling bias. Also, random sampling procedures are subject to bias if some elements of the selected sample decide not to participate in the research study. If questionnaires were sent to a random sample of nurses to examine their knowledge of malpractice issues in nursing, it is possible that nurses who possessed considerable knowledge of malpractice issues would be more likely to return the questionnaire than nurses with little knowledge of this subject.

After the discussion about various types of sampling procedures, it must be pointed out that nursing research studies involve voluntary subjects, regardless of the type of sampling procedure employed. Even if a random sampling method is used to select potential study subjects, the ethics of research requires that subjects must voluntarily agree to participate in research studies. Not all selected subjects may agree to participate in a study. The nurse researcher must always keep in mind that data are based on

Table 12–2 Sampling Error

Average pulse rates of a group of cardiac patients	66	80	59	70	71	
	71	63	70	74	55	
	70	65	67	92	83	
	67	79	66	80	72	$\mu = 71$
Random Sample #1	66, 59, 70, 55, 66			$\bar{x} = 63$		
Random Sample #2	80, 92, 83, 79, 80			$\bar{x} = 83$		
Random Sample #3	71, 71, 70, 64, 67			$\bar{x} = 71$		

μ = population mean; $\bar{x}$ = sample mean.

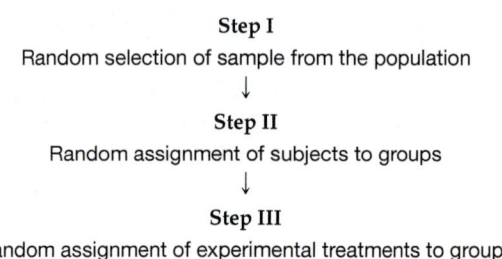

Figure 12–1 Randomization steps in experimental research.

voluntary responses. Unless all selected members of the sample actually participate in the research study, the potential for a biased sample is present.

Finally, a note of caution is presented about volunteers. **Volunteers** are subjects who approach the researcher asking to participate in the study. This type of sample is to be distinguished from a convenience sample, in which the researcher approaches the potential subjects and asks them to participate in a study. Volunteers may be greater risk takers than nonvolunteers. They also may be motivated to participate by monetary or other types of rewards.

Wewers and Ahijevych (1990) pointed out the differences between random samples and volunteer subjects. They studied the reactions of two groups of adult cigarette smokers to a smoking cessation campaign. One group was obtained through random telephone digit dialing; the other group was composed of volunteers who registered through the community lung association. The demographic characteristics, such as educational levels, were very different between the two groups. The volunteer group was found to be much more successful at attempting and maintaining cessation when compared to the randomly selected group. They confirmed that problems of generalizability exist when nonprobability samples are used in a study.

Randomization Procedures in Research

Random sampling and random assignment are two areas that seem to cause a great deal of confusion among beginning researchers. These two terms involve quite different aspects of the research process, but both are considered a type of randomization procedure. *Random sampling* involves the selection of a sample from the population. *Random assignment* involves the unbiased placement of subjects to either the experimental or control groups in a study. Random assignment is a necessary condition of a true experimental design. It seems important to discuss this concept again because of the tendency to confuse the two types of randomization procedures. Figure 12–1 depicts the threefold randomization process for experimental studies that would represent the ideal study procedure. First, subjects are randomly selected from the population. Next, subjects are randomly assigned to groups. Finally, experimental treatments are randomly assigned to the groups.

Critiquing the Sampling Procedure

The critiquer of a research study should be concerned with the study population and sample. A research article or report may include a separate section on the population and sample, but this information is usually contained in the methods section. It is generally easy to find the information about the sample, but the population from which the sample was selected may not be discussed.

The reader of a research report would like to know the group to which the investigator wishes to generalize the study results (target population) and the group from which the sample was selected (accessible population). To help the reader determine if the sample represents the accessible population, the report should describe the accessible population. The characteristics of the members of this group should be presented, such as average age, gender, and educational level. The size of the accessible population should also be presented. If a study had 100 subjects, the reader of the report would like to know if these 100 subjects represent merely a fraction of the accessible population or a large portion of this group.

The specific type of probability or nonprobability sampling method should be presented. Although probability sampling is the ideal, many nursing research studies use nonprobability samples. The reader should try to determine how the sample was obtained. Were the subjects volunteers, or were they approached and asked to participate in the study? The characteristics of the sample should be described.

The sample size is a very important area for critique. Many nursing studies have used small, nonrandom samples. If a small sample size was used, did the researcher present the rationale for the sample size? Was power analysis used to determine the sample size? Were you able to determine if some of the subjects dropped out of the study? The researcher has an obligation to point out this fact to the reader. Frequently, the reader is made aware of subject dropout when examining the tables. For example, a sample size of n = 58 that is presented in a table may not agree with the sample size of 60 mentioned in the methods section. Two subjects have mysteriously disappeared. Box 12–1 presents guidelines for critiquing the sampling section of a research report.

Box 12–1 Guidelines for Critiquing the Sampling Procedure

1. Is the target population identified?
2. Is the accessible population identified?
3. Was a probability or nonprobability sampling method used?
4. Is the specific sampling method named?
5. Is the sampling method described?
6. Is the sampling method appropriate for the study?
7. Are the demographic characteristics of the sample presented?
8. Is the sample size adequate?
9. Is the sample representative of the population?
10. Are potential sampling biases identified?
11. Is subject dropout discussed?

Summary

Populations are complete sets of people or objects that possess some common characteristic of interest to the researcher. The investigator wishes to generalize study findings to a target population, but generally is able to study only an accessible population. Studying entire populations is time-consuming and expensive. Samples, or subsets of the population, are usually studied in nursing research. A single member of the population is called an element, and these elements are chosen from a sampling frame, or listing of the population elements.

Samples are chosen through two types of sampling procedures: probability and nonprobability. Probability sampling, or random sampling, involves random selection of a sample from a population. The four types of probability sampling methods are simple, stratified, cluster, and systematic. Simple random sampling assures that each element of the population has an equal and independent chance of being chosen. A table of random numbers may be used to obtain a random sample, which is usually computer-generated. Stratified random sampling involves dividing the population into subgroups, then random samples are chosen from these groups. In proportional stratified sampling, samples are chosen from each stratum, and these samples are in proportion to the size of that stratum in the total population. When strata are unequal in size, disproportional stratified sampling may be used to assure adequate samples from each stratum. Cluster random sampling involves sampling from large groups called *clusters*. Individual members of clusters are selected in the final stage of the sampling process. Finally, in systematic random sampling every *k*th element of the population, such as every fifth element, is selected.

In nonprobability sampling, the sample elements are chosen by nonrandom methods. The types of nonprobability sampling methods are convenience, quota, and purposive. Convenience sampling, also called accidental or incidental, uses readily available people or objects. Snowball sampling, also called network sampling, is a type of convenience sampling in which subjects provide the names of other people they know who meet the criteria for the study. Quota sampling is similar to stratified random sampling, except that the desired number of elements for each stratum is selected through convenience sampling rather that random sampling. Purposive sampling, or judgmental sampling, involves handpicking of subjects based on the researcher's consideration or that of an expert as to the subjects being typical of the desired sample.

Longitudinal studies gather data from the same subjects several times to determine change associated with the passage of time. In a cohort study, a subgroup of the population is studied, frequently people in a similar age group. Cross-sectional studies examine several different groups that are thought to represent different age groups, time periods, or developmental states. Data are gathered at one point in time.

Generally, large samples are more representative of the population than small samples. As a rule, a sample size of 30 should be considered the minimum size for each group that is studied. Power analysis is a procedure that can be used to determine the optimum sample size for a study, particularly an experimental study.

Sampling error is the difference between data obtained from samples and data that would be obtained if an entire population was studied. This error is related to chance and not under the researcher's control. Sampling bias occurs when samples are not carefully selected by researchers. Volunteers are subjects who approach the researcher asking to participate in a study.

Randomization procedures in research involve random sampling and random assignment. Random sampling concerns selection of a sample from a population. Random assignment involves the unbiased assignment of subjects into groups in experimental studies.

Self-Test

Indicate if true or false
1. The best means of obtaining an unbiased sample of subjects in a community is to select a random sample of names from the telephone directory.
2. Nonprobability sampling means there is no probability that the subjects selected will constitute a biased sample.
3. Researchers generally study samples rather than populations.

4. A sampling frame is a listing of all elements of a population.

Indicate the type of sampling method used for each of the following examples in questions 5 through 10.

5. The clients in the hypertension clinics of two local hospitals are studied.
   A. Convenience
   B. Cluster
   C. Systematic random sampling
   D. Quota sampling
   E. Simple random sampling
   F. Snowball sampling

6. A total of 20 nursing service administrators are randomly selected from a random sample of 10 hospitals in the state.
   A. Convenience
   B. Cluster
   C. Systematic random sampling
   D. Quota sampling
   E. Simple random sampling
   F. Snowball sampling

7. To obtain mothers of children with cystic fibrosis, a researcher contacted one such mother who lived in her neighborhood and asked her if she knew any other mothers of children with cystic fibrosis.
   A. Convenience
   B. Cluster
   C. Systematic random sampling
   D. Quota sampling
   E. Simple random sampling
   F. Snowball sampling

8. Every fifth nurse is randomly selected from the mailing list of the American Nurses Association.
   A. Convenience
   B. Cluster
   C. Systematic random sampling
   D. Quota sampling
   E. Simple random sampling
   F. Snowball sampling

9. To determine the frequency of the recording of nursing diagnoses by nurses, a sample of 100 charts is randomly selected from all of the patients' charts during the previous year
   A. Convenience
   B. Cluster
   C. Systematic random sampling
   D. Quota sampling
   E. Simple random sampling
   F. Snowball sampling

10. The first 30 men and first 30 women who are admitted to the hospital for abdominal surgery during the time of the research study are asked to participate.
    A. Convenience
    B. Cluster
    C. Systematic random sampling
    D. Quota sampling
    E. Simple random sampling
    F. Snowball sampling

See answers to Self-Test in the Answer Section at the back of the book.

References

Adams, L. Y., Koop, P., Quan, H., & Norris, C. (2015). A population-based comparison of the use of acute healthcare services by older adults with and without mental illness diagnoses. *Psychiatric & Mental Health Nursing, 22*(1), 39–46. doi:10.1111/jpm.12169

Amini, K., Negarandeh, R., Ramezani-Badr, F., Moosaeifard, M., & Fallah, R. (2015). Nurses' autonomy level in teaching hospitals and its relationship with the underlying factors. *International Journal of Nursing Practice, 21*, 552–559. doi:10.1111/ijn.12210

Bryer, J., Cherkis, F., & Raman, J. (2013). Health-promotion behaviors of undergraduate nursing students: A survey analysis. *Nursing Education Perspectives, 34*(6), 410–415. doi:10.5480/11-614

Chen, H. C., & Lo, H. S. (2015). Nursing student satisfaction with an associated nursing program. *Nursing Education Perspectives, 36*(1), 27–33. doi:10.5480/13-1268

Choi, J., & Staggs, V. S. (2014). Comparability of nurse staffing measures in examining the relationship between RN staffing and unit-acquired pressure ulcers: A unit-level descriptive, correlational study. *International Journal of Nursing Studies, 51*, 1344–1352. http://dx.doi.org/10.1016/j.ijnurstu.2014.02.011

Cohen, J. (1988). *Statistical power analysis for the behavioral sciences* (2nd ed.). Hillsdale, NJ: Lawrence Erlbaum Associates.

Connelly, L. M. (2008). Research considerations: Power analysis and effect size. *Medsurg Nursing, 17*, 41–42. http://www.medsurgnursing.net/cgi-bin/WebObjects/MSNJournal.woa

Gaskin, C. J., & Happell, B. (2013). Power of mental health nursing research: A statistical analysis of studies in the International Journal of Mental Health Nursing. *International Journal of Mental Health Nursing, 22*, 69–75. doi:10.1111/j.1447-0349.2012.00845.x

Gaskin, C. J., & Happell, B. (2014). Power, effects, confidence, and significance: An investigation of statistical practices in nursing research. *International Journal of Nursing Studies, 51*, 795–806. http://dx.doi.org/10.1016/j.ijnurstu.2013.09.014

Gazarian, P. K. (2014). Nurses' response to frequency and types of electrocardiography alarms in a non-critical care setting: A descriptive study. *International Journal of Nursing Studies, 51*, 190–197. doi:10.1016/j.ijnurstu.2013.05.014

Lee, E. J., Kim, H. S., & Kim, H. Y. (2014). Relationships between core factors of knowledge management in hospital nursing organizations and outcomes of nursing performance. *Clinical Nursing, 23*, 3513–3524. doi:10.1111/jocn.12603

Lukewich, J., Edge, D. S., Tranmer, J., Raymond, J., Miron, J., Ginsburg, L., & VanDenKerkhof, E. (2015). Undergraduate baccalaureate nursing students' self-reported confidence in learning about patient safety in the classroom and clinical settings: An annual cross-sectional study (2010-2013). *International Journal of Nursing Studies, 52*, 930–938. doi:10.1016/j.ijnurstu.2015.01.010

Massive nurses' health study in seventh year, reports first findings on disease links in women. (1983). *American Journal of Nursing, 83*, 998–999. http://journals.lww.com/ajnonline/pages/default.aspx

Penders, Y., Albers, G., Deliens, L., Vander Stichele, R., & Van den Block, L. (2015). Awareness of dementia by family carers of nursing home residents dying with dementia: A post-death study. *Palliative Medicine, 29*(1), 38–47. doi:10.1177/0269216314542261

Petkovšek-Gregorin, R., & Skela-Savic, B. (2015). Nurses' perceptions and attitudes towards documentation in nursing. *Obzornik Zdravstvene Nege, 49*(2), 106–125. doi:10.14528/snr.2015.49.2.50

Polit, D. F., & Sherman, R. E. (1990). Statistical power in nursing research. *Nursing Research, 39*, 365–369. http://journals.lww.com/nursingresearchonline/pages/default.aspx

Poreddi, V., Pashapu, D. R., Kathyayani, B. V., Gandhi, S., El-Arousy, W., & Math, S. B. (2016). Nursing students' knowledge of child abuse and neglect in India. *British Journal of Nursing, 25*(5), 264–268. http://info.britishjournalofnursing.com/

Pradap, J. (2015). Effectiveness of planned teaching programme on knowledge regarding body mechanics among nursing students in selected nursing college of Mangalore taluk. *Asian Journal of Nursing Education & Research, 5*(2), 217–220. doi:10.5958/2349-2996.2015.00043.9

Roscoe, J. (1975). *Fundamental research statistics for the behavioral sciences* (2nd ed.). New York: Holt, Rinehart & Winston.

Shott, S. (1990). *Statistics for health care professionals*. Philadelphia: W. B. Saunders.

Suominen, T., Laakkonen, L., Lioznov, D., Polukova, M., Nikolaenko, S., Lipiäinen, L., . . .Kylma, J. (2015). Russian nursing students' knowledge level and attitudes in the context of human immunodeficiency virus (HIV) – a descriptive study. *BioMed Central Nursing, 14*(1). doi:10.1186/s12912-014-0053-7

Wewers, M. E., & Ahijevych, K. (1990). Differences in volunteer and randomly acquired samples. *Applied Nursing Research, 3*, 166–173. http://dx.doi.org/10.1016/S0897-1897(05)80140-5

Chapter 13
Measurement and Data Collection

Rose Nieswiadomy, PhD, RN, and Catherine Bailey, PhD, RN

Objectives

On completion of this chapter, you will be prepared to:

1. Differentiate among the four levels of measurement.
2. Compare data-collection methods and instruments.
3. Compare and contrast the concepts of reliability and validity.
4. Explain the factors and issues that impact data collection.

Introduction

Now the fun part of a research study begins. All of the preliminary phases of the study have been completed, and data collection is about to start. Many researchers are excited when they talk about the data-collection phase of their studies. This is the time when they get to interact with their study participants personally or through reading their responses on questionnaires. The real detective work begins.

In any study, the investigator must devise a way to examine or measure the concepts of interest. For example, anxiety could be measured in several ways, such as through galvanic skin response, pulse rates, or self-report questionnaires.

Measurement

An understanding of measurement principles is crucial in the data-collection phase of a study. Research variables must be operationally defined. As stated elsewhere, operational definitions indicate how variables will be observed or measured. An operational definition should not be confused with a conceptual definition, which is a dictionary definition of an abstract idea that is being studied by the researcher.

Measurement is the process of assigning numbers to variables. Ways to assign these numbers include counting, ranking, and comparing objects or events. Human beings have been using some type of measurement system throughout history. Probably fingers and toes were the first method of counting and keeping track of numbers. Measurement, as used in research, implies the quantification of information. This means that numbers are assigned to the data. Some qualitative studies gather data in narrative form, and numbers are not associated with these types of data. Thus, the narrative types of data that are collected from qualitative studies are not included in the concept of measurement as it is discussed in this book. However, you should know that if qualitative data were summarized and placed into categories, they would then fit the criteria for measurement. In the classic sense, measurement implies that some kind of comparison is made between pieces of information. Numbers are the means of comparing this information.

Level of Measurement

The types of mathematical calculations that can be made with data depend on the level of measurement of the data. The terms *level of measurement* and *measurement scale* are frequently used interchangeably. Four levels of measurement or measurement scales have been identified: nominal, ordinal, interval, and ratio.

While using the **nominal level of measurement**, objects or events are named or categorized. The categories must be distinct from each other (mutually exclusive categories) and include all of the possible ways of categorizing the data (exhaustive categories). There may be only two categories, or there may be many categories. Numbers are obtained for this type of data through counting the frequency or percentages of objects or events in each of the categories.

Examples of types of nominal data are gender, religious affiliation, marital status, and political party membership. The researcher could count the number of males and females in a study and report these as percentages or frequencies. No other mathematical operations could be performed with these data. You may have noticed that these types of variables are frequently assigned numbers on questionnaires, such as 0 for males and 1 for females. These numbers are only symbols used for data analysis purposes, and have no quantitative meaning.

Some types of nominal data may appear to contain what we call *real* numbers. Examples are Zip Codes and Social Security numbers. Actually, these numbers are symbols and can be placed only into categories. They should not be added or subtracted. The nominal level of measurement is considered the lowest level or least rigorous of the measurement levels.

Data that can be rank ordered as well as placed into categories are considered to be at the **ordinal level of measurement**. The exact differences between the ranks cannot be specified with this type of data. The numbers obtained from this measurement process indicate the order rather than the exact quantity of the variables. For example, anxiety levels of people in a therapy group might be categorized as mild, moderate, and severe. It would be appropriate to conclude that those individuals with severe anxiety are more anxious than those individuals with moderate anxiety. In turn, moderate anxiety sufferers in the group could be considered more anxious than group members with mild anxiety. You could not, however, determine the exact difference in anxiety levels of any individual within each of the categories. Frequency distributions and percentages are used with this type of data as well as some statistical tests.

Interval data consist of real numbers. **Interval level of measurement** concerns data that not only can be placed in categories and ranked, but also the distance between the ranks can be specified. The categories in interval data are the actual numbers on the scale, such as on a thermometer. If body temperature was being measured, a reading of 37°C might be one category, 37.2°C might be another category, and 37.4°C might constitute a third category. The researcher would be correct in saying that there is a 0.2°C difference between the first and second category, and between the second and third category. The researcher could even go one step further and find the average temperature reading.

Data collected at the ratio level of measurement are considered the highest or most precise level of data. **Ratio level of measurement** includes data that can be categorized and ranked; in addition, the distance between ranks can be specified, and what is referred to as a true or natural zero point can be identified. The zero point on the ratio scale means there is a total absence of the quantity being measured. The amount of money in your bank account could be considered ratio data because it is possible to be zero. Similarly, if a researcher wanted to determine the number of pain medication requests made by patients; it would be possible for some patients' requests to rank at the natural zero point because they request no pain medications. This type of data would be considered ratio data.

There is a debate about classifying some data as interval or ratio. For example, should weight be considered as interval or ratio data? Most authors classify weight as ratio data. However, when measuring humans, can someone have *no* weight?

Although it may be great fun to debate about whether a certain piece of data should be classified as interval or ratio, for research purposes it is really unimportant to distinguish between these two levels of measurement. The same statistical tests may be used with both types of data.

Converting Data to a Lower Level of Measurement

Data can always be converted from one level to a lower level of measurement, but not to a higher level. Interval and ratio data can be converted to ordinal or nominal data, and ordinal data can be converted to nominal data. For example, the number of requests by patients for pain medication could be converted to ordinal data. Requests could be categorized as follows: more than 10 requests per day, 5–10 requests per day, and 0–4 requests per day. This would be an instance of converting interval data to ordinal data. It would also be possible to change these data to nominal data by classifying the subjects into two groups: those with "no requests per day" and those with "1 or more requests per day." Rarely do researchers convert higher levels of data to lower levels, however, because precision is always lost. This means that this type of data ("1 or more requests per day") is not the most accurate reflection of the true value of the data. In this case, it could mean 2 or 20 requests per day.

Determining the Appropriate Level of Measurement

Now that you are familiar with the levels of measurement, you may wonder how one should determine which level of measurement to use in a study. If the researcher is very concerned about the precision of the data, the interval or ratio level of measurement should be selected when possible. If ranked or categorized data will be sufficient to answer the research questions or test the research hypotheses, ordinal data may be used. Finally, if categories of data are all that is called for, nominal data will be appropriate.

If the researcher were trying to determine the differences in the number of complications experienced by patients with diabetes who have varying blood glucose levels, accuracy would be very important. The two categories of elevated and nonelevated blood glucose levels (nominal data) would not be precise enough for making comparisons among the patients. The operational definition of the variable will determine the level of data that will be gathered.

Some variables, by their very nature, can be measured at only one level. For example, gender can be measured at only a nominal level. A person is either a male or a female. The main considerations in determining the level of measurement for data are (a) the level of measurement appropriate for the type of data that are being sought, and (b) the degree of precision desired when it is possible to consider the data at more than one level of measurement.

Data-Collection Process

There are five important questions to ask when the researcher is in the process of collecting data: Who? When? Where? What? How? Use the acronym WWWWH.

Who will collect the data? If the researcher is going to collect all of the data, this question is easy to answer. However, scientific investigations frequently involve a team of researchers. The decision will then need to be made about who will collect the data. Other people outside the research team may also be used in the data-collection phase; sometimes data collectors are paid for their services. Anytime more than one person is involved, assurances must be made that the data are being gathered in the same manner. Training will be needed for the data collectors, and checks should be made on the reliability of the collected data.

When will the data be collected? The determination will need to be made about the month, day, and sometimes even the hour, for data collection. Also, how long will data collection take? Frequently, the only way to answer this question is through a trial run of the procedure by the researcher. If questionnaires will be used, they should be pretested with people similar to the potential research participants, to determine the length of time for completion of the instrument. The decision may be made to revise the instrument if it seems to take too long for completion. Unfortunately, data collection usually takes longer than envisioned.

Where will the data be collected? The setting for data collection must be carefully determined. Optimum conditions should be sought. Having participants fill out questionnaires in the middle of the hallway while leaning against a wall would definitely not provide the optimum setting. Sometimes it is difficult to decide on the setting. If questionnaires are being used, a researcher might ask respondents to complete the questionnaire while the researcher remains in the same immediate or general area. This procedure will help ensure return of the questionnaires. If the participants happen to be tired or the room is too hot or too cold, the answers that are provided may not be valid. If respondents are allowed to complete the questionnaires at leisure, their answers may be more accurate. A disadvantage of using this procedure may be a reduction in the return rate of the questionnaires.

What data will be collected? This question calls for a decision to be made about the type of data being sought. For example, is the study designed to measure knowledge, attitudes, or behaviors? The type of data needed to answer the research questions or to test the research hypothesis should be the main consideration in data collection. If the researcher is concerned with the way crises affect people, the "what" of data collection becomes persons' behaviors or responses in crises.

How will the data be collected? Some type of research instrument will be needed to gather the data. This can vary from a self-report questionnaire to the most sophisticated of physiological instruments. Choosing a data-collection instrument is a major decision that should be made only after careful consideration of the possible alternatives.

Data-Collection Methods

The variable(s) of interest to the researcher must be measured in some fashion. This measurement is carried out through various data-collection methods. Data-collection methods are governed by several factors, including (a) the research question(s) or hypothesis (es), (b) the design of the study, and (c) the amount of knowledge available about the variable of interest.

There are many alternatives to choose from when deciding on a data-collection method. Physiological measures, observation methods, self-report questionnaires, interviews, attitude scales, psychological tests, and other types of data-collection methods may be selected. Questionnaires are probably the most frequently reported method of data collection in published nursing studies.

Many studies use more than one data-collection method. In fact, nursing studies are increasingly reporting the use of more than one method of measuring the variable(s) of interest. When several types of data-collection methods produce similar results, greater confidence in the study findings will occur.

Data-Collection Instruments

Research instruments, also called research tools, are the devices used to collect data. The instrument facilitates the observation and measurement of the variables of interest. The type of instrument used in a study is determined by the data-collection method(s) selected. If physiological data are sought, some type of physiological instrument will be needed. If observational data are needed to measure the variable of interest, some type of observational schedule or checklist will be called for. One area of the research over which the investigator has a great deal of control is in the choice of the data-collection instrument. Great care should be taken to select the most appropriate instrument(s).

USE OF EXISTING INSTRUMENTS While conducting a review of the literature on the topic of interest, a researcher may discover that an instrument is already available to measure the research variable(s). The use of an already tested instrument helps connect the present study with the existing body of knowledge on the variables. Of course, the instrument selected must be appropriate to measure the study variable(s).

Many research instruments are available for nurse researchers. Some of the best sources are published compilations of instruments. These compilations are particularly useful because they contain discussions of the instruments, such as the reliability and validity of the tools. In some cases, the instrument is printed in its entirety in these sources. If not, information is provided about where a copy of the tool can be obtained.

The oldest and most well-known sources of research instruments are the *Mental Measurement Yearbooks* (MMYs). There are currently 19 volumes; the first was published in 1938, and the most recent one published in 2014. To be reviewed in the MMY, a test must be commercially available, be published in the English language, and be new, revised, or widely used since it last appeared in the MMY series.

A very useful source for nurse researchers is *Instruments for Clinical Health-Care Research* edited by Frank-Stromborg and Olsen (2004). Another well-used source of instruments for nursing research has been the four-volume series originally edited by Strickland and Waltz (1988a, 1988b, 1990a, 1990b). These volumes, titled *Measurement of Nursing Outcomes*, are devoted to measurement of client outcomes as well as nursing performance outcomes. A more recent publication edited by Doran (2011) and titled *Nursing Outcomes: The State of the Science* provides a comprehensive and critical analysis of outcomes that are relevant and sensitive to nursing interventions. Some examples of outcomes provide analyses of functional status, self-care, symptom management, pain as a symptom outcome, adverse patient outcomes, patient satisfaction as a nurse-sensitive outcome, and mortality rate as a nurse-sensitive outcome (Doran, 2011).

Other important types of nursing-sensitive measures, such as unit or hospital-based measures of nurse staffing, nurse satisfaction, and patient outcomes have been included in the National Database of Nursing Quality Indicators (NDNQI), which was introduced by the American Nursing Association (ANA) (Doran, 2015). This database currently represents over 2000 hospitals in the United States, and provides information from data that are collected from chart reviews, prevalence surveys, incident reports, patient census, payroll and human resources and surveys of nurses in direct patient care roles (Press Ganey, 2015). The measures within the database are intended to help provide benchmarks or set standards that will allow comparisons between hospitals in terms of nursing care quality and patient outcomes (Doran, 2015).

Many of the existing instruments are copyrighted. The copyright holder must be contacted to obtain permission to use such an instrument. Sometimes this permission is given without cost, and other times the researcher has to pay for permission to use the instrument or purchase copies of the tool. Instruments developed in research projects supported by public funding generally remain in the public domain. Investigators have free access to these types of instruments.

If an existing instrument will be used, it may be desirable to contact the developer of the instrument to obtain information on its use in past research. This information is usually provided freely. Tool developers are generally pleased when other researchers want to use their creations. Frequently, the only request that will be made is that a copy of the study results and the data, particularly data on the reliability and validity of the instrument, be forwarded to the person who developed the instrument.

DEVELOPING AN INSTRUMENT If no instrument can be discovered that is appropriate for a particular study, the researcher is faced with developing a new instrument. Also, it may be possible to revise an existing instrument. Caution must be exercised when this approach to instrument development is used. If any items are altered or deleted, or new items added to an existing instrument, the reliability and validity of the tool might be altered. New reliability and validity testing will need to be conducted. Also, permission to revise the instrument will have to be obtained from the developer of the tool.

The development of a completely new instrument is a demanding task. Volumes of books have been written concerning tool development. Consult some of these sources for further information on this subject.

PILOT STUDIES One of the primary reasons a pilot study is conducted is to pretest a newly designed instrument. Whenever a new instrument is being used in a study, or a preexisting instrument is being used with people who have different characteristics from those for whom the instrument was originally developed, a pilot study should be conducted.

A pilot study is a small-scale trial run of the actual research project. A group of individuals similar to the proposed study subjects should be tested in conditions similar to those that will be used in the actual study. No set number of persons is needed for a pilot study. Factors such as time, cost, and availability of persons similar to the study subjects help determine the size of the pilot group. In an article published in *American Nurse Today*, Kilanowski (2011) discussed how the pilot phase of a research study helps with the development and use of instruments. The readability, accuracy, and comprehensibility of the questionnaire or scale items can be assessed. They can also be used to determine if they are valid measurements, measuring what they are intended to measure and also to determine if the instruments reliably measure the intended concept in different populations from which they were developed.

Criteria for Selection of a Data-Collection Instrument

Several criteria must be considered when deciding on a data-collection instrument; these include the practicality, reliability, and validity of the instrument.

Practicality of the Instrument

Before the researcher examines the reliability and validity of an instrument, questions should be asked about the practicality of the tool for the particular study being planned. The practicality of an instrument concerns its cost and appropriateness for the study population. How much will the instrument cost? How long will it take to administer the instrument? Will the population have the physical and mental stamina to complete the instrument? Are special motor skills or language abilities required of participants? Does the researcher require special training to administer or score the instrument? If so, is this training available? If a psychological instrument such as the Minnesota Multiphasic Personality Inventory (MMPI) will be used, is money available to purchase the instrument, and is someone available who is qualified to analyze the data? These are very important questions; the researcher must attend to the practicality of the instrument before considering the reliability and validity of the instrument.

Reliability of the Instrument

The researcher is always interested in collecting data that are reliable. The **reliability** of an instrument concerns its consistency and stability. If you are using a thermometer to measure body temperature, you would expect it to provide the same reading each time it was placed in a constant temperature water bath.

Regardless of the type of research, the reliability of the study instrument(s) is always of concern. Reliability needs to be determined whether the instrument is a mechanical device, a written questionnaire, or a human observer. The degree of reliability is usually determined by the use of correlational procedures. A correlation coefficient is determined between two sets of scores or between the ratings of two judges: The higher the correlation coefficient, the more reliable is the instrument or the ratings from the judges.

Although correlation coefficients can range between −1.00 and +1.00, correlation coefficients computed to test the reliability of an instrument are expected to be positive correlations. Correlation coefficients computed to test the reliability of an instrument are expected to be positive correlations. According to Polit and Beck (2008, 2012), it is risky to use an instrument with a reliability lower than .70. These authors have cautioned researchers to check for reliability as a routine step in all studies that involve observational tools, self-report measures, or knowledge tests because of their susceptibility to measurement errors.

Correlation coefficients are frequently used to determine the reliability of an instrument. However, when observers or raters are used in a study, the percentage or rate of agreement may also be used to determine the reliability of their observations or ratings.

In general, the more items that an instrument contains, the more reliable it will be. The likelihood of coming closer to obtaining a true measurement increases as the sample of items to measure a variable increases. If a test becomes too long, subjects may get tired or bored.

Be cautious about the reliability of instruments. Reliability is not a property of the instrument that, once established, remains forever. Reliability must continually be assessed as the instrument is used with different subjects and under different environmental conditions. An instrument to measure patient autonomy might be highly reliable when administered to patients while in their hospital rooms, but very unreliable when administered to these same patients while lying on a stretcher outside the operating room waiting for surgery.

Researchers should choose the most appropriate type of reliability for their particular studies. Three different types of reliability are discussed here: stability, equivalence, and internal consistency.

STABILITY RELIABILITY The **stability reliability** of an instrument refers to its consistency over time. A physiological instrument, such as a thermometer, should be very stable and accurate. If a thermometer were to be used in a study, it would need to be checked for reliability before the study began and probably again during the study (test-retest reliability).

Questionnaires can also be checked for their stability. A questionnaire might be administered to a group of people, and, after a time, the instrument would again be administered to the same people. If subjects'

Test-Retest Reliability

Test-retest reliability was one of the properties evaluated for the Walking Questionnaire (De Laat, Rommers, Geertzen & Roorda, 2012). This instrument is a patient-reported measure of activity limitations in walking in people with a lower limb amputation. The questionnaire was completed twice by the same 33 individuals. Test-retest reliability from the first testing time to the second testing time was 3 weeks. The mean scores for the first and second testing time were 52 and 55 respectively. The intraclass correlation coefficient was .73 indicating that the instrument provided satisfactory reliability.

responses were almost identical both times, the instrument would be determined to have high test-retest reliability. If the scores were perfectly correlated, the correlation coefficient (coefficient of stability) would be 1.00. The interval between the two testing periods may vary from a few days to several months or even longer. This period is a very important consideration when trying to determine the stability of an instrument. The period should be long enough for the subjects to forget their original answers on the questionnaire, but not long enough that real changes may have occurred in the subjects' responses.

If you were interested in developing a test to measure a personality trait, such as assertiveness, you might expect stability of responses. But because there has been a great deal of emphasis on assertiveness training in recent years, subjects might not score the same on an assertiveness test if the period between administrations is more than a few days. Many nursing studies are concerned with attitudes and behaviors that are not stable, and changes would be expected on two administrations of the same questionnaire. Stability over time (test-retest reliability), therefore, may not be the appropriate type of reliability for a research instrument when you anticipate a change among the respondents over time.

EQUIVALENCE RELIABILITY **Equivalence reliability** concerns the degree to which two different forms of an instrument obtain the same results, or two or more observers using a single instrument obtain the same results. **Alternate forms reliability** and **parallel forms reliability** are terms used when two forms of the same instrument are compared. **Interrater reliability** and **interobserver reliability** are terms applied to the comparisons of raters or observers using the same instrument. This type of reliability is determined by the degree to which two or more independent raters or observers are in agreement.

Interrater Reliability

A study was conducted to determine the interrater reliability of a tool used to assess pain among noncommunicative patients with an acquired brain injury (ABI) (Vink, Eskes, Lindeboom, van den Munckhof & Vermeulen, 2014). Ten hospitalized patients with an ABI with a minimum score of 5 on a Glasgow Coma Scale were filmed during tactile and noxious stimulation. Twenty-seven registered nurses observed the videos of the patients and rated them on four behavioral items (motor, verbal, and visual responses and facial expression) on a 4-point scale on the Nocieception Coma Scale (NCS) and also on three behavioral items (motor, verbal responses, and facial expressions) on the revised version, the NCS-R. All of the average-measure intraclass correlations for observations among the registered nurses on the NCS and NCS-R exceeded .80, indicating excellent interrater reliability.

When two forms of a test are used, both forms should contain the same number of items, have the same level of difficulty, and so forth. One form of the test is administered to a group of people; the other form is administered either at the same time or shortly thereafter to these same people. A correlation coefficient (coefficient of equivalence) is obtained between the two forms. The higher the correlation, the more confidence the researcher can have that the two forms of the test are gathering the same information. Whenever two forms of an instrument can be developed, this is the preferred means for assessing reliability. However, researchers may find it difficult to develop one form of an instrument, much less two forms.

INTERNAL CONSISTENCY RELIABILITY **Internal consistency reliability**, or scale homogeneity, addresses the extent to which all items on an instrument measure the same variable. This type of reliability is appropriate only when the instrument is examining one concept or construct at a time. This type of reliability is concerned with the sample of items used to measure the variable of interest.

If an instrument is supposed to measure depression, for example, all of the items on the instrument must consistently measure depression. If some items measure guilt, the instrument is not an internally consistent tool. This type of reliability is of concern to nurse researchers because of the emphasis on measuring concepts such as assertiveness, autonomy, and self-esteem. However, in the case of an instrument that contains subscales of an instrument, such as an instrument that measures anxiety in terms of the state of anxiety and the trait of anxiety, you could calculate the internal consistency of both subscales.

Before computers, internal consistency was tedious to calculate. Today, it is a simple process, and accurate split-half procedures have been developed. A common type of internal consistency procedure used today is the coefficient alpha (α) or Cronbach's alpha, which provides an estimate of the reliability of all possible ways of dividing an instrument into two halves. Think about that a minute. How many possible combinations of two halves could be made from a 30-item questionnaire? A lot.

Internal Consistency Reliability

Internal consistency reliability was used to evaluate the psychometric properties of the Vitality Scan, which is intended to determine possible signs of stagnation in one's functioning related to sustainable employability (Brouwers, Engels, Heerkens, & van der Beek, 2015). Coefficient alpha revealed an internal consistency reliability of 5 subscales with acceptable to good reliability (Cronbach's alpha 0.72–0.87).

Validity of the Instrument

The **validity** of an instrument concerns its ability to gather the data that it is intended to gather. The content of the instrument is of prime importance in validity testing. If an instrument is expected to measure assertiveness, does it, in fact, measure assertiveness? It is not difficult to determine that validity is the most important characteristic of an instrument.

The greater the validity of an instrument, the more confidence you can have that the instrument will obtain data that will answer the research questions or test the research hypotheses. Just as the reliability of an instrument does not remain constant, neither does an instrument necessarily retain its level of validity when used with other research participants or in other environmental settings. An instrument might accurately measure assertiveness in a group of participants from one cultural group. The same instrument might actually measure authoritarianism in another cultural group because assertiveness, to this group, means that a person is trying to act as an authority figure.

When attempting to establish the reliability of an instrument, all of the procedures are based on data obtained through using the instrument with a group of respondents. Conversely, some of the procedures for establishing the validity of an instrument are not based on the administration of the instrument to a group of respondents. Validity may be established through the use of a panel of experts, or an examination of the existing literature on the topic. Statistical procedures, therefore, may not always be used in trying to establish validity as they are when trying to establish reliability. When statistical procedures are used in trying to establish validity, they generally are correlational procedures.

Four broad categories of validity are considered here: face, content, criterion, and construct. Face and content validity are concerned only with the instrument that is under consideration. Criterion and construct validity are concerned with how well the instrument under consideration compares with other measures of the variable of interest.

FACE VALIDITY An instrument is said to have **face validity** when a preliminary examination shows that it is measuring what it is supposed to measure. In other words, on the surface or the face of the instrument, it appears to be an adequate means of obtaining the data needed for the research project. The face validity of an instrument can be examined through the use of experts in the content area, or through the use of individuals who have characteristics similar to those of the potential research participants. Because of the subjective nature of face validity, this type of validity is rarely used alone.

> ## Face Validity
>
> Chippendale (2015) sought to establish face validity of an Outdoor Falls Questionnaire that was formulated from the results of a qualitative study that explored the experience of older adults in their neighborhood in relation to a perceived outdoor fall risk and fall prevention strategies. Changes in the original questionnaire were based on a survey design expert's recommendations after a review of the questionnaire for language, structure, and order of questions.

CONTENT VALIDITY Content validity is concerned with the scope or range of items used to measure the variable. In other words, are the number and type of items adequate to measure the concept or construct of interest? Is there an adequate sampling of all the possible items that could be used to secure the desired data? There are several methods of evaluating the content validity of an instrument.

The first method is accomplished by comparing the content of the instrument with material available in the literature on the topic. A determination can then be made of the adequacy of the measurement tool in light of existing knowledge in the content area. For example, if a new instrument were being developed to measure the empathic levels of nurses in hospice settings, the researcher would need to be familiar with the literature on both empathy and the hospice setting.

A second way to examine the content validity of an instrument is through the use of a panel of experts, a group of people who have expertise in a given subject area. These experts are given copies of the instrument and the purpose and objectives of the study. They then evaluate the instrument, usually individually rather than in a group. Comparisons are made between these evaluations, and the researcher then determines if additions, deletions, or other changes need to be made.

A third method is used when knowledge tests are being developed. The researcher develops a test blueprint designed around the objectives for the content being taught and the level of knowledge that is expected (e.g., retention, recall, and synthesis).

The actual degree of content validity is never established. An instrument is said to possess some degree of validity that can only be estimated.

> ## Content Validity
>
> During the development of the Outdoor Falls Questionnaire, five content experts in geriatrics were asked to rate each question on relevance to outdoor falls on a four-point scale that ranged from "not relevant" to "very relevant" (Chippendale, 2015). The expert reviewers included two occupational therapists, a physical therapist, and two nurse practitioners. The majority of questions (22 out of 32) were considered either "quite relevant" or "very relevant". Feedback from the content experts was incorporated into a revised questionnaire. Eighty percent (n = 4) of the reviewers rated the overall questionnaire as "very relevant," while 20% (n = 1) rated the questionnaire as "quite relevant."

CRITERION VALIDITY Criterion validity is concerned with the extent to which an instrument corresponds to, or is correlated with, some criterion measure of the variable of interest. Criterion validity assesses the ability of an instrument to determine the research participants' responses at the present time or predict participants' responses in the future. These two types of criterion validity are called concurrent and predictive validity, respectively.

Concurrent validity compares an instrument's ability to obtain a measurement of participants' behavior that is comparable to some other criterion of that behavior. Does the instrument under consideration correlate with another instrument that measures the same behavior or responses? For example, a researcher might want to develop a short instrument that would help evaluate the suicidal potential of people when they call in to a suicide crisis intervention center. A short, easily administered interview instrument would be of great help to the staff, but the researcher would want to be sure this instrument was a valid diagnostic instrument to assess suicide potential. Responses received on the short instrument could be compared with those received when using an already validated, but longer, suicide assessment tool. If both instruments seem to be obtaining the essential information necessary to make a decision about the suicide potential of a person, the new, shorter instrument might be considered to have criterion validity. The degree of validity would be determined through correlation of the results of the two tests administered to a number of people. The correlation coefficient must be at least .70 to consider that the two instruments are obtaining similar data.

The second type of criterion validity, **predictive validity**, is concerned with the ability of an instrument to predict behavior or responses of subjects in the future. If the predictive validity of an instrument

Concurrent Validity

Two experienced nurses assessed 20 forensic mental health service patients with two tools that measure the risk of violence toward others during a stay and after discharge from a psychiatric hospital (Bjorkly, Eidhammer, & Selmer, 2014). The HCR-20 was developed to evaluate 20 key risk factors, while the HCR-20^{V3} (or Version 3) was revised to include a seven-step structure to guide risk management and the development of treatment and management strategies to mitigate risk. Pearson's r was used to calculate correlation coefficients for the association between the two versions of instruments. Concurrent validity testing revealed a significant correlation between the Version 2 and Version 3 concerning total scores for presence ($r = .58$, $p = 0.007$) and relevance ($r = .55$, $p = 0.007$).

is established, it can be used with confidence to discriminate between people, at the present time, in relation to their future behavior. This would be a very valuable quality for an instrument to possess. For example, a researcher might be interested in knowing if a suicidal potential assessment tool would be useful in predicting actual suicidal behavior in the future.

CONSTRUCT VALIDITY Of all of the types of validity, construct validity is the most difficult to measure. **Construct validity** is concerned with the degree to which an instrument measures the construct it is supposed to measure. A construct is a concept or abstraction created or "constructed" by the researcher. Construct validity involves the measurement of a variable that is not directly observable, but rather is an abstract concept derived from observable behavior. Construct validity is derived from the underlying theory that is used to describe or explain the construct.

Many of the variables measured in research are labeled constructs. Nursing is concerned with constructs such as anxiety, assertiveness, and androgyny.

One method to measure construct validity is called the **known-groups procedure**, in which the instrument under consideration is administered to two groups of people whose responses are expected to differ on the variable of interest. For example, if you were developing an instrument to measure depression, the theory used to explain depression would indicate the types of behavior that would be expected in depressed people. If the tool was administered to a group of supposedly depressed subjects and to a group of supposedly happy subjects, you would expect the two groups to score quite differently on the tool. If differences were not found, you might suspect that the instrument was not really measuring depression.

Construct Validity: Known Groups

A study was conducted to examine construct validity of the Individual Work Performance Questionnaire (IWPQ) among 1424 Dutch workers from three occupational sectors (Koopmans, Bernaards, Hildebrandt, de Vet, & van der Beek, 2014). One method of assessing the construct validity of the instrument was to use the "known-groups" technique or test discriminative validity. As predicted, there were significant differences in the IWPQ scores among workers who differed in job satisfaction and workers who differed in health. Workers high in job satisfaction showed higher task performance and lower counterproductive work behavior than persons low in job satisfaction. Persons with good overall health showed higher task performance and lower counterproductive work behavior than persons in poor overall health.

Another approach to construct validity is called **factor analysis**, a method used to identify clusters of related items on an instrument or scale. This type of procedure helps the researcher determine whether the tool is measuring only one construct or several constructs. Correlational procedures are used to determine if items cluster together.

Factor Analysis

Mansour (2015) tested the factor structure of the Health Care Professionals Patient Safety Assessment Curriculum Survey (HPPSACS) among 222 nursing students after they completed the program. The scale was composed of a 34-item scale survey and subscale. Twenty-three items assessed attitudes and comfort with skills contributing to patient safety; participants rated their level of agreement with each statement on a 5-point Likert scale (strongly agree = 1, strongly disagree = 5). The statistical analysis of the student responses led to the emergence of four factors, including willingness to disclose errors, recognition and management of medical errors, the perceived interprofessional context of patient safety, and the perceived support and understanding for improving patient safety.

Relationship between Reliability and Validity

Reliability and validity are closely associated. Both of these qualities are considered when selecting a research instrument. Reliability is usually considered first because it is a necessary condition for validity. An instrument cannot be valid unless it is reliable. However, the reliability of an instrument tells nothing about the degree of validity. In fact, an instrument can be very reliable and have *low* validity.

Reliability was considered first in this chapter's discussion of reliability and validity. In actuality, validity is often considered first in the construction of an instrument. Face validity and content validity may be examined, then some type of reliability is considered. Next, another type of validity may be considered. The process is not always the same. The type of desired validity and the type of reliability are decided, then the procedures for establishing these criteria for the instrument are determined. A word of caution about using the term *established* in regard to reliability and validity of instruments: Strickland (1995), in an editorial in the *Journal of Nursing Measurement*, stated that reliability and validity cannot be established because there is always an error component in measurement. She wrote that it is more correct to use terms like "supported," "assessed," or "prior evidence has shown" (p. 91).

Utilizing the Data

Variations are usually expected in data that are collected from participants in a study. If the researcher did not expect to find some type of variation in the data, there would probably be no interest in conducting the study. Ideally, the variations or differences that are found are real rather than artificial. Every researcher must recognize that some error component is likely to exist in the data that are obtained, especially when the data are being collected from human beings, and the degree of control that can be placed on the research situation is limited. Data-collection errors can arise from instrument inadequacies, instrument administration biases, environmental variations, and temporary subject characteristics during the data collection process.

Sources of Error in Data Collection

Instrument inadequacies concern the items used to collect data and the instructions to participants that are contained within the instrument, such as a questionnaire. Are the items appropriate to collect the data that are being sought? Do the items adequately cover the range of content? Will the order of the items influence subjects' responses? Are the items and the directions for completing items clear and unbiased?

Even when there are no errors in the research instrument, biases or errors may occur in the administration of the instrument. Is the instrument administered in the same fashion to all participants? Are observers collecting data in the same manner?

Environmental conditions during data collection can also influence the data that are gathered. Is the location for data collection the same for all participants? Are conditions such as temperature, noise levels, and lighting kept consistent for all participants?

Finally, the characteristics of the participants during data collection can be a source of error in research data. Are there any personal characteristics of the participants, such as anxiety levels, hunger, or tiredness, influencing responses? This source of error may be called transitory personal factors.

Preparing Data for Analysis

Once data have been gathered, this information must be prepared for analysis. If a computer will be used to analyze data, it is very important that the data are in a form that facilitates entry into the computer. Quantitative data, such as age and weight, may be entered directly into the computer. Qualitative data, such as information obtained from open-ended questions, will need to be transferred into data that the computer can understand if computer analysis will be used. It is important to have data ready for speedy entry, and not be shuffling pieces of paper searching for data. Data coding should be considered, and decisions about missing data made before data entry begins.

Many nurse researchers with personal computers and statistical software packages are able to do much of their data analysis on their own. Some researchers visit a statistician after their data are collected to find out what to do with their data. This is not the proper way to use the statistician's talents. The time to seek help is in the early planning stages of a study. Cirrincione, Smith, and Pang (2014) have recommended that the role of a statistician should be that of a collaborator throughout clinical trials. Thus, a statistician can not only help to determine which instruments, methods of data collection, and statistical analysis are most appropriate for the researcher's study purposes, but also assist with determining which study design and sample size will most effectively ensure outcomes that will lead to valid conclusions.

Critiquing Data-Collection Procedures

It is important for the reader of a research report to determine if the measurement and collection of data has been conducted appropriately. This may be a very difficult task because the reader will not get to see the instruments. Even when questionnaires are used, they are rarely contained in the research article or report.

However, there are some guidelines that may be used and some questions that may be asked (Box 13–1) when critiquing the data-collection section of a research report.

The reader first tries to find a section in the research report where the measurement and collection of data are reported. The information sought concerns who collected the data, when the data were collected, where the data were collected, what data were collected, and how the data were collected.

A determination is made of the level of measurement that would be appropriate to test the research hypothesis (es) or answer the research question(s). For example, if compliance with diabetic regimen was the dependent variable, has the researcher used a physiological measure of compliance, or has the patient been asked to self-report compliance?

The research instruments should be described clearly and thoroughly. Information should be provided about the reliability and validity of the instruments. The types and degree of reliability and validity should be reported.

Finally, the results of the pilot study should be reported. If a pilot study was not conducted, the rationale for failure to do so should be discussed.

Box 13–1 Guidelines for Critiquing the Data-Collection Procedures

1. Did the research report provide information on who collected the data, when the data were collected, where the data were collected, what data were collected, and how the data were collected?
2. Was the appropriate level of measurement used to measure the research variables?
3. Was there a section in the research report where the data-collection instruments were described?
4. Was the description of the instruments thorough?
5. Had the instrument(s) been used previously?
6. Had the instrument(s) been tested for reliability?
7. If so, what type of reliability was assessed, and was there sufficient evidence to indicate that the instrument(s) was (were) reliable?
8. Had the instrument(s) been tested for validity?
9. If so, what type of validity was assessed, and was there sufficient evidence to indicate that the instrument(s) was (were) valid?
10. Was a pilot study conducted using the instruments?

Summary

Measurement is the process of assigning numbers to variables. The four levels of measurement are nominal, ordinal, interval, and ratio. Nominal level of measurement produces data that are named or categorized. Ordinal level of measurement categorizes and ranks the data. The distance between the ranks can be specified with interval level of measurement. In addition to these characteristics, ratio level of measurement specifies a true zero point.

Five important questions need to be answered concerning the data-collection process: Who will collect the data? When will the data be collected? Where will the data be collected? What data will be collected? How will the data be collected?

There are many alternatives to choose from when selecting a data-collection method. These methods include physiological measures, observational methods, questionnaires, interviews, attitude scales, and psychological tests. The devices used to collect data are called the research instruments or tools. The researcher may use an existing instrument or develop a new instrument.

A pilot study should be conducted whenever a new instrument is being developed or when a preexisting instrument is being used with people who have different characteristics from those for whom the instrument was originally developed.

Factors to be considered when choosing a data-collection instrument are the practicality, reliability, and validity of the instrument. The **practicality** of an instrument concerns its cost and appropriateness for the population. The reliability of an instrument determines its consistency and stability. Validity concerns the ability of the instrument to gather the data that it is intended to gather.

Types of reliability are stability, equivalence, and internal consistency. The stability reliability of an instrument refers to its consistency over time and is usually determined by test-retest procedures. Equivalence reliability concerns the degree to which two forms of an instrument obtain the same results or two or more observers obtain the same results when using a single instrument. Alternate forms reliability and parallel forms reliability are terms used when two forms of the same instrument are compared. Interrater reliability or interobserver reliability is the degree of agreement on ratings or observations made by independent judges. Internal consistency reliability addresses the extent to which all items on an instrument measure the same variable.

Types of validity are face, content, criterion, and construct. Face validity measures the degree to which an instrument appears, on the surface, to measure the variable of interest. Content validity is concerned with the scope or range of items used to measure the variable. Criterion validity considers the degree to which an instrument correlates with some criterion measure on the variable of interest. Two types of criterion validity are concurrent and predictive. Concurrent validity compares data obtained through the use of a new instrument with data gathered through the use of an existing instrument that measures the same variable. Predictive validity examines the ability of an instrument to predict behavior of subjects in the future. Finally, construct validity concerns the measurement of a variable that is not directly observable, but rather a construct or abstract concept derived from observable behavior. Two types of construct validity are the known-groups procedure and factor analysis.

Reliability and validity are closely associated. Reliability is a necessary condition for validity. However, an instrument can be reliable and not valid.

Errors associated with data-collection can arise from (a) instrument inadequacies, (b) instrument administration biases, (c) environmental variations, and (d) temporary subject characteristics during the data-collection process.

The researcher must prepare data for analysis. In many studies, nurse researchers use statistical consultants early in the project as well as in the data-analysis phase.

Self-Test

1. Which is an example of mutually exclusive categories that are grouped according to age?
   A. 10 to 20 years of age; 21 to 30 years of age; 31 to 40 years of age; 41 to 50 years of age
   B. ages of: 10 to 20; 20 to 30; 30 to 40; 40 to 50; 50 to 60.
   C. older than 10 years old; younger than 20 years; older than 30 years, younger than 50 years
   D. preschool age, kindergarten age, grade school age, high school age

2. Select the answer that provides the best example of the highest level of measurement for pain.
   A. Pain is mild, moderate, or severe.
   B. Pain is absent or pain is present.
   C. Pain is a 5 on a scale of 0 to 10.
   D. Pain is described as stabbing, sharp, or dull.
3. Select a valid example of a concept that describes the ratio level of measurement
   A. the temperature of water
   B. the amount of money in a bank account
   C. a baby's age at birth
   D. the baby's weight at birth
4. A concern that data collectors will be trained to collect the data is necessary to:
   A. promote reliability of data collection from participant to participant.
   B. promote validity of the use of the instruments.
   C. promote the correct level of measurement use.
   D. promote the statistical analysis of the data.
5. Identify a type of outcome measure that is sensitive to nursing interventions:
   A. physical therapy
   B. infection
   C. symptom management
   D. addiction
6. Which type of instrument reliability would be appropriate for measuring a single participant's ability that is expected to remain the same over time?
   A. construct reliability
   B. stability reliability
   C. interrater reliability
   D. internal consistency reliability
7. What are some characteristics of a construct? A construct is:
   A. an abstract concept that can be directly observed.
   B. a concrete concept that can be directly observed.
   C. composed of items that are directly related to each other.
   D. an abstract concept that is not directly observable.
8. Which test of construct validity would demonstrate how related items in an instrument cluster together?
   A. factor analysis
   B. predictive validity
   C. concurrent validity
   D. known groups validity
9. Which type of data-collection information should be included in the research report?
   A. biographical information on the authors of the study
   B. a description of the data collection instruments
   C. a list of the statisticians who analyzed the data
   D. the marital status of the participants who answered the questions on the surveys
10. What other data-collection information should be reviewed in a research article?
    A. Did the instrument developer provide permission to report on the validity of the instrument?
    B. Was the instrument tested for reliability in the current sample?
    C. How old is the instrument?
    D. How many others have used this instrument for this study purpose?

See answers to Self-Test in the Answer Section at the back of the book.

References

Bjorkly, S., Eidhammer, G., & Selmer, L. E. (2014). Concurrent validity and clinical utility of the HCR-20V3 compared with the HCR-20 in Forensic Mental Health Nursing: Similar tools but improved method. *International Association of Forensic Nurses, 10*(4), 234–242. doi:10.1097/JFN.0000000000000047

Brouwers, L. A., Engels, J. A., Heerkens, Y. F., & van der Beek, A. (2015). Development of a Vitality Scan related to workers' sustainable employability: A study assessing its internal consistency and construct validity. *BioMed Central Public Health, 15,* 551. doi:10.1186/s12889-015-189-z

Chippendale, T. (2015). Development and validity of the Outdoor Falls Questionnaire. *International Journal of Rehabilitation Research, 38,* 263–269. doi:10.1097/MRR.0000000000000115.

Cirrincione, C. T., Smith, E. M. L., & Pang, H. (2014). Methodological considerations in the design and implementation of clinical trials. *Seminars in Oncology Nursing, 30*(1), 74–79. doi.org/10.1016/j.soncn.2013.12.011

De Laat, F. A., Rommers, G. M., Geertzen, J. H., & Roorda, L. D. (2012). Construct validity and test-retest reliability of the walking questionnaire in people with lower limb amputation. *Archives of Physical Medicine Rehabilitation, 93,* 983–989. doi:10.1016/j.apmr.2011.11.030

Doran, D. M. (2015). Outcomes research. In S. Grove, J. Gray, & N. Burns (Eds.), *Understanding nursing research: Building an evidence-based practice* (pp. 466–499). St. Louis, MO: Elsevier.

Doran, D. M. (Ed.). (2011). *Nursing outcomes: The state of the science.* Sudbury, MA: Jones & Bartlett Learning.

Feider, L. L., & Mitchell, P. (2009). Validity and reliability of an oral care practice survey for the orally intubated adult critically ill patient. *Nursing Research, 58,* 374–377. doi: 10.1097/NNR.0b013e3181b4b3d1

Frank-Stromborg, M., & Olsen, S. (Eds.). (2004). *Instruments for clinical health-care research* (3rd ed.). Boston: Jones & Bartlett Learning.

Kilanowski, J. (2011). Pilot studies: Helmsman on the ship of research design. *American Nurse Today, 6*(4). http://www.americannursetoday.com/pilot-studies-helmsman-on-the-ship-of-research-design/

Koopmans, L., Bernaards, C. M., Hildebrandt, V. H., de Vet, H. C. W., & van der Beek, A. J. (2014). Construct validity of the Individual Work Performance Questionnaire. *Occupational and Environmental Medicine, 56*(3), 331–337. doi:10.1097/JOM.0000000000000113

Mansour, M. (2015). Factor analysis of nursing students' perception of patient safety education. *Nurse Education Today, 35,* 32–37. doi:10.1016/j.nedt.2014.04.020

Polit, D., & Beck, C. T. (2008). *Nursing research: Principles and methods* (8th ed.). Philadelphia: Lippincott Williams & Wilkins.

Polit, D. F., & Beck, C. T. (2012). *Nursing research: Generating and assessing evidence for nursing practice* (9th ed.). Philadelphia: Wolters Kluwer | Lippincott Williams & Wilkins.

Press Ganey. (2015). Nursing special report: The influence of nurse work environment on patient, payment and nurse outcomes in acute care settings. http://pressganey.com/solutions/clinical-quality/nursing-quality

Strickland, O. L. (1995). Can reliability and validity be "established?" *Nursing Measurement, 3,* 91–92. http://www.springerpub.com/journal-of-nursing-measurement.html

Strickland, O. L., & Waltz, C. F. (Eds.). (1988a). *Measurement of nursing outcomes: Vol. 1. Measuring client outcomes.* New York: Springer.

Strickland, O. L., & Waltz, C. F. (Eds.). (1988b). *Measurement of nursing outcomes: Vol. 2. Measuring nursing performance: Practice, education, and research.* New York: Springer.

Strickland, O. L., & Waltz, C. F. (Eds.). (1990a). *Measurement of nursing outcomes: Vol. 3. Measuring clinical skills and professional development in education and practice.* New York: Springer.

Strickland, O. L., & Waltz, C. F. (Eds.). (1990b). *Measurement of nursing outcomes: Vol. 4. Measuring client self-care and coping skills.* New York: Springer.

Vink, P., Eskes, A. M., Lindeboom, R., van den Munckhof, P., & Vermeulen, H. (2014). Nurses assessing pain with the Nocieception Coma Scale: Interrater reliability and validity. *Pain Management Nursing, 14*(4), 881–887. http://dx.doi.org/10.1016/j.pmn.2014.01.004

Chapter 14
Data-Collection Methods

Rose Marie Nieswiadomy, PhD, RN, and Sharon Souter, RN, PhD, CNE

 Objectives

On completion of this chapter, you will be prepared to:

1. Summarize the constuction of questionnaires as a data-collection method.
2. Explain the important concepts in using interviews as a data-collection method.
3. Explain the important concepts in using observation as a data-collection method.
4. Compare the characteristics and implications of the Likert and the Semantic Differential attitude scales.
5. Explain roles of physiological and psychological data-collection methods.
6. Compare and contrast other types of data-collection methodologies.

Introduction

"Would you mind filling out this short questionnaire?" You have probably received such a request. Surveys or polls in which questionnaires are used are a common occurrence in our society. You may have walked in the opposite direction at the mall when you saw someone taking a poll.

Questionnaires are one of the most common data-collection methods used by nurse researchers. Other data-collection methods include interviews, observational methods, and various physiological and psychological measures. Try not to be confused by the wide variety of data-collection methods. Once you have had experience in critiquing and helping plan research studies, you will be able to select the most appropriate data-collection methods. As you read about the various methods presented in this chapter, try to envision a research project that might call for each type of data-collection method discussed.

Questionnaires

A **questionnaire** is a self-report instrument. Questionnaires come in a variety of formats and delivery options. Most questionnaires seek a subject's response to questions pertaining to their beliefs or thoughts about a certain subject. Some questionnaires are short, with three-to-five responses required, while others are lengthy and may require paragraph-length responses.

Many people mistakenly believe that developing a good questionnaire is a fairly easy task. Oppenheim (1966) wrote, "The world is full of well-meaning people who believe that anyone who can write plain English and has a modicum of common sense can produce a good questionnaire" (p. vii). This is definitely not true. Many questionnaires have been used only one time because they were poorly constructed and did not obtain the type of data for which they were designed. Many literature resources are available for use in the construction of questionnaires and some sources provide questionnaires for future use that have demonstrated reliability and validity. Also, help can be sought from experts in the area of questionnaire construction.

Questionnaires may be used to measure knowledge levels, opinions, attitudes, beliefs, ideas, feelings, and perceptions, as well as to gather factual information about respondents. Of course, the validity of the data obtained through this method is governed by the respondents' willingness or ability to provide accurate information. Nevertheless, questionnaires are extremely important in nursing research and may be the only method of obtaining data on certain human responses. Each one of you will probably be involved in the construction of a questionnaire at some time during your career. More presentations of nursing research are derived from questionnaires than any other methods of data collection.

Overall Appearance of Questionnaire

The old saying that "first impressions are lasting impressions" may hold true as potential research participants scan a study questionnaire. Remember, a spell-check software program cannot differentiate between words like *hear* and *here*, and *seam* and *seem*. Researchers must always proof their questionnaires.

There are many methods of duplicating questionnaires, but it is important to use a high-quality printing process and paper. Questionnaires should be neat in appearance, grammatically correct, and error-free. The spacing of questions is important. A questionnaire that has a cluttered or crowded appearance may be difficult and confusing for the respondent to complete. Adequate margins and spacing of the questions are needed. It may be better to add another page to the questionnaire rather than crowding too many questions on one page. Keep in mind, however, that if the questionnaire seems too long, potential respondents may become discouraged and discard the questionnaire or fail to answer all the questions.

Language and Reading Level of Questions

A questionnaire should be written in the respondents' preferred language (e.g., English, Spanish) and appropriate for the knowledge and reading level of the least-educated respondents.

A survey of adult literacy levels was conducted in 2003 by the National Center for Education Statistics. This survey included a component on health literacy. Health literacy was reported at four levels: Below Basic, Basic, Intermediate, and Proficient. The majority (53%) of respondents had "Intermediate" health literacy, 22% had "Basic" health literacy, and 14% had "Below Basic" health literacy, with only 11% being "Proficient" in health literacy. Adults with "Below Basic" or "Basic" health literacy were less likely than adults with higher health literacy to obtain health information from written sources, such as newspapers, magazines, books, brochures, or the Internet. They were more likely to obtain health information from radio and television. (For more information on this topic, go to the website dedicated to the National Assessment of Adult Literacy on the National Center for Education Statistics website.)

Shields, McDonald, McKenzie, and Gielen (2015) assessed the health literacy levels of 450 parents of children in an emergency department. The focus of the study was to describe how literacy levels influence health communication interventions that are designed to improve safety knowledge among urban families. The researchers found that 38% of participants had marginal or inadequate health literacy. Following an analysis of the readability of the patient education materials in a pediatric ophthalmology practice, the researchers suggested that online patient resources should be written between a 3rd and 7th grade level for sufficient patient comprehension (John, John, Hansberry, & Guo, 2015). Many formulas are available that determine the reading level of various printed materials, including the Flesch Reading Ease, Fog, Flesch-Kincaid Grade Level, and Simple Measure of Gobbledygook (SMOG). The Flesch Reading Ease formula examines the average length of sentences and number of syllables per word. It provides a number from 0 to 100, with a higher score indicating an easier reading level. The Fog formula is similar to the Flesch Reading Ease formula in that it examines sentence and syllable lengths. A score of 5 is assigned to material that is considered readable; a score of 20 is assigned to material that is very difficult. The Flesch-Kincaid Grade Level formula provides a U.S. school grade level. For example, a score of 8.2 means that an average student in the eighth grade would understand the material. SMOG is a readability formula that estimates the years of education needed to understand a written passage, and looks at the number of multisyllable words.

The readability level of the first paragraph in this section was assessed, and the Flesch Reading Score was reported to be 41 (the higher the score, the easier is the passage to read). The Flesch-Kincaid Grade Level (FKGL) score was 12th grade.

Flesch-Kincaid Grade Level scores were calculated for 67 oral health education brochures from 11 dental clinics across Tasmania, Australia (Barnett, Hoang, & Furlan, 2016). Fourteen brochures that were supplied by the government health department were considered to be appropriate for 4th to 11th grade readers. Twenty-two brochures from commercial sources ranged from grades 3 to 13, while 22 brochures from professional associations ranged from grades 5 to 10. The brochures that were appropriate for lower reading levels had fewer words and less professional jargon.

Other researchers studying the grade readability level of 260 online patient-education materials from the American Academy of Orthopedic Surgeons (AAOS) identified the proportion of the online material that exceeded the recommended (sixth grade) and mean (eighth grade) reading levels (Eltorai, Sharma, Wang, & Daniels, 2015). With the use of Flesch-Kincaid formula that was built into the Microsoft Word software, the researchers reported that the readability level of the AAOS education materials was at grade 9.2. Two hundred and fifty-one (97%) pieces of the material had a readability score above the sixth grade level; of those, 210 (81%) had a readability score above the eighth grade level, which is the average reading level of U.S. adults. The researchers concluded that most of the online patient-education material from the AAOS had readability levels that are far too advanced for many patients to comprehend.

Length of Questionnaire and Questions

The length of a questionnaire may influence respondents' willingness to participate in a study. Although research results are inconclusive on the length of a questionnaire most likely to be returned, generally speaking, short questionnaires are more likely to be returned than long ones. It would probably be advisable to limit the required completion time to 10 minutes or less, which means the questionnaire should probably not be longer than two or three pages.

Questions should be kept as short as possible. Keep in mind that the purpose of the questions is to seek data and not to test the respondents' reading ability and tenacity. A desirable length for a question is less than 20 words. A question may need to be divided into two questions if the length becomes excessive, or the question asks the respondent to consider more than one idea at a time.

Wording of Questions

The most difficult aspect of questionnaire construction is the actual wording of individual questions. Here are some general guidelines:

1. *State questions in an affirmative rather than a negative manner*
   Negative words, such as *never*, can be overlooked, and the respondent will answer the exact opposite of an intended response. Students often complain about the use of negative wording in questions. You are now going to have revealed to you a well-kept secret of teachers. Questions are written this way because it is much easier to write *one* incorrect answer and *three* correct answers for a question than it is to write *three* plausible incorrect responses and *one* correct response.
2. *Avoid ambiguous questions*
   Ambiguous questions contain words that have more than one meaning or can be interpreted differently by various people. Examples of such words are *many, usually, few, often, large, several*, and *generally*.
3. *Avoid double negative questions*
   It is difficult for respondents to reply to a question like this: "Don't you disagree with the idea that …"
4. *Questions should contain neutral wording*
   Any question that implies the type of answer to be given may result in biased responses. Consider the following question: "Do you believe that smoking is a disgusting habit?" The desired answer is quite obvious. Even if you think that smoking is a disgusting habit, you would not want to bias the answers of respondents. Examples of a neutrally worded question, a subtly biased question, and a completely biased question follow:
   A. What is your opinion about cigarette smoking? *(neutral)*
   B. Would you say that you are against cigarette smoking? *(subtly biased)*
   C. You do not believe that people should smoke cigarettes, do you? *(completely biased)*
5. *Avoid double-barreled questions*
   Double-barreled questions ask two questions in one. An example of such a question might be, "Do you plan to pursue a master's degree in nursing and seek an administrative position upon graduation?" When a question contains "and," it is quite likely that two questions are being asked rather than one.

Types of Questions

There are many ways to categorize questions. This section examines these categories of questions: demographic, closed-ended, open-ended, contingency, and filler questions. These types of questions are not mutually exclusive. For example, a demographic question could be written as an open-ended or a closed-ended question.

DEMOGRAPHIC QUESTIONS **Demographic questions** gather data on the characteristics of the sample. These characteristics, sometimes called **demographic variables** or **attribute variables**, include such factors as age, educational background, and religious affiliation. Nearly every questionnaire seeks some kind of demographic data. These data are used to describe the study sample. Also, these data may be statistically analyzed to examine relationships between respondents' characteristics and other variables of interest in the study.

CLOSED-ENDED QUESTIONS The most structured questions are **closed-ended questions**, those in which the respondents are asked to choose from given alternatives. There may be only two alternatives, as in a true-or-false question, or many, as in a checklist type of question where respondents are asked to check all items that apply to them. Other types of closed-ended questions include multiple choice questions and matching questions.

When closed-ended items are used on a questionnaire, the response categories must be collectively exhaustive and mutually exclusive. **Collectively exhaustive categories** means that all possible answers are provided, and **mutually exclusive categories** means that there is no overlap between categories. The following example demonstrates categories that are collectively exhaustive and mutually exclusive.

How many apples do you eat each week?
_____ A. None
_____ B. 1–2
_____ C. 3–4
_____ D. More than 4

The following question *violates* the rule concerning collectively exhaustive categories:

Please check your highest level of education:
_____ A. Elementary
_____ B. High school
_____ C. College

How would subjects who had not completed elementary school respond? Other categories are needed to cover all possible answers that respondents might provide. Sometimes researchers find a quick solution to this problem by adding an "other" category. A blank is provided beside the word *other* for respondents' answers.

The researcher also must provide answers that are mutually exclusive. A respondent should be able to check only one response from among a set of alternatives. The following is a sample question that *violates* this rule:

Please check the length of time that you have dieted:
_____ A. 1–4 weeks
_____ B. 4–8 weeks
_____ C. 8–12 weeks
_____ D. More than 12 weeks

Did you notice the overlap between the categories? A respondent's answer to the preceding question may well depend on the amount of weight loss. If a woman has been on a diet for 4 weeks and is feeling guilty because she has lost only 2 pounds, the 1- to 4-weeks category might be checked, rather than the 4- to 8-weeks category.

OPEN-ENDED QUESTIONS The researcher asks respondents to complete questions in their own words in **open-ended questions**. Essay and fill-in-the-blank are types of open-ended questions. Open-ended questions may be used in combination with closed-ended questions. After the closed-ended item is presented, a space may be provided for respondents to answer in their own words.

CONTINGENCY QUESTIONS Questionnaire items that are relevant for some respondents and not for others are called **contingency questions**. The determination of whether respondents should answer certain questions is dependent, or contingent, upon their answers to other questions. For example, a researcher might want to determine if a client has been satisfied with the type of nursing care received during previous hospitalizations. If the client has not been hospitalized previously, an answer could not be provided to this particular question.

1. Have you ever been hospitalized before?
_____ Yes $\longrightarrow$ How would you rate the care you received during your *last* hospitalization?
_____ Poor _____ Fair _____ Good
_____ No

2. ...

The arrow indicates that respondents who answer "Yes" also should answer the question on the right. Respondents who answer "No" will continue downward on the questionnaire.

FILLER QUESTIONS Occasionally, the researcher wishes to decrease the emphasis on the specific purpose of the study to avoid the tendency for respondents to provide answers they believe the researcher is seeking. **Filler questions** are items in which the researcher has no direct interest but are included on a questionnaire to reduce the emphasis on the specific purpose of other questions. For example, if the main purpose of a study was to gain information concerning patients' perceptions of the nursing care they had received, the researcher might include other questions about the food they had been served, visiting hours, and so forth. Patients might answer more honestly if a few questions about the nursing care they had received were scattered in among a lot of other questions.

Placement of Questions

All questions about a certain topic should be grouped together. Also, demographic questions, which ask for factual information about the respondents, should be grouped together. There is much discussion about the order or placement of questions in certain areas of the questionnaire, such as at the beginning or at the end. Demographic questions are frequently placed at the beginning of a questionnaire because these types of questions are easy to answer and may encourage the respondent to continue with the questionnaire. However, the researcher may choose to place the demographic questions at the end of the questionnaire in the belief that some demographic questions, such as those asking for income or age, may be threatening to the respondents.

Cover Letter

A cover letter should accompany all mailed questionnaires and is helpful anytime a questionnaire is administered. The letter should be brief and contain the following information:

1. Identification of the researcher and any sponsoring agency or person
2. Purpose of the research
3. How the participant was selected
4. Reason the respondent should answer the questionnaire
5. Length of time to complete the questionnaire
6. How data will be used or made public
7. Deadline for return of questionnaire
8. An offer to inform the respondent of the results of the study
9. Contact phone number, mailing address, or email address
10. Personal signature of the researcher

The cover letter is extremely important and may be the single most important factor in motivating respondents to complete questionnaires. Consider what approach or what information would impress you the most and make you want to complete the questionnaire.

Completion Instructions

Information on how to complete the questionnaire must be clear and concise. If all questions are to be answered using the same type of format, a general set of instructions may be written at the top of the questionnaire. Frequently, however, several different types of questions are included on the instrument, and instructions need to precede each type of question. It is very helpful to provide the respondent with an example of the appropriate way to respond to a particular type of question.

Distribution of Questionnaires

There are many methods of distributing questionnaires. They may be given to potential respondents in a one-to-one contact, such as might occur when the nurse researcher distributes instruments to hospitalized patients. Researchers may hand out questionnaires to students in a classroom or distribute questionnaires to members of an organization as they enter a meeting room. Questionnaires also may be placed in a container in a given location where potential respondents can take one if they so desire. The internet has opened up a valuable new method for distributing questionnaires and collecting data. SurveyMonkey is an online software program designed for the creation of questionnaires that is very inexpensive and easy to use. Despite language barriers, electronic surveys offer an efficient way to reach respondents across international borders.

Factors Influencing Response Rates

One serious disadvantage of questionnaires is the frequent low return rate. If you were to mail a survey to a random sample of people listed in a phone book, you would probably not receive a return rate greater than 20%. Factors that positively influence response rates include the following:

1. Mailing at a time other than holiday seasons or popular vacation times
2. Hand-addressed outer envelopes
3. Personal signature of the researcher on the cover letter
4. Information in the cover letter that motivates respondents
5. Neatness and clarity of the instrument
6. Ease of completion of the instrument
7. Time to complete the instrument does not exceed 10 to 15 minutes
8. Guarantee of anonymity
9. Inclusion of a preaddressed, stamped envelope
10. An incentive, such as a small cash payment or an instant coffee sample to drink while completing the questionnaire

Medical students were recruited to respond to survey questions that described their attitudes associated with mental illness, its causes, and changes in attitudes about the mental illness as they progressed through their education (Chiles, Stefanovics, & Rosenheck, 2016). The participants of the study were effectively incentivized to join the study with an offer of $20 for completion of the survey.

Advantages of Questionnaires

1. Questionnaires are a quick and generally inexpensive means of obtaining data from a large number of respondents.
2. Testing for reliability and validity is easier than for many other research instruments.
3. The administration of questionnaires is less time-consuming than interviews or observation research.
4. Data can be obtained from respondents in widespread geographical areas.
5. Respondents can remain anonymous.
6. If anonymity is assured, respondents are likely to provide honest answers.

Disadvantages of Questionnaires

1. Mailing of questionnaires may be costly.
2. Response rate may be low.

3. Respondents may provide socially acceptable answers.
4. Respondents may fail to answer some of the items.
5. There is no opportunity to clarify items that may be misunderstood by respondents.
6. Respondents must be literate.
7. Respondents must have no physical disability that would deter them from completing a questionnaire.
8. Respondents may not be representative of the population.
9. Undeliverable mail.

Interviews

The phone rings and you answer it. A voice on the other end of the line says, "Hello, I'm conducting a research study on _____. It will take only 5 to 10 minutes of your time, and the information you provide will be very important to the results of this study." Have you ever received such a call? If so, did you provide information or did you hang up the phone? If you have received such a call or have participated in a study in which interviews were conducted, you are already familiar with some of the material on interviews.

An **interview** is a method of data collection in which an interviewer obtains responses from a subject in a face-to-face encounter, through a telephone call, or, today, through an Internet connection. Interviews are used to obtain factual data about people, as well as to measure their opinions, attitudes, and beliefs about certain topics. Information is provided here about how to conduct interviews because it is possible that you will be a data collector sometime even if you never serve as a principal investigator.

Types of Interviews

Interviews can be unstructured or structured. However, most interviews range between the two ends of the continuum. For simplification in discussion, interviews are categorized here as unstructured, structured, and semistructured.

In **unstructured interviews**, the interviewer is given a great deal of freedom to direct the course of the interview. Unstructured interviews are conducted more like a normal conversation, and topics are pursued at the discretion of the interviewer. Unstructured interviews are particularly appropriate for exploratory or qualitative research studies in which the researcher does not possess enough knowledge about the topic to develop questions in advance of data collection. The interviewer may start the interview with a broad opening statement like, "Tell me what it was like for you after your husband had his heart attack." Depending on how the spouse responds to this opening question, further questions are formulated. **Probes** are additional prompting questions that encourage the respondent to elaborate on the topic being discussed. When accurate comparisons between subjects are not a critical issue, unstructured interviews produce more in-depth information on subjects' beliefs and attitudes than can be obtained through any other data-gathering procedure.

Structured interviews involve asking the same questions, in the same order, and in the same manner of all respondents in a study. Structured interviews are most appropriate when straightforward factual information is desired. The interviewer uses an interview schedule that has been planned in detail because one of the main purposes of this type of interview is to produce data that can be compared across respondents. Interviewers must try to remain very objective during the interview and avoid unnecessary interactions with respondents.

Most interviews fall somewhere in between the structured and the unstructured types of interviews. In **semistructured interviews**, interviewers are generally required to ask a certain number of specific questions, but additional probes are allowed or even encouraged. Both closed-ended and open-ended questions are included in a semistructured interview. In this type of interview, data are gathered that can be compared across all respondents in the study. In addition, individualized data may be gathered that will provide depth and richness to the findings.

Interview Instruments

Data obtained in interviews are usually recorded on an instrument referred to as an interview schedule. The **interview schedule** contains a set of questions to be asked by the interviewer and space to record the respondents' answers.

Respondents' answers can be entered directly on the interview schedule or recorded on a separate coding sheet, such as one that can be tallied by the use of a computer or grading machine. Data obtained from an interview also can be recorded on audiotapes or videotapes. Some researchers believe the written recording of responses jeopardizes rapport and reduces the amount of eye contact that can be established between the interviewer and the interviewee. Also, through tape-recording devices, the total interview process can be captured, and the interviewer is free to observe the respondents' behavior. However, respondents may be reluctant to give permission to be taped. Written permission is required, and the permission form should indicate how the information will be used and how confidentiality will be maintained.

Telephone interviews involve the collection of data from subjects through the use of phone calls, rather than in face-to-face meetings. This data-collection method is a quick and inexpensive means of conducting interviews. Another advantage of telephone interviews is that the respondents' anonymity can be protected. However, several disadvantages are associated with telephone interviews. Many people have unlisted numbers. Some people have caller IDs installed on their phones; they may not answer the phone if they do not recognize the caller's phone number. Many people use cell phones, and it is difficult to obtain their phone numbers. Another disadvantage of phone interviews is that the interviewer cannot observe nonverbal responses of participants.

Interview Questions

The difficulty in developing good items for a questionnaire has been discussed. You might think that questions for an interview would be much simpler to construct because the interviewer will be present to explain any unclear items. This may be true to some extent, especially for unstructured interviews. Even items for an unstructured interview, however, must be given thoughtful consideration. Once the data are collected, it is too late to add, subtract, or alter questions.

Items must be clear, unambiguous, and short. When questions are long or complex, it may be difficult to ask them orally. If items cannot be simplified, it may be advantageous to print these questions on cards and have subjects read them before they respond. Of course, this procedure would require that subjects could read.

There are two basic categories of questions: open-ended and closed-ended. Both types of questions were described in the section on questionnaires.

Interviewer Training

The investigator of a study in which interviews will be conducted has the responsibility to provide training for all interviewers who will collect data during the study. The training must be quite rigorous. The research investigator should continue to work closely with the interviewers throughout the study.

During the training session(s), the researcher should provide interviewers with a description of the study and its purpose. General procedures are discussed, and the interview schedule is reviewed in detail. The purpose of each question is pointed out, and the meanings of all words are clarified. The process of recording information must be explicitly communicated. Special attention should be given to the use of probes, and any variations that will be allowed in the interview process should be discussed.

Interviewer training should be carried out in groups, so all interviewers receive the same instructions. Role-playing of interviews helps the interviewer gain some appreciation of what the actual interviews will be like. Each interviewer should role-play both the interviewer's part and the respondent's part. By acting as a respondent, the interviewer gains a greater insight into the experience of potential study participants.

Timing and Setting for Interviews

Choosing the most appropriate time for conducting an interview can present a real challenge. If home interviews are conducted, the interviewer should try to determine when respondents would be at home. In past years, interviewers found many women at home during the daytime. This is not true today, as women have increased their presence in the workforce.

If hospitalized patients are to be interviewed, the nurse researcher should become familiar with hospital routines and procedures to determine the most convenient times for interviews. Routines to be considered are patient care activities, visiting hours, and physicians' rounds.

Regardless of the setting, the interviewer should attempt to seek as much privacy as possible for the interview. The respondent and interviewer should be alone, and interruptions should be avoided. The television or radio should be turned off.

Interviewer Guidelines

Although each interview is unique, some guidelines are presented here that can be followed in most circumstances. The guidelines will be presented in three phases: before the interview, during the interview, and after the interview.

Before the interview is conducted, the interviewer should introduce herself or himself to the potential participants. The purpose of the study should be explained. Potential participants should be told how they were chosen and how the information will be used. Each person should be told how long the interview will last.

Once the person has agreed to the interview, the interviewer should ensure a comfortable interview atmosphere. Participants should be seated in a comfortable position or lying down, as in some hospital interviews. Unnecessary noises must be controlled as much as possible. The interviewer should use language that is clearly understood and should talk in a conversational tone. Participants should be informed that there are no right or wrong answers. No pressure should be applied for answers. Sensitive questions should be left until the end of the interview, when rapport may be more fully established.

After the interview has concluded, participants should be asked if they have any questions. Further explanations of the study may be made at this time. Common courtesy dictates that people be thanked for their participation in the study. In some studies, compensation may be provided. Anytime compensation is provided, the possibility of biased data must be considered. Finally, the interviewer should indicate how study participants may obtain the results of the study.

Influence of Interviewers on Respondents

In face-to-face interviews, the interviewer may have a great deal of influence on the outcome. In nonexperimental research, this phenomenon is referred to as the Rosenthal effect. In experimental studies, it is referred to as the experimenter effect. Studies have shown that certain characteristics of the interviewer, such as ethnic background, age, gender, manner of speaking, and clothing, influence the answers provided by respondents. In telephone interviews, the interviewer's verbal mannerisms, such as tone of voice and dialect, may be a positive or a negative factor in soliciting cooperation from respondents.

First impressions are very important in face-to-face interviews. If an appointment has been made for the interview, punctuality should be maintained. Interviewers should be neat in appearance, courteous, friendly, and relaxed. Flashy jewelry should be avoided as well as any item that would identify the interviewer with some social group or organization. It is desirable for interviewers to possess similar demographic characteristics and dressing styles as the respondents.

Advantages of Interviews

1. Responses can be obtained from a wide range of individuals.
2. The response rate is high.
3. Most of the data obtained are usable.
4. In-depth responses can be obtained.
5. Nonverbal behavior and verbal mannerisms can be observed.

Disadvantages of Interviews

1. Training programs are needed for interviewers.
2. Interviews are time-consuming and expensive.
3. Arrangements for interviews may be difficult to make.
4. Respondents may provide socially acceptable responses.
5. Respondents may be anxious because answers are being recorded.
6. Respondents may be influenced by the interviewers' characteristics.
7. Interviewers may misinterpret nonverbal behavior.

Observation Methods

Although observations can be made through all of the senses, generally speaking, **observation research** is concerned with gathering data through visual observation. Nurses are well-qualified to conduct observation research because they observe clients in healthcare settings nearly every day. The researcher must decide what behaviors will be observed, who will observe the behaviors, what observational procedure will be used, and what type of relationship will exist between the observer and the subjects.

Determining Behaviors to be Observed

The research question or study hypothesis should determine the behaviors that will be observed. Psychomotor skills can be evaluated, such as the ability of clients with diabetes to perform insulin injections. Personal habits, such as smoking and eating behaviors, might be of interest. Nonverbal communication patterns, such as body posture or facial expressions, are frequently observed. The types of observations that are of interest to nurse researchers are quite numerous.

Research Observers

If the researcher decides to use other people to collect or help collect data, training sessions are necessary. It is generally preferable to have more than one observer so estimates of the reliability of the data can be made. Human error is quite likely to occur in visual observations. Interrater reliability is the degree to which two or more raters or observers assign the same rating or score to an observation.

Observation Procedures

The researcher must determine how and when observations will be made. The degree of structure of the observations and the period for gathering data must be considered.

STRUCTURED AND UNSTRUCTURED OBSERVATIONS   Observations may range from very structured to very unstructured observations. Most observations lie somewhere in between these two ends of the continuum. **Structured observations** are carried out when the researcher has prior knowledge about the phenomenon of interest. The data-collection tool is usually some kind of checklist. The expected behaviors of interest have been placed on the checklist. The observer needs to indicate only the frequency of occurrence of these behaviors. In **unstructured observations**, the researcher attempts to describe events or behaviors as they occur, with no preconceived ideas of what will be seen. This requires a high degree of concentration and attention by the observer. Frequently, a combination of structured and unstructured observations is used in research. The observation guide or instrument is designed with some preconceived categories identified, but the observer is also instructed to record any additional behaviors that may occur. This combination of structured and unstructured observations provides the quantitative and qualitative types of data that have become important to nurse researchers.

EVENT SAMPLING AND TIME SAMPLING   Observation research may be classified as either event sampling or time sampling. **Event sampling** involves observation of an entire event. **Time sampling** involves observations of events or behaviors during certain specified times. If a researcher were interested in determining the ability of nursing students to perform catheterization procedures correctly, event sampling probably would be most appropriate because the entire procedure would need to be observed. If the area of interest was territorial behaviors of families in intensive care unit waiting rooms, it might be more appropriate to conduct time-sampling observations. Some initial trial observation periods probably would be useful to help determine when observations should be made during the 24-hour day. Also, the researcher might select random times to observe family members.

Relationship between Observer and Subjects

There are four ways to categorize observation research according to the relationship between the observer and the subjects: (a) nonparticipant observer (overt), (b) nonparticipant observer (covert), (c) participant observer (overt), and (d) participant observer (covert).

As a **nonparticipant observer (overt)**, the observer openly identifies that she or he is conducting research and provides subjects with information about the types of data that will be collected. This type of observer might wear a laboratory coat, carry a clipboard and pen, and be clearly identified as a researcher.

The **nonparticipant observer (covert)** is one who does not, before the beginning of data collection, identify herself or himself to the subjects who are being observed. Generally, this type of research is not ethical. Except for instances of public behavior, observation research should be conducted only when permission has been obtained from those who will be the subjects of the study, or with the consent of appropriate persons, such as family members when children are being observed. Public behavior research might involve observations of the number of people who have their seat belts fastened while driving on the highway. This type of observation would be ethical.

Nurse researchers must not abuse their privilege as nurses by covertly observing the behaviors of clients. Researchers may contend that concealed observations are necessary because subjects will alter their behavior if they know they are being observed. People may initially change their behavior, but if an adjustment period is allowed, they will generally respond as they normally would.

Such devices as hidden cameras and one-way mirrors may be used as long as subjects are fully informed about them. Therapy groups are frequently observed, with the members' permission, by observers in an adjoining room that contains a one-way mirror.

In some research studies, the observer becomes involved in interactions with the participants. This interaction may be overt or covert. The **participant observer (overt)** becomes involved with participants openly and with the full awareness of those people who will be observed. Margaret Mead conducted many of her famous anthropological field research studies in this manner. She lived with the people, such as the Samoans, and observed their behaviors in their day-to-day living. The participant observer (overt) role is used frequently in qualitative research.

In contrast, as a **participant observer (covert)**, the observer interacts with the participants and observes their behavior without their knowledge. This type of observer might be disparagingly called a "plant" or "spy" by people who find out the real purpose of the researcher's behavior. There are very few situations in which this type of observation is ethical.

The Role of the Nurse versus the Researcher

Nurse researchers frequently have difficulty in maintaining the role of researcher in observation studies. For example, consider the situation in which a nurse researcher is sitting in a patient's room observing his or her behavior after some treatment procedure. Will the nurse researcher sit silently and continue with the planned observations if the patient seems to be in pain, if the room seems to be too warm, or if the bottle of intravenous fluid is almost empty? It is hoped not. The client's welfare should always take precedence over the gathering of research data. However, if the researcher varies from the guidelines for the data-collection procedure, the accuracy of the data may be in question.

In an editorial statement about the key partnership requirements between clinical practice and research, Rathman (2016) reminded readers that nursing practice is supported by evidence and guided by theory. Rathamn Regardless of the practice area, nurses encounter gaps in evidence that provide a basis for potential research. Nurses need to participate in all areas of nursing as nurses develop practice guidelines to aid in their basis for practice.

Attitude Scales

Attitude scales are self-report data-collection instruments that ask respondents to report their attitudes or feelings on a continuum. Attitude scales are composed of a number of related items, and respondents are given a score after the item responses are totaled. Respondents' attitudes may be compared by examining the scores that are obtained for each person or each group. The most commonly used attitude scales are the Likert scale and the semantic differential scale.

Likert Scale

The **Likert scale** was named after its developer, Rensis Likert. This scale usually contains five or seven responses for each item, ranging from strongly agree to strongly disagree. Figure 14–1 provides an example of a Likert scale.

Nursing Diagnosis Questionnaire

Please read the following items and indicate your agreement or disagreement by checking the appropriate category.

SD = Strongly disagree
D = Disagree
U = Uncertain
A = Agree
SA = Strongly agree

	SD	D	U	A	SA
1. Nursing diagnoses should be written on all nursing care plans.	___	___	___	___	___
2. The use of nursing diagnoses enables nurses to be autonomous health care professionals.	___	___	___	___	___
3. The medical diagnosis is more important in determining clients' health care needs than is the nursing diagnosis.	___	___	___	___	___
4. Nursing care should be based on the nursing diagnosis.	___	___	___	___	___
5. Nurses waste valuable time in trying to formulate nursing diagnoses.	___	___	___	___	___
6. The term *nursing diagnosis* is a popular phrase that will soon become forgotten.	___	___	___	___	___

Figure 14–1 Example of a Likert scale

Some researchers prefer to eliminate the uncertain category and force respondents into some form of agreement or disagreement with the items. When the uncertain option is eliminated, however, respondents may be forced to select answers that are really not their choice.

An approximately equal number of positively and negatively worded items should be included on a Likert instrument. Respondents are then required to read each question carefully. They will not be able to rapidly complete an instrument by checking *one* category of responses all the way through the instrument.

If five responses are used, scores on each item generally range from 1 to 5. A score of 1 is usually given to "strongly disagree," 2 to "disagree," 3 to "uncertain," 4 to "agree," and, finally, 5 to "strongly agree." Negatively worded items are reverse scored: "Strongly disagree" responses to negative items would receive a score of 5, rather than 1. If 20 items were included on an instrument, the total score could vary from 20 to 100.

Although data from a Likert scale are generally at the ordinal level of measurement, some statistical texts indicate that arithmetic operations may be performed with this type of data and, therefore, the more powerful parametric statistical tests may be used in analyzing the data.

Likert Scale

Flood and Commendador (2016) surveyed baccalaureate nursing students' perceptions of their cultural competency following the integration of a transcultural nursing thread throughout the curriculum. The survey consisted of five sections: training, cross-cultural experiences, resources, specialty areas, and personal and professional characteristics. A 5-point Likert scale was used to measure items that addressed perceptions of preparedness of caring for patients from cultures different from their own. Students rated their responses on a scale of 1 to 5. The lowest number (1) of the scale indicated "very unprepared" and the highest number (5) meant "very well prepared"

Semantic Differential Scales

Although not as commonly used as the Likert scale, the semantic differential is a useful attitude scale for nurse researchers. The **semantic differential** asks subjects to indicate their position or attitude about some concept along a continuum between two adjectives or phrases that are presented in relation to the concept being measured. The technique was developed by Osgood, Suci, and Tannenbaum (1957) to measure the psychological meaning of concepts. They used the term *semantic differential* to indicate that the difference in subjects' attitudes could be compared by examining their responses in "semantic space" or attitudinal space.

Study participants usually are asked to describe or evaluate a particular situation or experience. This technique also may be used to evaluate a setting, a person, a group, or an educational course. The positions along the continuum or scale are assigned numerical values. The number of positions on the continuum varies from five to nine, with seven being used commonly. Scores are derived much the same way as in the Likert procedure. Figure 14–2 presents an example of a semantic differential scale.

The semantic differential scale is generally easier for subjects to complete than a Likert scale. However, subjects may not understand the adjectives that are used on a semantic differential scale, or may become bored with the format of the items and select the middle scale position throughout the entire instrument.

Semantic Differential

Kleiss (2016) was interested in assessing the utility and reliability of a multidimensional patient experience questionnaire to review patient experience pre and post magnetic resonance scan. Kleiss developed a multidimensional semantic differential questionnaire to measure four independent factors reflective of patients' subjective experiences along four variables: a) evaluation/valence, (b) potency/control, (c) activity/arousal, and (d) novelty. A group of 60 patients used the questionnaire to assess pre-scan expectations and post-scan experiences. Results suggest more positive evaluation/valence, higher potency/control, and lower activity/arousal for post-scan ratings compared to pre-scan expectations. Ratings of novelty were neutral in both the pre-scan and the post-scan conditions. Subsequent analysis suggested that internal consistency for some concepts could be improved by replacing several specific rating scales. The researcher reported that evidence supports the utility and reliability of a multidimensional semantic questionnaire for measuring these patient experiences in an actual clinical setting.

Evaluation of Clinical Instructor

Each item below concerns characteristics of instructors. Words are presented in pairs and represent opposite characteristics. Please place a (✓) above the line on the scale at the place which you believe comes the closest to describing your evaluation of the instructor.

Example:
Kind ____ ✓ ____ ____ ____ ____ Unkind

1. Friendly ____ ____ ____ ____ ____ ____ Unfriendly
2. Sensitive ____ ____ ____ ____ ____ ____ Insensitive
3. Praises ____ ____ ____ ____ ____ ____ Criticizes
4. Caring ____ ____ ____ ____ ____ ____ Uncaring
5. Flexible ____ ____ ____ ____ ____ ____ Inflexible
6. Helpful ____ ____ ____ ____ ____ ____ Unhelpful

Figure 14–2 Example of a semantic differential scale

Physiological and Psychological Measures

Physiological measures involve the collection of physical data from subjects. These types of measures are generally more objective and accurate than many of the other data-collection methods. It is much more difficult for subjects to provide biased data on physiological measures, intentionally or unintentionally, than on self-report measures.

One of the greatest advantages of physiological measures is their precision and accuracy. One of the greatest disadvantages is that special expertise may be necessary to use some of these devices. Another disadvantage is that the presence of certain data-collection instruments may adversely influence the subjects. For example, the process of applying the equipment to measure a person's blood pressure may, in fact, cause the blood pressure readings to be elevated.

In today's nursing research, many studies involve the use of physiological variables. To evaluate the effectiveness of physiological and behavioral variables that accurately assess and measure acute pain response in infants, Hatfield and Ely (2015) used facial expression and body movements and heart rate and oxygen saturation to determine levels of acute pain. To evaluate the physiological effects of older adults upon interacting with a companion robot, Robinson, McDonald, and Broadbent (2015) used blood pressure readings before, during, and after interaction with the robot to determine the degree of positive response.

Increasing numbers of published studies are reporting data that have been collected from both physiological measures and self-report measures. The use of multiple data-collection instruments provides a more valid measure of a variable than when only one of these types of instruments is employed.

Psychological Tests

Researchers have devised many methods to assess the personality characteristics of people. Personality inventories and projective techniques are two of these methods.

PERSONALITY INVENTORIES **Personality inventories** are self-report measures used to assess the differences in personality traits, needs, or values of people. These inventories seek information about a person by asking questions or requesting responses to statements that are presented. Scores are then derived for each person for the trait being measured. Many of the personality inventories have preprinted scoring guides that allow comparisons between subjects and also allow comparisons with a "norm" or "average" group. Because these devices are self-reports, they are accurate to the extent that subjects respond honestly to the items.

Some of the more commonly used personality inventories are the Minnesota Multiphasic Personality Inventory (MMPI), Edwards Personal Preference Schedule (EPPS), and Sixteen Personality Factor Questionnaire (16 PF). The MMPI contains 550 affirmative statements that require an answer of True, False, or Cannot Say. This test is composed of 10 subdivisions, including areas such as depression, paranoia, and hysteria. The MMPI has been used with people considered normal and those with psychological problems. The EPPS contains 15 scales that measure concepts such as autonomy and dominance. The 16 PF measures personality dimensions such as reserved versus outgoing, practical versus imaginative, and relaxed versus tense.

PROJECTIVE TECHNIQUE One of the criticisms of self-report psychological measures is that they may elicit socially acceptable answers or answers desired by the researcher, rather than the true feelings or attitudes of the subjects. A data-collection method believed to be more accurate in gathering psychological data is the projective method. In a **projective technique**, a respondent is presented with stimuli designed to be ambiguous or to have no definite meaning. Then, the person is asked to describe the stimuli or to tell what the stimuli appear to represent. The responses reflect the internal feelings of the subjects that are projected onto the external stimuli.

Probably the most famous of all the projective measures is the Rorschach Inkblot Test. Respondents are presented with cards that show designs that are actually inkblots rather than true pictures or drawings. One person might interpret a card to be two figures dancing; another might describe the same scene as two people fighting. Of course, only specialists should interpret this type of data.

Another commonly used projective test is the Thematic Apperception Test (TAT). The TAT consists of a set of pictures, and individuals are asked to tell a story relating what they think is happening in the pictures. Projective tests are particularly useful with small children because of their limited vocabularies. Children may be given dolls and asked to arrange the dolls in a particular setting that is provided by the researcher. Children also may be given finger paint, crayons, or clay to use in telling a story.

Projective Techniques

A study of 7- to 12-year-old Korean and Korean American children used a projective technique to describe their emotional reactions to illness and hospitalization (Park, Foster, & Cheng, 2009). The children were presented with vignettes about being sick, going to the doctor, and being hospitalized. When responding to the vignettes, the children expressed stressful emotions through words that indicated being scared, worried, nervous, frightened, and afraid.

Other Data-Collection Methods

Q Sort

The **Q sort**, also called Q methodology, is a means of obtaining data in which subjects sort statements into categories according to their attitudes toward, or rating of, the statements. Q sorts may be used to identify perspectives and to gain a better understanding of diverse viewpoints (Zabala & Pascual, 2016). Participants receive cards or pieces of paper with a number of words or statements written on them. The researcher predetermines the number of items the participants are to place into each category or pile. This forced-choice arrangement usually calls for piles to be distributed in the form of a bell-shaped curve. If 100 items were being used, the distribution might look like this:

$$1 \quad 4 \quad 11 \quad 21 \quad 26 \quad 21 \quad 11 \quad 4 \quad 1$$

The respondents are asked to arrange the items from left to right in front of them according to their attitude toward, or rating of, the items. The first pile should contain the item about which the person has the most positive attitude or strongest belief about its importance to the topic of interest; the last pile on the right should contain the item about which the person has the most negative attitude or weakest belief about the item's importance. The other piles will contain items of varying intensity of attitudes or beliefs. This type of data-collection procedure may present a difficult task for respondents. Therefore, clear instructions must be provided.

Q Sort

Yeun et al. (2016) were interested in studying the stress family care providers feel while caring for family members undergoing hemodialysis (HD). Q-methodology was undertaken because it integrates quantitative and qualitative research methods. A convenience sample of 33 primary caregivers of HD patients participated. Forty selected Q-samples were obtained from each participant and their choices were classified into a forced normal distribution using a nine-point grid. Data was analyzed using a pc-QUANL program.

Delphi Technique

The term **Delphi technique** is used to describe a data-collection technique that employs several rounds of questions to seek a consensus on a particular topic from a group of experts. The technique received its name from the famous Greek oracle at Delphi. As you may remember, the ancient Greeks sought answers to important questions from the deities. The purpose of this data-collection method is to obtain group consensus from the panel of experts without bringing this group together in a face-to-face meeting. This type of procedure is appropriate to examine the opinions, beliefs, or future predictions of knowledgeable people on some special topic of interest.

A classic Delphi study was conducted by Lindeman (1975). The purpose of this study was to determine priorities for future clinical nursing research. Of the 433 leaders in nursing originally contacted, 341 experts responded to all four rounds of questionnaires. The results indicated that the most important priority for clinical nursing research was the development of valid and reliable indicators of quality nursing care. Other important areas were identified as (1) effective ways to decrease the psychological stress experienced by patients, (2) means of enhancing the quality of life for the aged, and (3) interventions to manage pain.

Delphi

A mixed method two-stage Delphi technique was employed to identify and achieve consensus about the elements needed for the success of health-promotion practices that were delivered by registered nurses (RNs) in primary healthcare in eastern Finland (Maijala, Tossavainen, & Turunen, 2016). The participants agreed that a health-promoting organizational culture and the need for nurses' health orientation were the main elements necessary for the success of health-promotion practices in primary healthcare.

Visual Analogue Scale

The **visual analogue scale** (VAS) presents subjects with a straight line drawn on a piece of paper. The line is anchored on each end by words or short phrases that represent the extremes of some phenomenon, such as pain. Subjects are asked to make a mark on the line at the point that corresponds to their experience of the phenomenon. Frequently, the line is 100 mm in length, which simulates a 0 to 100 rating scale. From their review of the literature, Huang, Wilkie, and Berry (1996) concluded that the VAS is a "simple, reliable, reproducible, valid, and sensitive tool" (p. 370).

If you are trying to photocopy a VAS for use in a study, the length of the line may change slightly (lengthen) during the photocopying process and you will not end up with a 100-mm line. The VAS line may be drawn either horizontally or vertically on the paper. Some authors have suggested that the vertical scale is easier for subjects to use (Flaherty, 1996). It appears to be universally recognized that the bottom of a vertical scale is low, and the top of a vertical scale is high. On the other hand, not all cultural groups view the far left on a horizontal scale as indicating a low score and the far right as indicating a high score.

The VAS is being used with increasing frequency in nursing research studies. It has been found to be particularly useful with patients who are experiencing discomfort, such as nausea, pain, fatigue, or shortness of breath.

Visual Analogue Scale

Blauwhoff-Buskermolen et al. (2016) employed the use of the Anorexia/Cachexia Subscale (A/CS) of the Functional Assessment of Anorexia/Cachexia Therapy (FAACT) questionnaire and the visual analog scale (VAS) to study appetite as a portion of the assessment of anorexia in patients with cancer. The aim of the study was to obtain cutoff values for these instruments. The study results led the researchers to suggest cutoff values of ≤37 for the FAACT-A/CS and ≤70 for the VAS.

Preexisting Data

Nurse researchers have available a wealth of data that may be used for research. As a data-collection method, preexisting data involves the use of existing information that may not have been collected for research purposes. Sources of existing data include records from agencies and organizations such as hospitals and the U.S. government.

Many large databases are available that are valuable to nurse researchers. Secondary analysis of these data sets can be the focus of an investigator's entire research program. Large data sets are available from federal and state agencies and associations for a small fee, or even free. These large data sets offer researchers the opportunity to test new hypotheses or answer research questions.

The Agency for Healthcare Research and Quality (AHRQ) is the health services arm of the U.S. Department of Health and Human Services (HHS). It is the nation's leading federal agency for research on health quality, costs, outcomes, and patient safety. This agency sponsors the Healthcare Cost & Utilization Project (HCUP). HCUP has put together databases of patient-level information, which have been gathered from state organizations, hospital associations, private data organizations, and the federal government. For more information visit the website for U.S. Department of Health and Human Service, Agency for Healthcare Research and Quality (AHRQ).

There are many local sources of data for nurse researchers. These include local public health departments, churches, and professional organizations. Personal documents, such as diaries and letters, may be examined, as well as almanacs and professional journals.

Diaries

Hinsliff-Smith and Spencer (2016) employed the use of diaries in a qualitative healthcare research study to identify the phenomena involved in early breastfeeding. The diaries permitted the participants to enter unstructured, narrative accounts of their experiences. The results suggest that using diaries was a valid and useful tool for capturing the desired phenomena. The researchers reported that the use of diaries has relevance for healthcare researchers who are interested in capturing real-life experiences. However, due to the challenges associated with diaries, Hinsliff-Smith and Spencer recommended that researchers focus on diary management, including diary structure, format, and support for participants throughout the study period.

Critiquing Data-Collection Methods

In an earlier chapter of this book, some general critiquing guidelines were presented concerning the data-collection process reported in a research report. The specific data-collection methods used also need to be critiqued. Box 14–1 presents some general guidelines for critiquing data-collection methods, and some specific questions to ask about questionnaires and interviews.

If a questionnaire was used in a study, sufficient information should be provided to enable the reader to determine if the tool was appropriate for use in the study. The manner in which the questionnaire was developed, the reliability and validity of the instrument, the number of questions, how the instrument was scored, and the range of possible scores should be presented.

When an interview has been used, the reader needs information about how long the interviews took, who conducted the interviews, and how the interviewers were trained.

Observation research requires that the reader be able to determine how observations were made, who made the observations, and how data were recorded. Were subjects aware that they were being observed?

If physiological instruments were used, the accuracy of these data-collection measures needs to be addressed. Does it appear that the researcher had the expertise to use these instruments?

The researcher may have used a psychological data-collection method, such as an attitude scale or a personality test. The reader will need to determine the appropriateness of these instruments and the qualifications of the researcher to use them.

The reader may not be familiar with data-collection methods such as the Delphi technique or Q sort that are mentioned in research articles. It would be advisable to consult research textbooks to learn more about the data-collection methods cited in research reports.

Box 14–1 Guidelines for Critiquing Data-Collection Methods

General Criteria
1. Were the data-collection methods described thoroughly?
2. Were the data-collection methods appropriate to test the research hypotheses or answer the research questions?
3. Was a self-report or psychological method used when a physiological method might have gathered more valid data?
4. How many methods were used to collect data? If only one method was used, would the study have benefited from more than one method?

Questionnaires
1. Was information provided on the number of questions, the length of the questionnaire, and how long it would take to complete the questionnaire?
2. Was the response rate provided for the return of the questionnaires?
3. Were sampling biases discussed?
4. Was anonymity or confidentiality assured?

Interviews
1. Was information provided on how long the interview would take?
2. Was information provided about training for the interviewers?
3. Was confidentiality assured?

Other Methods
1. Was the specific method identified (e.g., semantic differential)?
2. Was the rationale for use of the method presented?
3. Was the instrument described in detail?
4. Was the scoring method clearly discussed?

Summary

A questionnaire is a self-report instrument. Factors to consider in constructing questionnaires are overall appearance, language and reading level, length of questionnaire and questions, wording of questions, types of questions, and placement of questions.

Ambiguous questions contain words that have more than one meaning. Double-barreled questions ask two questions in one. Demographic questions concern subject characteristics. These subject characteristics are called demographic variables or attribute variables. Closed-ended questions are very structured, and respondents are asked to choose from given alternatives. The term *collectively exhaustive categories* indicates that a category is provided for every possible answer. Mutually exclusive categories are categories that are uniquely distinct; no overlap occurs between categories. Open-ended questions enable respondents to answer questions in their own words. Contingency questions are items that are relevant for some respondents and not for others. Filler questions are items in which the researcher has no direct interest, but are included on a questionnaire to reduce the emphasis on the specific purpose of other questions.

A cover letter should accompany all mailed questionnaires. Questionnaires may be distributed in a one-to-one contact, through group administration, through a mailing system, or through the Internet. Response rates of questionnaires are frequently low. There are many advantages and disadvantages in using questionnaires as a method of data collection.

An interview is a data-collection method in which an interviewer obtains responses from a subject in a face-to-face meeting or from telephone interviews. Data are recorded on an interview schedule or may be tape recorded. Unstructured interviews contain open-ended questions and are appropriate for exploratory studies in which the researcher possesses little knowledge of the study topic. Probes are additional prompting questions that encourage the respondent to elaborate on a certain topic. Structured interviews are made up of closed-ended questions and are generally used to obtain straightforward factual information. Semistructured interviews contain both open-ended and closed-ended questions. The majority of interviews are of the semi-structured type.

Observation research gathers data through visual observations. In structured observations, the expected behaviors are predetermined, and the frequency of occurrence is noted during data collection. In unstructured observations, the researcher describes events or behaviors as they occur, with no preconceived ideas of what will be seen. Event sampling involves observation of an entire event, whereas time sampling involves observation of events or behaviors during certain specified times.

As a nonparticipant observer (overt), the observer openly identifies that research is being conducted. The nonparticipant observer (covert) does not identify herself or himself as a researcher. This type of observation is quite likely to be unethical. The participant observer (overt) becomes involved with participants openly and with the full awareness of those who will be observed in their natural settings. In contrast, the participant observer (covert) interacts with individuals and observes their behavior without their knowledge. Again, this type of observation may be unethical.

Physiological measures involve the collection of physical data from study participants. These measures are generally quite accurate.

Attitude scales ask respondents to report their attitudes or feelings on a continuum. The scales are composed of a number of related items, and respondents are given a score after the item responses are totaled. The Likert scale and the semantic differential are two commonly used attitude scales.

Personality inventories are self-report measures that seek information about someone's personality traits, needs, or values by requesting responses to statements that are presented.

In a projective technique, individuals are presented with stimuli designed to be ambiguous. Responses reflect internal feelings of the subjects that are projected on the external stimuli.

When a Q sort is used, participants are asked to sort statements into categories according to their attitudes toward, or rating of, the statements. The statements are written on cards or pieces of paper, and the participants are asked to arrange the items in piles according to the intensity of their attitudes or beliefs about the items.

A Delphi technique uses several rounds of questionnaires to seek consensus on a particular topic from a group of experts. This procedure is appropriate for examining the opinions, beliefs, or future predictions of knowledgeable people on a topic of interest.

The visual analogue scale (VAS) presents subjects with a straight line drawn on a piece of paper. Respondents are asked to make a mark on the line at the point that corresponds to their experience of pain, for example. The line may be drawn either horizontally or vertically.

Preexisting data are data from records of agencies or organizations such as hospitals, the U.S. government, and public health departments. Large data sets are available to nurse researchers for secondary analysis. Also, diaries, letters, almanacs, and professional journals may be examined.

Self-Test

1. Which is an advantage of an interview method of data collection versus a questionnaire?
   A. Data are less expensive to obtain.
   B. The collected data tend to be more complete.
   C. Data collectors do not need to be trained.
   D. Data may be collected more easily from a widespread geographical area.
2. A researcher wants to determine future priorities for research in psychiatric nursing. The participants will be clinical specialists in psychiatric nursing. Which data-collection method would probably be used?
   A. projective technique
   B. observation method
   C. delphi technique
   D. semantic differential
3. Which data-collection method is most likely to prevent participants from providing socially acceptable responses to questions?
   A. attitude scale
   B. projective technique
   C. self-report questionnaire
   D. interview

Choose the letter of the data-collection method that matches the method described in statements 4 to 8.

4. Presents statements to which respondents indicate level of agreement or disagreement along a continuum.
   A. semantic differential
   B. projective technique
   C. Q sort
   D. Likert scale
   E. Delphi
5. Contains sets of bipolar adjectives; asks respondents to select a point on a scale between two adjectives.
   A. semantic differential
   B. projective technique
   C. Q sort
   D. Likert scale
   E. Delphi
6. Participants are asked to place statements into categories according to their attitudes toward or rating of the statements.
   A. semantic differential
   B. projective technique
   C. Q sort
   D. Likert scale
   E. Delphi
7. Subjects are asked to look at pictures and tell what meaning the pictures have for them.
   A. semantic differential
   B. projective technique
   C. Q sort
   D. Likert scale
   E. Delphi

8. Leaders in critical care nursing are asked to identify research priorities for critical care nursing in the next 5 years.
   A. semantic differential
   B. projective technique
   C. Q sort
   D. Likert scale
   E. Delphi

See answers to Self-Test in the Answer Section at the back of the book.

References

Barnett, T., Hoang, H., & Furlan, A. (2016). An analysis of the readability characteristics of oral health information literature available to the public in Tasmania, Australia. *BMC Oral Health, 16*(1), 35. doi:10.1186/s12903-016-0196-x

Blauwhoff-Buskermolen, S., Ruijarok, C., Ostelo, R. W., de Vet, H. C., Verheul, H. M., de van der Schueren, M. A., & Langius, J. A. (2016). The assessment of anorexia in patients with cancer: Cut-off values for the FAACT-A/CS and the VAS for appetite. *Supportive Care in Cancer, 24*(2), 661–666. doi:10.1007/s00520-015-2826-2

Chiles, C., Stefanovics, E., & Rosenheck, R. (2016). Attitudes of students at a U.S. medical school toward mental illness and its causes. *Applied Psychiatry.* (In press.)

Eltorai, A. E. M., Sharma, P. Wang, J., & Daniels, A. H. (2015). Most American Academy of Orthopaedic Surgeons' online patient education material exceeds average patient reading level. *Clinical Orthopaedics and Related Research, 471*, 1181–1186. doi:10.1007/s11999-014-4071-2

Flaherty, S. A. (1996). Pain measurement tools for clinical practice and research. *American Association of Nurse Anesthetists, 64*, 39. http://www.aana.com/newsandjournal/Pages/aanajournalonline.aspx

Flood, J. L., & Commendador, K. A. (2016). Undergraduate nursing students and cross-cultural care: A program evaluation. *Nurse Education Today, 36*, 190–194. doi:10.1016/j.nedt.2015.10.003

Hatfield, L. A., & Ely, E. A. (2015). Measurement of acute pain in infants: A review of behavioral and physiological variables. *Biological Research for Nursing, 17*(1), 100–111. http://brn.sagepub.com/

Hinsliff-Smith, K., & Spencer, R. (2016) Researcher perspectives from a study of women's experiences of breastfeeding. *Nurse Researcher, 23*, 3, 13–17. http://dx.doi.org/10.7748/nr.23.3.13.s4

Huang, H., Wilkie, D. J., & Berry, D. L. (1996). Use of a computerized digitizer to score and enter visual analogue scale data. *Nursing Research, 45*, 370–372. http://journals.lww.com/nursingresearchonline/pages/default.aspx

John, A. M., John, E. S., Hansberry, D. R., Thomas, P. J., & Guo, S. (2015). Analysis of online patient education materials in pediatric ophthalmology. *American Association for Pediatric Ophthalmology and Strabismus, 19*(5), 430–434. doi:http://dx.doi.org/10.1016/j.jaapos.2015.07.286

Kleiss, J. A. (2016, April 5). Preliminary development of a multidimensional semantic patient experience measurement questionnaire. *Health Environments Research & Design.* http://her.sagepub.com/ doi:10.1177/1937586716636841

Lindeman, C. (1975). Delphi survey of priorities in clinical nursing research. *Nursing Research, 24*, 434–441. http://journals.lww.com/nursingresearchonline/pages/default.aspx

Maijala, V., Tossavainen, K., & Turunen, H. (2016). Health promotion practices delivered by primary health care nurses: Elements for success in Finland. *Applied Nursing Research, 30*, 45–51. doi:http://dx.doi.org/10.1016/j.apnr.2015.11.02

Oppenheim, A. (1966). *Questionnaire design and attitude measurement.* New York: Basic Books.

Osgood, C., Suci, G., & Tannenbaum, P. (1957). *The measurement of meaning.* Urbana: University of Illinois Press.

Park, J., Foster, R., & Cheng, S. (2009). Language used by Korean and Korean American children to describe emotional reactions to illness and hospitalization. *Transcultural Nursing, 20,* 176–186. doi:10.1177/1043659608330060

Rathman, L. D. (2016). A key partnership: Clinical practice and research. *Heart & Lung, 45*(3), 165. http://dx.doi.org/10.1016/j.hrtlng.2016.02.009

Robinson, H., McDonald, B., & Broadbent, E. (2015). Physiological effects of a companion robot on blood pressure of older people in residential care facility: A pilot study. *Australian Journal on Aging, 34*(1), 27–32. doi:10.1111/ajag.12099

Shields, W. C., McDonald, E. M., McKenzie, L. B., & Gielen, A. G. (2015). Does health literacy level influence the effectiveness of a kiosk-based intervention delivered in the pediatric emergency department? *Clinical Pediatrics, 29*(5), 628–634. doi:10.1097/PEC.0b013e31828e9cd2

Yeun, E. J., Bang, H. Y., Kim, E. J., Jeon, M., Jang, E. S., & Ham, E. (2016). Attitudes toward stress and coping among primary caregivers of patients undergoing hemodialysis: A Q-methodology study. *Hemodialysis International.* doi:10.1111/hdi.12404

Zabala, A., & Pascual, U. (2016) Bootstrapping Q methodology to improve the understanding of human perspectives. *PLoS ONE, 11*(2): e0148087. doi:10.1371/journal.pone.0148087

PART V Data Analysis

Chapter 15
Descriptive Statistics

Rose Nieswiadomy, PhD, RN; Jo-Ann Stankus, PhD, RN,
and Peggy Mancuso, PhD, RN

 Objectives

On completion of this chapter, you will be prepared to:

1. Summarize the key concepts related to statistical symbols and classification.
2. Compare the four classifications of descriptive statistics.
3. Discuss how measures of relationships differ from the other three classifications of descriptive statistics.

Introduction

Many students are intimidated by the very idea of statistics. Statistics can be a daunting subject, especially as you progress into more complex processes. If you are an individual who tries to avoid anything involving mathematics, rest assured that only minimal math skills are necessary to understand the material here. All that is needed is basic mathematical knowledge and logical thinking. Does that make you feel better? Rather than understanding each of the various statistical tests, it is much more important that you are familiar with the types of data you or someone else has collected and the types of statistical tests that might be appropriate for these data. Also, you do not need to know how to calculate statistics. It is quite unlikely you will ever have to hand compute any statistical formulas.

The word *statistics* is derived from the Latin word for state. In the mid-18th century, the term was used in a political context to describe the resources of states and kingdoms. The term is used much more broadly today, and statistics are used by many disciplines. Statistics, as a singular noun, is a branch of knowledge used to summarize and present numerical data. As a plural noun, statistics are numerical characteristics of samples. The purpose of statistics is to enable researchers to collect and analyze data and make meaningful evaluations of those data.

This chapter presents a review of the statistical concepts associated with descriptive statistics. If you need more information, many statistics textbooks are available. One that may be of particular interest to you is *Statistics for the Terrified* by Kranzler (2010). In addition, some free statistical textbooks can be found online.

Key Concepts in Statistics

When discussing numerical characteristics of populations, the word **parameter** is used. When discussing numerical characteristics of samples, the term **statistics** is used. An easy way to recall this information is to remember that population and parameter both begin with a *p*, and sample and statistics both begin with an *s*. Different symbols are used to depict parameters and statistics.

Statistical Symbols

Greek letters such as mu (μ) are used to designate population parameters; English letters such as s and SD are used to indicate sample statistics. When you encounter these symbols in descriptions of research studies and in tables that accompany studies, you will be able quickly to determine which types of data are being reported.

	Population Symbols	Sample Symbols
Mean	μ	M, $\bar{X}$
Standard deviation	ρ	s, SD
Variance	σ^2	s^2, SD^2

In many research articles, words are used instead of symbols. A recent review of the literature revealed that words and letters rather than symbols are frequently used to depict both population parameters and sample statistics. For example, in reviewing some recent research articles, the words *mean* or *average* and the letter *M* were found more frequently to indicate the mean rather than the X with a bar. The sixth edition of the American Psychological Association's *Publication Manual* (2010) includes helpful guides and tables explaining how various statistical tests and mathematical functions are presented in scholarly work.

Classifications of Statistics

There are two broad classifications of statistics—descriptive and inferential. **Descriptive statistics**, very simply defined, are those statistics that organize and summarize numerical data gathered from samples. **Inferential statistics** are concerned with populations and use sample data to make an inference about a population. Inferential statistics help the researcher determine if the difference found between two groups, such as an experimental and a control group, is a real difference or only a chance difference that occurred because an unrepresentative sample was chosen from the population. Any time that sample data are used to estimate the characteristics of a population, there is a chance the estimate will be inaccurate. Inferential statistics are used to determine the likelihood that the sample chosen for a study is actually representative of the population.

Descriptive Statistics

Descriptive statistics allow the researcher to examine the characteristics, behaviors, and experiences of study participants (Norwood, 2010). There are many different ways to categorize descriptive statistics. In this book, they are divided into four classifications: (a) measures to condense data, (b) measures of central tendency, (c) measures of variability, and (d) measures of relationships.

Measures to Condense Data

When the researcher is faced with analyzing a large amount of data, some method is needed to condense the data into a more understandable form. **Measures to condense data** are statistics used to summarize and condense data. Some of the various ways to condense or summarize the data include frequency distributions, graphic presentations, and percentages.

FREQUENCY DISTRIBUTIONS One of the simplest ways to present data is through frequency distributions. Frequencies are obtained by counting the occurrence of values or scores represented in the data. Frequency distributions are appropriate for reporting all levels of data (nominal, ordinal, interval, and ratio). In a frequency distribution, all values or scores are listed, and the number of times each one appears is recorded. Values may be listed from highest to lowest or from lowest to highest.

It is helpful to use the familiar slash method of recording frequencies: Four vertical lines (or forward slashes: ////) are listed for the first four occurrences of a score, and a slash line (horizontal line or backward slash: — or \) is used to indicate the fifth occurrence. This procedure is repeated until all scores are recorded.

Frequency distributions present useful summaries of data. For example, the reader will get a much clearer picture of students' scores on a test or the pulse rates of a group of patients.

If the range of scores in a frequency distribution is small, say less than 20, each score may be listed individually, as in Table 15–1. When the range of scores is large, it may be helpful to group the scores before counting frequencies, as is seen in Table 15–2.

Groups of scores in a frequency distribution are called **class intervals**. These intervals are arbitrarily chosen to depict the data in the most meaningful way. Class intervals may be in units of 3, 5, 10, and so forth. The intervals must be exhaustive (include all possible values) and mutually exclusive (no overlapping of categories). Of course, when data are grouped, some information is lost. Consider the following examples:

EXAMPLE A		EXAMPLE B	
Score	Frequency	Score	Frequency
20	3	20–22	14
21	5		
22	6		
	14		

Table 15–1 Frequency Distribution of Respiration Rates

Respiration	Rate Tallies	Frequency
14	///	3
15	//	2
16	////	5
17	////	4
18	///	3
19	//	2
20	/	1
		20

Table 15–2 Frequency Distribution of Pulse Rates

Pulse Rate	Tallies	Frequency
56–60	//	2
61–65	//	2
66–70	////	5
71–75	//// //	7
76–80	//// ///	8
81–85	//// ////	10
86–90	//// //	7
91–95	////	5
96–100	////	4
		50

In Example A, you can determine exactly how many people received a score of 20, 21, or 22. In Example B, you are able to determine only that 14 people scored between 20 and 22. This loss of information is the price that is paid when data are summarized into groups or classes.

Frequency distributions may be described according to their shape. Distribution shapes may be characterized as either symmetrical or nonsymmetrical. **Symmetrical distributions** are those in which both halves of the distribution are the same. If the left half of the distribution were folded over the right half, the two halves would match. **Nonsymmetrical distributions**, also called **skewed**, are those in which the distribution has an off-center peak. If the tail of the distribution points to the right (Figure 15–1), the distribution is said to be **positively skewed**; if the tail points to the left (Figure 15–2), the distribution is said to be **negatively skewed**. An example of a variable that tends to be positively skewed is personal income. A lot of people have small or middle incomes, and a few people have large incomes. An example of a negatively skewed distribution would be the age of people who have chronic illnesses. A few young and middle-age men and women have chronic illnesses, but many more elderly people have chronic conditions.

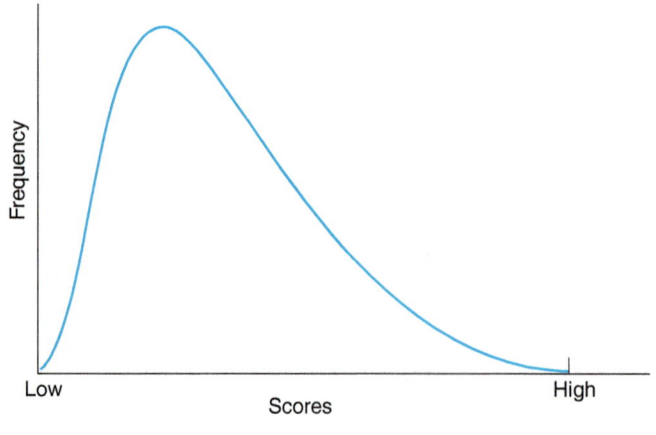

Figure 15–1 Positively skewed distribution

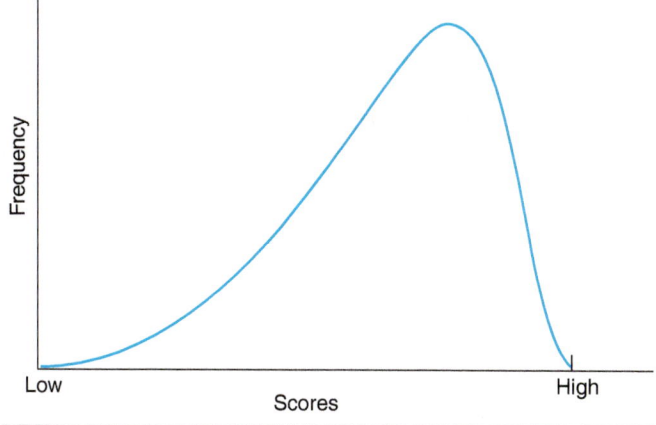

Figure 15-2 Negatively skewed distribution

A theoretical frequency distribution of particular importance in statistics is the normal distribution. The **normal distribution** is a symmetrical distribution that has one central peak or set of values in the middle of the distribution. The **normal curve** is a bell-shaped curve that graphically presents a normal distribution (see Figure 15–3). The normal curve is sometimes called the Gaussian curve because Carl Gauss developed the concept of the normal distribution.

As with all graphic presentations of frequency distributions, the values of the distribution are placed on the horizontal axis, and the frequencies of the values are placed on the vertical axis. The one difference in this type of graph compared with a histogram or frequency polygon is that the vertical axis is usually not displayed. The actual frequency of the values is therefore not depicted on the graph of a normal curve.

Normal is a mathematical rather than a medical or psychological term, and used in the sense that a normal distribution is frequently found in many happenings in nature. Such variables as height and weight are normally distributed in the population. For example, most people are of average height. There are a few very short and a few very tall people, but most people are within a few inches of each other in height.

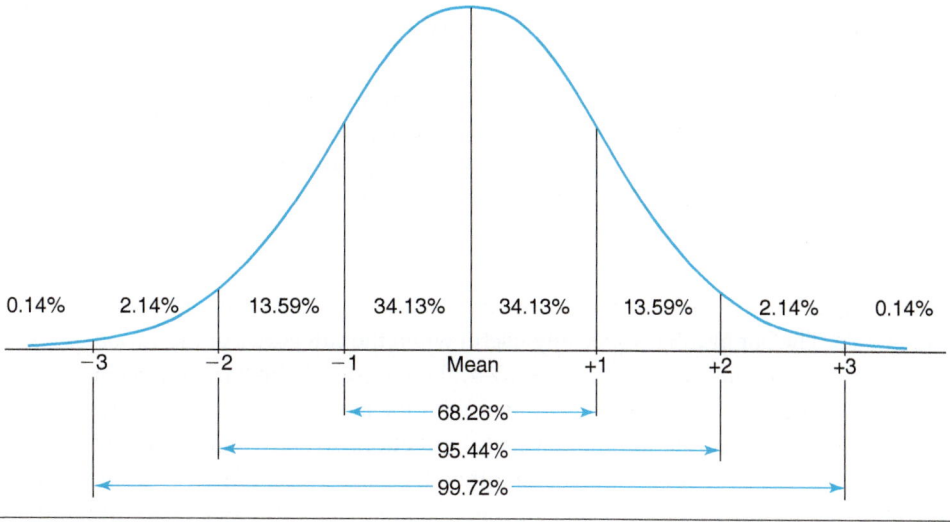

Figure 15-3 Normal curve

For a frequency distribution to approximate the normal curve, a fairly large number of values are needed. However, the normal curve can be closely approximated with sample sizes of at least 30 (Roscoe, 1975; Shott, 1990). Some inferential statistical methods are based on the assumption that what is being measured follows a normal curve distribution. A sample size of 30 can sometimes indicate value measures that are normally distributed. However, a research question might require a much larger sample than 30 to be able to generalize the results obtained from the sample to the population of interest. In this case, it would be wise to do a power analysis to determine the best sample size for a specific research question. Power analysis measurements are based upon the strength of the relationships among the variables addressed in the research questions.

The characteristics of the normal curve include the following:

1. It is bell shaped, with a symmetrical distribution, and the maximum height is the mean.
2. The mean, median, and mode are the same value.
3. Most of the values cluster around the mean.
4. A few values occur on both extreme ends of the distribution curve.
5. The point where the curve begins to grow faster horizontally than vertically is called an *inflection point* and lies at 1 SD (standard deviation) above and 1 SD below the mean.
6. The tails of the curve never touch the base because the distribution is theoretical rather than empirical.

In the normal curve, 50% of the values lie on the left half of the distribution, and 50% lie on the right half. Other percentages can be determined by assessing the distances of various values from the mean. For example, 34.13% of the area under the curve lies between the mean and +1 SD from the mean. Because the distribution is symmetrical, 34.13% of the area under the curve lies between the mean and −1 SD from the mean. Therefore, 68.26% of the distribution lies within ±1 SD from the mean, 95.44% of the distribution lies within ±2 SD from the mean, and 99.72% lies within ±3 SD of the mean. Although theoretically the curve never touches the base, nearly 100% of the values lie between −3 SD and +3 SD. Only 0.14% of the values lie above +3 SD and 0.14 % below −3 SD. Figure 15–3 depicts the areas under the normal curve.

The percentages under the normal curve may be thought of as probabilities. These probabilities are usually stated in decimal form. For example, 34.13% of the area under the normal curve lies between the mean and +1 SD. When this percentage is converted to a decimal, it becomes .3413. The probability that a value in a normal distribution lies between the mean and +1 SD is .3413. The probability that a value lies above +1 SD is .1587 (.5000 − .3413 = .1587). An understanding of probabilities is very important when considering inferential statistics and this topic is discussed in other chapters in this textbook.

GRAPHIC PRESENTATIONS Data may be presented in a graphic form that makes the frequency distribution of the data readily apparent. Graphic presentations also have a visual appeal that may cause the reader to analyze the data more closely than would be the case if a written description of the data were presented. Various graphic displays are appropriate according to the level of measurement of the variable to be presented. A graphic display is called a *figure*.

Bar Graph   A **bar graph** is a figure used to represent a frequency distribution of nominal data and some types of ordinal data. The bar graph is especially useful when the categories of the variables are qualitative rather than numerical. As you can see in Figure 15–4, the lengths of the bars represent the frequency of occurrence of the category. Bar graphs may be drawn with the bars extending in a horizontal direction (as in Figure 15–4) or with the bars extending in a vertical direction. To show that the data being represented are separate categories, the bars do not touch each other. Data are presented on only one variable in a bar graph. In Figure 15–3, the variable is "reasons for missed clinic appointments." Each of the reasons given by the respondents represents a separate category of the variable being measured.

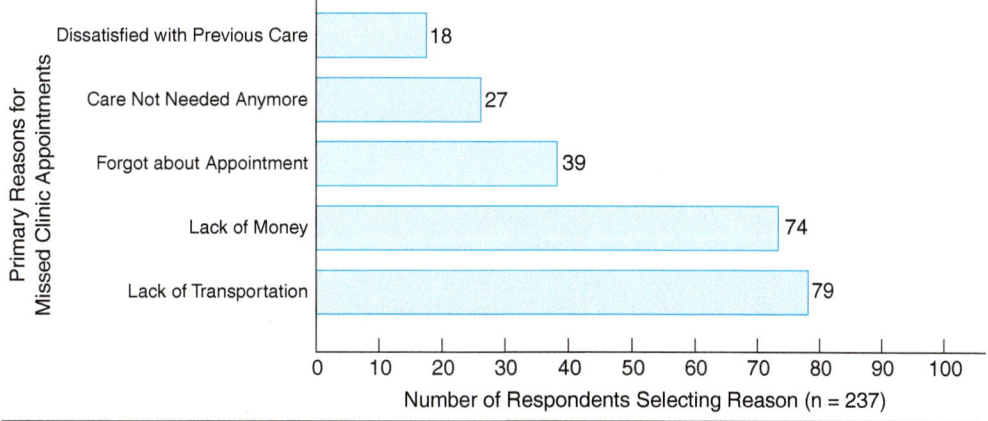

Figure 15–4 Bar graph of reasons for missed clinic appointments

Histogram   A **histogram** is a graph that uses bars to represent the frequency distribution of a variable measured at the ordinal, interval, or ratio level (Figure 15–5). Data are presented on only one variable in a histogram. The bars in a histogram are of equal width and touch each other to indicate that data are being presented on a continuum. The width of the bar represents the size of the class interval. The height of the bar represents the frequency of occurrence of each class interval. To construct a histogram, two axes are drawn: a vertical axis and a horizontal axis. The vertical axis is called the *ordinate,* and the horizontal axis the *abscissa.* Beginning at 0, the ordinate axis is marked off in equal intervals up to the highest possible frequency of the category being measured. The abscissa is marked off with the class intervals or categories of the variable. For good graphic proportions, the vertical axis is generally drawn about two-thirds the length of the horizontal axis.

Frequency Polygon   A **frequency polygon** is a graph that uses dots connected with straight lines to represent the frequency distribution of ordinal, interval, or ratio data (Figure 15–6). A dot is placed above the midpoint of each class interval; these dots are then connected. Although not strictly correct, it is customary to bring the distribution down to the horizontal axis by adding a 0 frequency at each end of the distribution.

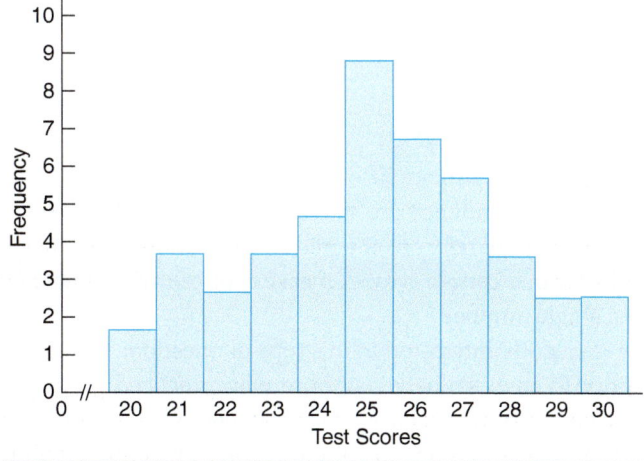

Figure 15–5 Histogram of test scores

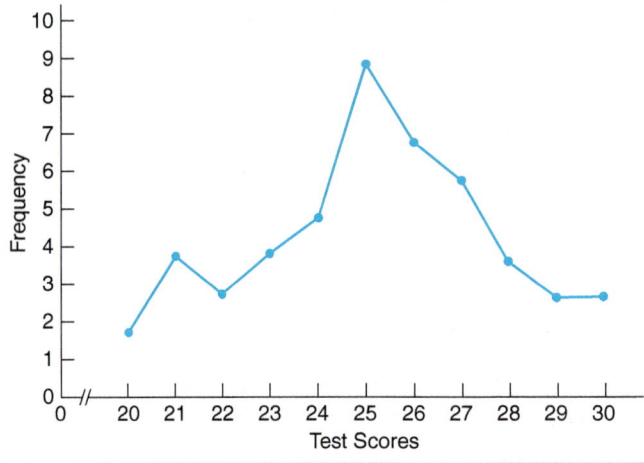

Figure 15–6 Frequency polygon of test scores

As is the case with histograms, the class intervals of the variable are represented on the horizontal axis of the frequency polygon, and the frequencies of the class intervals are represented on the vertical axis. The height of each dot indicates the frequency of a particular class interval.

PERCENTAGES A **percentage** is a statistic that represents the proportion of a subgroup to a total group, expressed as a percentage ranging from 0 to 100. A percentage is the number of parts per 100 that a certain portion of the whole represents. The size of the total group on which a percentage is based should be reasonably large for the percentage to be a useful or valid statistic. The minimum number for the computation of percentages should be at least 20. This number assures that each element in a group represents only 5% of the total group. To illustrate the need for fairly large numbers of scores or values when computing percentages, consider the following example. A friend comes up to you and says, "I just heard that they conducted a survey, and 60% of the students interviewed said they thought another year should be added to our educational program." If you were a student in the program, your first instinct might be to go find the traitors and give them a piece of your mind. First, however, it would be wise to ask how many students were interviewed. If told that only five students were interviewed, you would probably not consider the sample to be very representative of the student population and not worry about the survey's results.

Measures of Central Tendency

In many cases, the condensing of data will not be of as much interest or importance as the average value of a distribution. **Measures of central tendency** are statistics that describe the average, typical, or most common value for a group of data. *Central* refers to the middle or average value; *tendency* refers to the general trend of the numbers to cluster in a certain way. A measure of central tendency summarizes a frequency distribution by the use of a single number.

Nurse researchers are frequently interested in this type of question: "What is the average level of anxiety of nursing students prior to an exam between those who practiced progressive relaxation before the exam compared with those who did not practice progressive relaxation?" Of course, the frequency distribution of the anxiety scores would be of interest, but the average anxiety level would provide a much more exact indication of any difference that might exist in the anxiety levels of the two groups.

Although average is frequently used to indicate the arithmetic mean, there are also two other measures of central tendency: the mode and the median. The level of measurement of the data determines which measure of central tendency should be used in presenting the average value of a set of data.

MODE The **mode**, sometimes abbreviated as *Mo*, is the category or value that occurs most often in a set of data under consideration. It may be thought of as the most representative category or value in the group. The mode is determined by visually analyzing and counting data.

The mode is the only measure of central tendency appropriate for nominal data. When the data are only categories rather than actual numbers, as is the case with nominal data, the category with the greatest frequency is called the **modal class**. For example, if a sample was composed of 50 nurses, 40 occupational therapists, 35 dental technicians, and 30 physical therapists, the modal class would be nurses.

The mode may also be reported for ordinal, interval, or ratio data. In the following distribution of scores, the mode is 13 because it appears twice and the other six numbers only appear once:

16   15   13   13   12   9   6   4

If the distribution of the values is symmetrical in a frequency distribution, the mode is the same value as the median and the mean. A set of data with one value that occurs most frequently is called **unimodal**. If two values have the same high frequency, the distribution is called **bimodal**. If more than two values have the same high frequency, the distribution is said to be **multimodal**. Although the mode is an interesting statistic, it is rarely reported in the literature because it is only a crude estimate of the average value of the data.

MEDIAN The **median**, sometimes abbreviated as *Md* or *Mdn*, is the middle score or value in a group of data. With interval and ratio data, the median divides the frequency distribution of the data in half. If the number of scores or values is uneven, the median is the middle value. If the number of scores is even, the median is the midpoint between these two middle values and is found by averaging these two values. Consider the following examples:

Uneven Numbers of Scores		Even Number of Scores	
16 15 13 13	50% of values	16 15 13 13	50% of values
12	Median	(12.5)	Median
9 6 4 3	50% of values	12 9 6 4	50% of values

The median is appropriate for ordinal, interval, and ratio data. When ordinal data are analyzed, the average category can be identified. For example, if anxiety levels were classified as mild, moderate, severe, and panic, the average category might be moderate. When percentiles are being calculated, the median is the 50th percentile. If grouped data from a frequency distribution are being used, a formula is needed to compute the median. One of the most valuable qualities of the median is that it is not influenced by extreme values. The median is frequently used in reporting average income because extremely high or low incomes do not affect the median, as would be the case if the mean were calculated.

MEAN The **mean**, sometimes abbreviated as M or presented as $\overline{X}$ (X-bar), is the average sum of a set of values found by adding all values and dividing by the total number of values. This measure of central tendency is also called the arithmetic mean. Whereas the mode and median indicate the position of certain values in a distribution, the mean considers all of the values as a whole.

The mean is appropriate for interval and ratio data. It is considered the most stable measure of central tendency for these levels of data if the distribution is normal. If the distribution is not normal and extreme values are present, the mean will not present an accurate picture of the distribution. As mentioned under the discussion of the median, if average income were reported as the mean, a few extremely wealthy people could make the rest of us appear rich.

The symbol for a sample mean is M or $\overline{X}$, and the symbol for the population mean is μ. The mean is figured in the following manner:

$$\overline{X} = \frac{\Sigma X}{N}$$

where X = score; Σ = a summation sign, indicating that all scores are added; and N = total number of scores.

$$\begin{array}{c} 16 \\ 15 \\ 13 \\ 13 \\ 12 \\ 9 \\ 6 \\ \underline{4} \\ \Sigma X = 88 \end{array}$$

$$\overline{X} = \frac{\Sigma X}{N} = \frac{88}{8} = 11$$

Measures of Variability

Measures of variability describe the spread of scores in a distribution of values. Although measures of central tendency are very important, sometimes it may be of more interest to know how spread out the values are in a distribution. Consider the following pulse rates:

Group A	Group B
80	100
79	90
78	80
78	70
75	50
$\Sigma X = 390$	$\Sigma X = 390$
$\overline{X} = 78$	$\overline{X} = 78$

As you can see, the mean of both groups of pulse rates is the same. However, pulse rates of people in Group A are homogeneous, or alike, whereas pulse rates of people in Group B are heterogeneous, or dissimilar. This information would be very important because the arithmetic mean is not as appropriate to use in describing Group B or to use in comparing the two groups of pulse rates. The most common measures of variability are range, percentile, standard deviation, variance, and z-scores.

RANGE The distance between the highest and lowest value in a group of values or scores is called the **range**. The range is the simplest measure of variability. It is presented as a single number. Frequently, the word range is used incorrectly to indicate the lowest and highest values. For example, you might hear this statement: "The scores ranged from 40 to 60." Although this type of statement is fairly common, technically the range for these scores is 20 (60 − 40 = 20). The range is a measure that can be used to gain a quick picture of the dispersion of the data. The range has limited usefulness because one extreme score can change the range drastically.

To correct for the influence of extreme scores or values, the interquartile range (IQR) may be reported. The **interquartile range** contains the middle half of the values in a frequency distribution

$$IQR = Q^3 - Q^1$$

where Q_3 = the point below which three-fourths of the distribution lies, and Q_1 = the point below which one-fourth of the distribution lies. The **semiquartile range** (SQR) is found by dividing the interquartile range in half: SQR = IQR/2.

PERCENTILE A **percentile** is a datum point below which lies a certain percentage of the values in a frequency distribution. If you score at the 80th percentile on a test, it means that 80% of the other students received lower scores. You might also say that 20% of the other students scored higher (depending on whether you are an optimist or a pessimist).

The median of a frequency distribution lies at the 50th percentile. Percentile is a common statistic used to allow people to compare their performance with that of others. Raw scores, or untreated data, are transformed into percentile ranks. Most basic statistics books give instructions for how to calculate percentiles.

Percentiles are used a great deal in the assessment of infants and children. Imagine you read a child's chart and find that, for his age group, he is at the 95th percentile in height and the 15th percentile in weight. What would you expect the physical appearance of this child to be like in height and weight? Tall and skinny, right?

An anxiety test used frequently in nursing research is the State-Trait Anxiety Inventory by Spielberger (1983). Spielberger views state anxiety as a current feeling of emotional and physical uneasiness, whereas trait anxiety refers to an individual's basic tendency to be anxious and is considered a relatively stable personality trait. The test booklet that accompanies this anxiety test provides information about the test and furnishes percentile ranks for groups on which the test was normed. The lowest possible score is 20 and the highest possible score is 80 on the two scales that measure state and trait anxiety. You might think that an average anxiety score would be 50, which is halfway between 20 and 80. Not so. A raw score of 50 on the state anxiety scale is at the 82nd percentile when compared with a group of female college students who were used in establishing norms for the test. A score of 66 is at the 99th percentile.

STANDARD DEVIATION The standard deviation is the most widely used measure of variability when interval or ratio data are obtained. This statistic describes how values vary about the mean of the distribution. The word standard is used to mean average. The **standard deviation**, abbreviated SD or s, is a measurement that indicates the average deviation or variation of all the values in a set of values from the mean value of those data. Like the arithmetic mean, the standard deviation takes into consideration all the values in a distribution. The actual definition of the standard deviation is a little bit difficult to understand. Mathematically, the standard deviation is equal to the square root of the sum of the squared deviations about the mean divided by the total number of values. Were you able to follow that statement?

You may wonder when you would ever use the SD in nursing. I am sure that all of you are familiar with critical pathways. They are useful in planning care for a group of patients with the same condition and who have a predictable course of recovery. If, for example, the SD for length of stay (LOS) for a group of patients with a certain serious condition is 5.2 days, it might be very difficult to develop a critical pathway. It appears there may be too much variability in recovery time for one plan of care to be suitable for all patients with this condition.

VARIANCE The **variance** is a measure that is used in several inferential statistical tests. Mathematically, the variance is equal to the sum of the squared deviations about the mean divided by the total number of values. This definition may seem complex, but squared values allow the mathematician to account for both positive and negative numbers. The standard deviation is the square root of the variance or, in other words, the variance is the standard deviation squared. The variance is reported less frequently because the variance is not in the same unit of measurement as the variable being examined, as is the case with the standard deviation, which is the square root of the variance.

Z-SCORES A **z-score** is a standard score that indicates how many SDs from the mean a particular value lies. A z-score is called a standard score because it is interpreted in relation to SD units above or below the mean. This is the formula for calculating z-scores:

$$z = \frac{X - \overline{X}}{s}$$

where z = z-score, X = score or value,
$\overline{X}$ = mean of scores or values, and s = standard deviation.

The z-score is a very useful statistic for interpreting a particular value in relation to the other values in a distribution. Also, z-scores allow you to compare the performance of someone on nonequivalent tests. If a score is 1 SD above the mean, it has a z-score of 1. Consider the following example. You received a raw score of 92 on a test with 110 questions. The mean raw score was 98, and the SD was 3. How well did you score on the test compared with others who took the examination?

$$\frac{92 - 98}{3} = \frac{-6}{3} = -2.0$$

You did not do too well. Your z-score is −2.0. This means that only 2.28% of the group scored lower than you did. Review Figure 15–3 again, and you will see that 2.14% of the values lie between −2 SD and −3 SD, and .14% of the values lie beyond −3 SD. Thus, 2.28% of the values lie beyond −2 SD (2.14 + .14 = 2.28). Tables are available in statistical texts if you wish to determine the percentage of a distribution above and below any given z-score.

Measures of Relationships

So far, the material in this chapter has been concerned with the analysis of data on one variable at a time. The frequency distributions that were discussed might be referred to as univariate frequency distributions. In nursing research, however, we are frequently concerned with more than one variable. **Measures of relationships** concern the correlations between variables. As you recall, a correlation concerns the extent to which values of one variable (X) are related to values of a second variable (Y). You might want to determine if there is a correlation between the amount of time spent with a patient and the number of requests for pain medication made by that patient. A record might be made of the total time nurses spent in a patient's room during a given time period of the day and the number of requests for pain medication made by the patient during that same time period. These data would be gathered on a group of patients. You would want to know if these two values seemed to vary together. When the time spent with the patient increased, did the number of requests for pain medications increase or decrease? There are several ways to examine a relationship such as this. Correlation coefficients, scatter plots, and contingency tables, along with various types of correlational procedures, are discussed here.

Correlation Coefficients

Correlations are computed through pairing the value of each subject on one variable (X) with the value on another variable (Y). You may recall from the earlier discussion of correlational studies that the magnitude and direction of the relationship between these two variables is presented through a measurement called a correlation coefficient. The correlation coefficient can vary between −1.00 and +1.00. These two numbers represent the extremes of a perfect relationship. A correlation coefficient of −1.00 indicates a perfect negative relationship, whereas +1.00 indicates a perfect positive relationship, and 0 indicates the absence of any relationship. Correlation coefficients are frequently symbolized by the letter r.

An $r = +.80$ indicates that as the value of one variable (X) increases, the value of the other variable (Y) tends to increase. It also means that as the value of one variable decreases, the value of the other variable tends to decrease. In other words, a positive relationship means the values of the two variables tend to increase or decrease together. Although a plus sign has been included to show a positive relationship (+.80), the sign is usually not included, and the assumption is made that the relationship is positive if no sign is present (.80). An $r = -.80$ denotes a negative (inverse) relationship and indicates that as the value one variable increases, the value of the other variable tends to decrease.

A positive relationship might be found between anxiety levels and pulse rates. As anxiety levels go up, pulse rates go up. A negative relationship might be found between anxiety levels and test scores. As anxiety levels go up, test scores go down.

Whereas the sign of the correlation coefficient shows the direction or nature of the relationship (positive or negative), the size of the correlation coefficient indicates the magnitude or strength of the relationship. An $r = .80$ denotes a stronger relationship than an $r = .60$. Also, an $r = -.50$ indicates a stronger relationship than an $r = -.40$. Remember, the sign only indicates the direction of the relationship.

Generally, correlation coefficients are calculated on measurements obtained from each subject on two variables. Correlation coefficients, however, may be calculated on the measurements of one variable that are obtained from two groups of matched subjects, such as fathers and sons. A researcher might want to determine if there is a relationship between the height of fathers and their sons. Correlation coefficients can also be used to measure reliability. For example, the reliability of an instrument can be determined by examining subjects' scores at Time 1 versus scores at Time 2. This is called test-retest reliability.

Caution must be exercised in interpreting correlations. *It cannot be emphasized too much that correlation does not equate with causation.* If a strong positive relationship is found between anxiety levels and pulse rates, you should not conclude that the anxiety levels *caused* the pulse rates to go up. It is possible that the pulse rates increased then the anxiety levels increased, or that some other variable caused the pulse rates to rise and also increased anxiety. Another example would be reading level and shoe size in a population of elementary school children. Although there may be a strong correlation between the larger shoe size and a higher reading level in this age group, having larger feet does not cause an increase in reading level.

You may wonder how to determine if a correlation is weak or strong. Does $r = .30$ indicate a mild or a moderate relationship? There are no set criteria to evaluate the actual strength of a correlation coefficient. The nature of the variables being studied will help determine the strength of the relationship. Correlations between psychosocial variables rarely exceed .50. Roscoe (1975) wrote, "a correlation of .70 between scholastic aptitude in the first grade and grade point average in college would be phenomenal" (p. 101). He cautioned, however, that a correlation of .70 between two tests that were supposedly equivalent would be too low.

The coefficient of determination is a statistic that should be calculated after the computation of a correlation coefficient. The **coefficient of determination** is obtained by squaring the correlation coefficient (r^2) and is interpreted as the percentage of variance shared by the two variables. The coefficient of determination for an $r = .50$ would be .25 ($.50 \times .50 = .25$), which would then be multiplied by 100 and read as 25%.

Suppose a correlation of .60 were obtained between anxiety scores and pulse rates. The coefficient of determination would be .36, which would mean that these two variables share a common variance or overlap of 36%. If you knew a person's anxiety score, you would have 36% of the information needed to predict that person's pulse rate. Because the coefficient of determination is reversible, you would have 36% of the information needed to predict that person's anxiety level if you knew his or her pulse rate. Of course, you would still be lacking 64% of the knowledge needed to predict one of these variables based on knowledge of the other variable. Table 15–3 displays the percentage of variance explained by different correlation coefficients. An $r = .708$ is necessary before 50% of the variance is explained. Perhaps researchers will begin to report this statistic more often because the coefficient of determination gives a much clearer picture of the value of a correlation coefficient than the tests of significance of correlation coefficients, discussed later. It is possible for a very low correlation coefficient, such as .20 or even lower, to be statistically significant when a large sample size is used. Only 4% of the shared variance of two variables is explained by a correlation coefficient of .20. If the coefficient of determination is not presented in a research article in which correlation coefficients are presented, you can quickly do the calculation yourself.

SCATTER PLOTS A **scatter plot**, also called a **scatter diagram** or a **scattergram**, is a graphic presentation of the relationship between two variables. The graph contains variables on an X axis and a Y axis. The X variable is plotted on the horizontal axis; the Y variable is plotted on the vertical axis. The scatter plot is a visual device that can be used to eyeball a correlation between two variables. The magnitude of the relationship as well as the direction of the relationship can be determined.

Pairs of scores are plotted on a graph by the placement of dots to indicate where each pair of Xs and Ys intersects. For a positive correlation, the lowest score or value for each variable is placed at the lower left corner of the graph. Values increase as they go up the vertical axis and as they go toward the right on the horizontal axis. If the dots seem to be distributed from the upper left corner down toward the lower right corner, a negative correlation is said to exist.

Table 15–3 Percentage of Variance Explained by Correlations

Coefficient (r)	Coefficient of Determination (r^2)	Percentage of Variance Explained
.950	.9025	90
.850	.7225	72
.750	.5625	56
.708	.5013	50
.650	.4225	42
.550	.3025	30
.450	.2025	20
.350	.1225	12
.250	.0625	6
.150	.0225	2

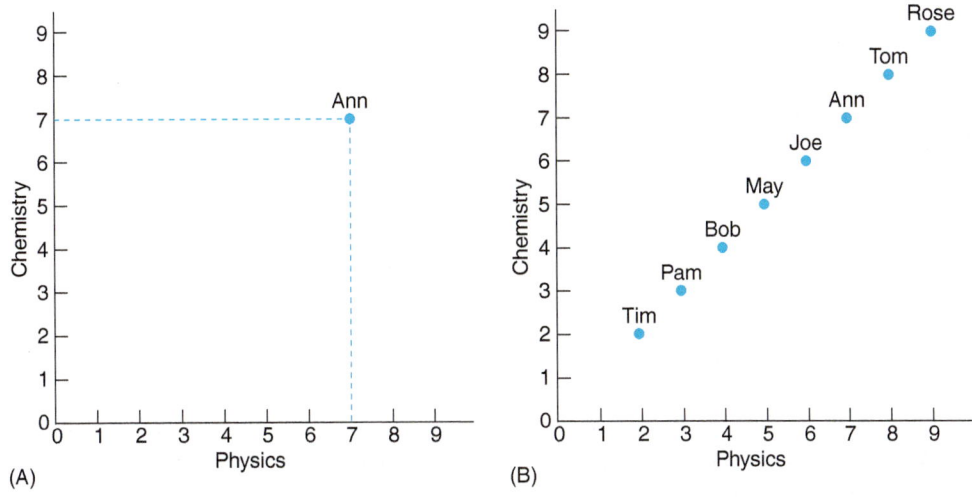

Figure 15–7 Scatter plots of chemistry and physics test scores for one student (A) and for eight students (B)

Examine Figure 15–7. This graph depicts chemistry and physics examination scores. One student's score is plotted on the graph (Figure 15–7A). As can be seen, the student, Ann, scored a 7 on both tests. If each student receives the same score on both tests (5 and 5, 6 and 6), a perfect positive correlation is said to exist, and the dots would all fall on a straight line drawn from the lower left corner of the graph to the upper right corner. Figure 15–7B shows the placement of the dots for 8 students' scores (Note the name of the person who scored the highest.).

Generally you will not find a perfect correlation as seen in Figure 15–7B. Figure 15–8 depicts varying degrees of correlations. The closer the dots are to a straight line, the higher is the correlation. When the dots are scattered all over the graph, it indicates that no relationship exists between the two variables.

CONTINGENCY TABLES If data are nominal or categorical, relationships cannot be depicted on a scatter plot. No actual scores are available for nominal data; rather the frequencies of the occurrences of the categories are presented. A **contingency table**, also called a cross-tabulation table, is a visual means of displaying the relationship between sets of nominal data. For example, the researcher might wish to determine if a relationship exists between gender and exercise behavior. Table 15–4 depicts the data that were gathered on 50 male and 50 female subjects.

The data from Table 15–4 seem to indicate that more men than women participate in regular exercise programs. The chi-square statistic can be calculated to determine if there is a significant relationship between these variables. If a significant relationship is found, the researcher cannot conclude that gender causes one to participate in an exercise program. The reason for the existence of the relationship would still remain unknown.

Table 15–4 is called a 2 × 2 table because there are two variables and each variable has two categories. If exercise had been divided into three categories, such as never exercises, occasionally exercises, and frequently exercises, the table would have been called a 2 × 3 table.

TYPES OF CORRELATIONAL PROCEDURES There are many different correlational procedures. The determination of the appropriate correlation procedure is dependent upon the level of data (nominal,

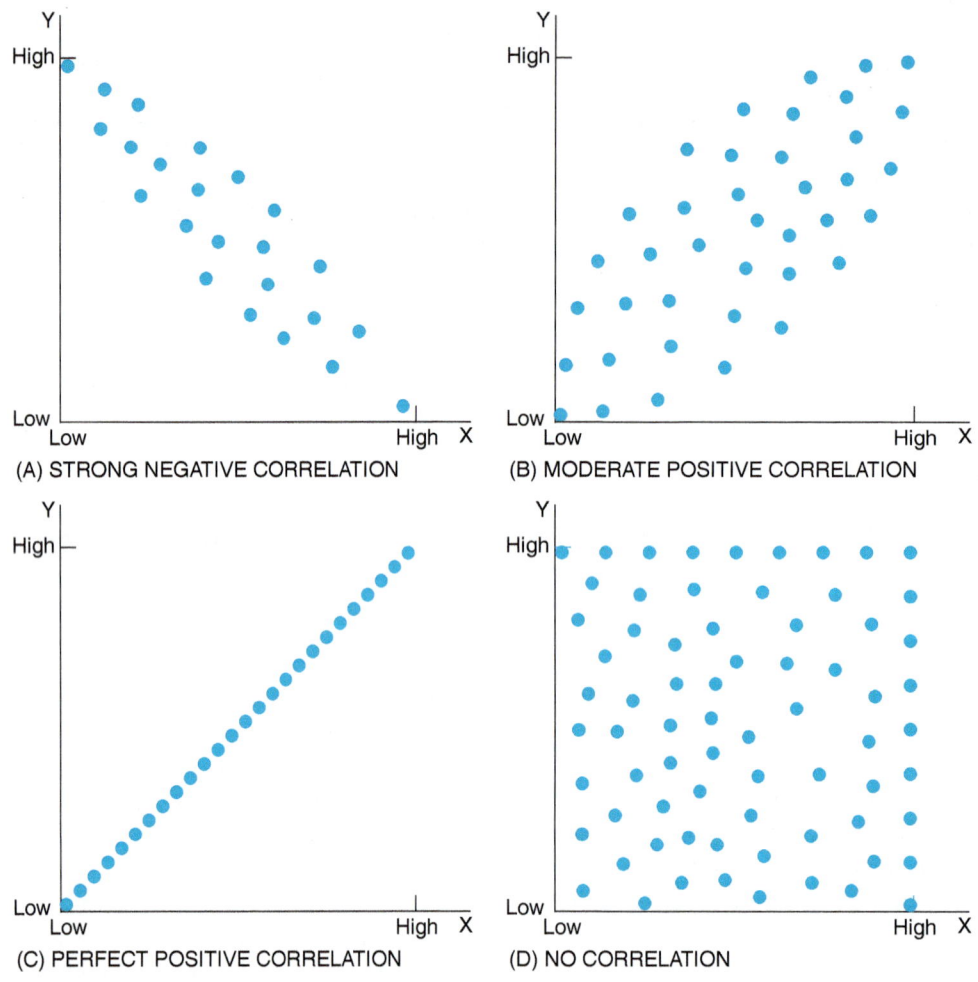

Figure 15–8 Scatter plots of correlations

Table 15–4 Example of Contingency Table

	Exercise Regularly	Do Not Exercise Regularly	Total
Males	35	15	50
Females	10	40	50
Total	45	55	100

ordinal, interval, or ratio) of the variables being correlated. The researcher should select the correlation procedure that is appropriate for the lowest level of data.

Pearson *r* The most common correlational procedure used in nursing research when both sets of data are at the interval or ratio level is the Pearson product-moment correlation (Pearson *r*), symbolized by the letter *r*.

Pearson r

The Pearson r test was used by Lin, Liao, Chen, and Fan (2012) to study the relationships between job stress, poor sleep quality and self-perceived health status among 266 nurses from four hospitals in Taiwan. There was a significant correlation between job stress and reported poor sleep quality (meaning the greater the job stress, the poorer the sleep quality) ($r = 0.34$, $p < .001$); a moderately negative, significant correlation between job stress and self-perceived health status (meaning the greater job stress, the poorer self-perceived health) ($r = -0.36$, $p < .001$); and a moderately positive significant correlation was found between poor sleep quality and self-perceived health (meaning the poorer sleep quality, the poorer the self-perceived health status) ($r\ -0.37$, $p < .001$).

Spearman Rho   The Spearman rho is the correlational procedure commonly used with ordinal data. It is symbolized by r_s, r_{rho}, or rho. Although this correlational procedure is used less frequently than the Pearson r because it is not as powerful a procedure, many published research studies present the Spearman rho because at least some of the data were gathered at the ordinal level.

Spearman Rho

Inkpen, Parker, and Kirby (2012) examined the relationship between self-reported manual wheelchair capacity and performance from manual wheelchair users with an average of over ten years of experience. Some of the data were not normally distributed; therefore, the Spearman rho correlation coefficient was used. A positive relationship (.853, $p = .000$) was found between wheelchair capacity and performance scores.

Correlational procedures for nominal data   Finally, several correlational procedures are appropriate for nominal data: contingency coefficient, phi coefficient, and Cramer's V. These correlations depend on the chi-square (χ^2), explored later.

Sometimes researchers gather two levels of data in a correlational study. For example, a researcher might study the correlation between anxiety levels and pulse rates. Anxiety levels might be measured at the ordinal level (panic anxiety, high anxiety, moderate anxiety, and mild anxiety), whereas pulse rates are measured at the interval level (numerical pulse rates). The researcher would be forced to use the Spearman rho rather than the Pearson r. In other words, the researcher must select the correlational statistic that is appropriate for the lowest level of data. If a correlation were being examined on two sets of data that were gathered at the ordinal and nominal levels of measurement, a statistical procedure would be used that is appropriate for nominal data, which is the lower of these two levels of measurement.

Intraocular Method of Data Analysis

The researcher should always use the so-called intraocular method when analyzing data. This is a humorous term used to indicate that you should eyeball your data. Many mistakes could be avoided in data analysis if the researcher's eyes and common sense were used. For example, imagine the following group of scores were obtained: 78, 79, 80, 76, and 74. When the average is calculated, it is found to be 68. The intraocular method should tell the researcher that a mistake has been made in calculation. After glancing at the data, an estimate should be made of the results of data analysis. This procedure provides a checks-and-balances system that frequently pays off in the detection of an error in calculations or an error in the data entry process.

Critiquing Descriptive Statistics in Research Reports

It is often difficult for the beginning reader of research reports to critique the statistical content of these reports. The reader may not have taken a basic statistics course. Even if such a course was completed, the content may have been forgotten or misunderstood. Therefore, many consumers of research are hesitant to examine the study statistics in a research report.

It is desirable to have some background in statistics before reading research reports. However, the background knowledge needed to critique most reports is not extensive. Knowledge of a few statistical concepts goes a long way toward helping the reader understand data analysis presented in research articles and other types of research reports. Box 15–1 lists some guidelines for critiquing descriptive statistics.

Box 15–1   Guidelines for Critiquing Descriptive Statistics

1. What types of descriptive statistics are included in the research report?
2. Were the descriptive statistics appropriate for the level of measurement of the variable(s)?
3. Were measures of central tendency and variability both presented?
4. Do the descriptive statistics clearly present the demographic characteristics of the subjects?
5. Are the descriptive statistics clearly presented in the text? In tables and graphs?
6. Do the descriptive statistics presented in the text agree with those presented in the tables?

The first task is to identify the various descriptive statistics that were used to analyze data. Nearly every research study uses descriptive statistics to present the demographic characteristics of the sample. For example, the ages, educational levels, and incomes of the subjects may be presented through descriptive statistics. If the mean was used to present the average income, the reader should try to determine if the median would have been a more appropriate measure of central tendency. This would be true if some of the subjects reported extremely high or low incomes.

The level of measurement of each variable should be determined, if possible, then a decision made about the appropriateness of the descriptive statistics reported. Was gender treated as a nominal variable or reported as an interval variable? It makes no sense to see gender reported as an average of 1.2. This might occur if the researcher had assigned a value of 1 to women and 2 to men and did not relay this information to the statistician who analyzed the data. The best way to determine the level of measurement for variables is to search for the researcher's operational definitions. These are frequently found in the discussion of the instruments used in the study.

Were the descriptive data presented both in the text of the report and in tables and graphs? If so, do the data agree? If the data were not presented in tables or graphs, would the use of these methods of reporting data have made the material more easily understood?

Descriptive statistics should be presented in a manner that can be understood by the average practicing nurse. If this is not done, the results of the study will not be considered for implementation in practice.

Summary

Statistics is a branch of knowledge used to summarize and present numerical data. Numerical characteristics of populations are called parameters; numerical characteristics of samples are called statistics.

Statistics can be classified as descriptive and inferential. Descriptive statistics are those that organize and summarize numerical data from populations or samples. Inferential statistics are concerned with populations and use sample data to make an inference about a population. Types of descriptive statistics are (a) measures to condense data, (b) measures of central tendency, (c) measures of variability, and (d) measures of relationships.

Measures to condense data are statistics that summarize and condense data. Included in this category are frequency distributions, graphic presentations, and percentages. Frequency distributions are used with all levels of data. Groups of scores in a frequency distribution are called class intervals.

Distribution shapes can be classified as symmetrical or nonsymmetrical. Symmetrical distributions are those in which both halves of the distribution are the same. Nonsymmetrical distributions, also called skewed distributions, are those in which the distribution has an off-center peak. The tail of the distribution points to the right in a positively skewed distribution and to the left in a negatively skewed distribution. The normal distribution is a symmetrical distribution that has one central peak or set of values in the center of the distribution. The normal curve is a bell-shaped curve that graphically presents a normal distribution. The distribution is symmetrical, with 50% of the values contained on the left half of the curve and 50% on the right half. Approximately 68% of the distribution of a normal curve lies within ±1 SD of the mean. Approximately 95% of the distribution lies within ±2 SD of the mean, and about 99% lies within ±3 SD of the mean.

Graphic presentations include bar graphs, histograms, and frequency polygons. A bar graph is used to depict nominal data and some types of ordinal data. A histogram and a frequency polygon are used to display ordinal, interval, and ratio data.

A percentage is a statistic that represents the proportion of a subgroup to a total group, expressed as a percentage ranging from 0 to 100.

Measures of central tendency are used to describe the average value of a set of values. The mode is the category or value that occurs most often in a set of data. Modal class is the category of nominal data with the greatest frequency. A frequency distribution that contains one value that occurs more frequently than any other is called unimodal. If two values have the same high frequency, the distribution is bimodal. If more than two values have the same high frequency, the distribution is multimodal.

The median is the middle score or value in a group of data, and the mean is the average sum of a set of values.

Measures of variability describe how spread out the values are in a distribution of values. Measures of variability are range, percentile, standard deviation, variance, and *z*-score. The range is the distance between the highest and lowest value in a group of values. The interquartile range contains the middle half of the values in a frequency distribution. The semiquartile range is found by dividing the interquartile range in half. A percentile is a data point below which lies a certain percentage of the values in a frequency distribution. The standard deviation is a measure that indicates the average deviation or variability of all the values from the mean of a set of values. The standard deviation is the most widely used measure of variability when interval or ratio data are described. The variance is the standard deviation squared. A ***z*-score** is a standard score that indicates how many SDs from the mean a particular value lies.

Measures of relationships are concerned with the correlation between variables. Correlation coefficients, scatter plots, and contingency tables are means of presenting correlations.

The magnitude and direction of a relationship between two variables is presented through a correlation coefficient that varies between −1.00 and +1.00. The coefficient of determination is a statistic obtained through squaring a correlation coefficient. This statistic is interpreted as the percentage of variance shared by two variables.

A scatter plot, also called a scatter diagram or a scattergram, is a graphic presentation of the relationship between two variables. Pairs of scores are plotted on a graph by the placement of dots to indicate where each pair of Xs and Ys intersects.

A contingency table is a means of displaying the relationship between two sets of nominal data. No actual scores are presented; rather, the table includes the frequencies of occurrence of the categories.

The most common correlation procedures used in nursing research are the Pearson product-moment correlation (Pearson r) and the Spearman's rho. The Pearson r is used with interval and ratio data, and Spearman's rho is used with ordinal data. Three common correlational procedures used with nominal data are the contingency coefficient, phi, and Cramer's V.

Self-Test

1. What symbol is most frequently used for the standard deviation of a sample?
   A. SD
   B. Σ
   C. μ
   D. X

2. Identify the mode of the following group of vision test results: 20/20; 20/30; 20/40; 20/30; 20/50; 20/40; 20/100; 20/30.
   A. 20/20
   B. 20/30
   C. 20/40
   D. 20/100

3. Which measure of central tendency would most appropriately describe the average pulse rates of a group of hospitalized patients?
   A. mode
   B. median
   C. mean
   D. correlations

4. The standard deviation is a measure of:
   A. skewness.
   B. correlation.
   C. central tendency.
   D. variability.

5. A person's score is 2.5 standard deviations above the mean on a test. This means that:
   A. all of the scores on the test are high.
   B. this person's score is unusually high compared with the other scores of the test.
   C. an error has been made in recording the score.
   D. this score is 25% higher than the mean.

6. Which statement is true?
   A. The most reliable and accurate measure of central tendency is the mode.
   B. The standard deviation indicates how spread out the scores are in a distribution.
   C. The type of graph that shows the relationship between two variables is a histogram.
   D. The range of a group of scores is figured by adding the highest and lowest numbers.

7. A correlation coefficient is used to determine if:
   A. X comes before Y.
   B. X causes Y.
   C. X and Y are different.
   D. X and Y vary together.

8. Which correlation coefficient would indicate the strongest relationship between anxiety and the ability to concentrate?
   A. $r = .30$
   B. $r = -.30$
   C. $r = -.50$
   D. $r = -1.30$

9. As a nurse researcher conducting a research study with a group of children, you discover that the average weight of the subjects is at the 90th percentile for their age. Which statement would be correct?
   A. The subjects are not eating enough.
   B. The subjects are 90% above the average weight for their age.
   C. The subjects are 90% below the average weight for their age.
   D. The subjects are well above the average weight for their age.
10. The researcher wants to describe a central measure of the incomes of research participants from an urban area. Which is considered the best descriptive statistic for this purpose?
    A. mode
    B. median
    C. mean
    D. correlation

See answers to Self-Test in the Answer Section at the back of the book.

References

American Psychological Association. (2010). *Publication manual of the American Psychological Association* (6th ed.). Washington, DC: Author.

Inkpen, P., Parker, K., & Kirby, L. (2012). Manual wheelchair skills capacity versus performance. *Archives of Physical Medicine and Rehabilitation, 93*, 1009–1013. doi:10.1016/j.apmr.2011.11.027

Kranzler, J. H. (2010). *Statistics for the terrified* (5th ed.). Upper Saddle River, NJ: Pearson.

Lin, S.-H., Liao, W.-C., Chen, M.-Y., & Fan, J.-Y. (2012). The impact of shift work on nurses' job stress, sleep quality and self-perceived health status. *Nursing Management, 22*, 604–612. doi:10.1111/jonm.12020

Norwood, S. (2010). *Research essentials: Foundation for evidence-based practice.* Upper Saddle River, NJ: Pearson.

Roscoe, J. (1975). *Fundamental research statistics for the behavioral sciences* (2nd ed.). New York: Holt, Rinehart & Winston.

Shott, S. (1990). *Statistics for health care professionals.* Philadelphia: W. B. Saunders.

Spielberger, C. (1983). *Manual for the state-trait anxiety inventory.* Palo Alto, CA: Consulting Psychologists Press.

Chapter 16
Inferential Statistics

Rose Nieswiadomy, PhD, RN; Jo-Ann Stankus, PhD, RN;
and Peggy Mancuso, PhD, RN

 Objectives

On completion of this chapter, you will be prepared to:

1. Summarize the two broad purposes of statistics.
2. Discuss the three factors affecting choice of statistical measures.
3. Describe statistical tests commonly used in nursing studies.

Introduction

The material in this chapter is not really difficult to understand, but if you have not been exposed to this type of material before or did not absorb the content during a statistics class, you may think it is difficult. If so, learning this content can be a rewarding challenge. I hope your efforts will gain you a greater appreciation of the value of statistics in making decisions about data obtained in research studies. You may also be able to use your knowledge of statistics in many areas of nursing.

Descriptive statistics (discussed elsewhere) are used to present the characteristics of samples or populations. This chapter discusses inferential statistics, which use sample data to make decisions or inferences about a population. Even though the researcher obtained the data from samples, the researcher is interested in applying these findings to the designated population.

Inferential statistics are based on the laws of probability. The word *chance* is used in discussing probability. Other terms that are sometimes used interchangeably in the literature are *sampling error* and *random error*. All inferential statistical tests are based on the assumption that chance (sampling error, random error) is the only explanation for relationships that are found in research studies. For example, *if one group of participants scores higher than another group on a test, the basic assumption is made that the difference is related to chance.* Reread that sentence several times. The concept of chance is used throughout this chapter. A researcher wants to demonstrate that chance is *not* the reason for the relationships found in research.

The larger the difference found between groups, the lower the probability that the difference occurred by chance. In other words, the groups really are different on the variable being measured. The same can be said of tests that examine the significance of correlations: The larger the correlation between variables measured on members of the sample, the greater the likelihood is that the variables are, in fact, correlated in the population.

Inferential statistics are based on the assumption that the sample was randomly selected. When a random sample is selected, each member of the population has an equal chance of being selected. At this point, you may be wondering how inferential statistics can be useful because random samples are sometimes difficult to obtain. Some of the reasons for using nonprobability samples (or samples that are not randomly selected) involve time, money, and ethical issues. Spatz and Johnston (1984) presented the rationale for the use of inferential statistics with nonrandom samples. "Usually, the results based on samples that are unsystematic (but not random) are true for other samples from the same population" (p. 162). Shott (1990) stated that it is appropriate to make a statistical inference from a nonrandom sample to the population, as long the researcher does not deliberately select a biased sample. Other researchers have agreed that inferential statistics may be used with nonrandom samples, but cautioned the researcher to be conservative in interpreting study findings.

The use of a nonrandom sample greatly reduces the ability to generalize study results. You can now better understand the need for replication studies in nursing. Agreement among the findings of several similar studies conducted with nonrandom samples allows for conclusions to be derived from the data that are similar to the conclusions that could be made if one large random sample had been used.

Purposes of Inferential Statistics

The two broad purposes of inferential statistics are to estimate population parameters from sample data and to test hypotheses. The second purpose has been of more interest to nurse researchers because hypotheses are often tested in nursing research studies. However, estimating population parameters, which involve determining confidence intervals, is also an important purpose of inferential statistics.

A distinguishing point between the two purposes concerns the time of data collection. The estimation of population parameters is considered after the data are collected, whereas the testing of hypotheses is considered before data collection. Hypotheses are formulated before the data collection begins. Of course, the decision to support or not support the hypothesis is made after the data are analyzed.

Estimating Population Parameters

To estimate population parameters from sample data, an understanding of sampling error and sampling distribution is necessary. Whenever a sample is chosen to represent a population, there is some likelihood that the sample will not accurately reflect the population. Even when a true random sample is chosen, the sample may not be an average or representative sample. Sampling error occurs when the sample does not accurately reflect the population. Examine the example in Table 16–1. The table contains pulse measurements on a population of 20 subjects. The mean pulse rate for the population is 71. One sample of five subjects drawn from the population is shown to have an average pulse rate of 71. Another sample of five subjects has an average pulse rate of 63, and still another sample has an average pulse rate of 83. These last two samples demonstrate what sampling error means. The pulse rates of these two samples of subjects do not accurately reflect the average pulse rate of the population.

An interesting phenomenon may be observed about sampling error. The majority of the samples chosen from a population will accurately reflect the population. In the previous example, if an infinite number of separate samples were chosen from the population, the majority of the mean pulse rates of these samples would be close to the population average pulse rate of 71. Most of the samples would have average rates such as 69, 70, 71, 72, and 73. A few samples would have average rates that were quite different from the population mean, like the previously mentioned 63 and 83. The phenomenon in which sample values tend to be normally distributed around the population value is known as the **central limit theorem**.

Table 16–1 Frequency Distribution of Pulse Rates

Pulse Rate	Tallies	Frequency
56–60	//	2
61–65	//	2
66–70	////	5
71–75	//// //	7
76–80	//// ///	8
81–85	//// ////	10
86–90	//// //	7
91–95	////	5
96–100	////	4
		50

Whenever a large number of sample values are arranged in a frequency distribution, those values will be normally distributed even if the original population of values was not normally distributed. This may be hard to believe, but it has been demonstrated to be true if the sample size is fairly large. The sampling distribution of the mean approximates the normal curve when samples contain 100 or more observations or values. Sample sizes as small as 30 are generally considered to be adequate to ensure the sampling distribution of the mean will closely approximate the normal curve (Shott, 1990).

A theoretical frequency distribution, based on an infinite number of samples, is called a **sampling distribution**. This distribution is said to be theoretical because you never actually draw an infinite number of samples from a population. Instead, decisions are made based on one sample. The concept of sampling distributions, however, is used over and over in inferential statistics. The researcher works with one sample, but inferential statistics are based on the idea of what would occur if the researcher had actually drawn an infinite number of samples from one population. You may want to reread that sentence again. The reason the concept of sampling distributions is difficult for some people to understand is that it deals with "what ifs" rather than actual data. Sampling distributions are based on mathematical formulas and logic. You will never have to calculate or plot out sampling distributions. Statisticians determined what these theoretical distributions were years ago.

Every inferential statistical test is based upon the concept of sampling distributions, and each test has its own particular set of sampling distributions that are referenced when analyzing the data obtained in a study. The sampling distribution of the mean is a sampling distribution used quite often in inferential statistical tests.

Sampling Distribution of the Mean

When scores or values are normally distributed, approximately 68% of the values lie between ±1 SD and the mean, and approximately 95% lie between ±2 SD and the mean. To be exact, 95% of the values in a normal distribution lie between ±1.96 SD from the mean. That figure of 1.96 will become more important as you read on in this discussion about the use of inferential statistics to estimate population parameters, but it will be even more important during the discussion of hypothesis testing.

Let us discuss the theoretical sampling distribution of the mean. The standard deviation of any sampling distribution is called the standard error (rather than the standard deviation). The standard deviation of the sampling distribution of the mean is called the **standard error of the mean** ($s_{\bar{x}}$). The term *error* indicates that when a theoretical sampling distribution of the mean is used to estimate a population mean, some error is likely to occur in this estimate. The smaller the standard error of the mean, the more confidence you can have that the mean from a sample is an accurate reflection of the population mean. How can you tell how much error is likely to exist in your estimate of the population mean based on only one sample? A simple formula allows you to calculate the $s_{\bar{x}}$.

$$s_{\bar{x}} = \frac{SD}{\sqrt{n}}$$

where SD = standard deviation of sample and n = sample size.

Suppose 25 subjects have taken a test. Their average raw score is 70. The standard deviation is 10. Plug these data into the formula for $s_{\bar{x}}$.

$$s_{\bar{x}} = \frac{10}{\sqrt{25}} = \frac{10}{5} = 2$$

The standard error of the mean ($s_{\bar{x}}$) is 2. You can now determine there is approximately a 68% likelihood that the population mean lies between 68 and 72 (70 ± 2). Also, there is about a 95% likelihood that the population mean lies between 66 and 74 (70 ± 4).

Confidence Intervals

Although the value of a sample mean may be chosen as the value that is most likely to be the actual population mean, most researchers are not very comfortable with this choice. As you recall, any one sample chosen from a population may or may not be an accurate representation of the population. Researchers establish a range of values within which the population parameter is thought to occur. A **confidence interval** (CI) is a range of values that, with a specified degree of probability, is thought to contain the population value. Confidence intervals contain a lower and an upper limit. The researcher asserts with some degree of confidence that the population parameter lies within those boundaries.

Suppose a nurse researcher named Joan wishes to determine how knowledgeable the nurses in her state are about legal responsibilities in their practice. A test is located (or she develops one) that measures knowledge of legal issues in nursing practice. Joan is able to obtain the mailing list for all the 10,000 registered nurses in her state. When she examines her financial situation, the cost of mailing a questionnaire to all of the nurses does not fit in her budget. She decides to select a random sample of 100 nurses from the list. Let us assume all 100 of the nurses return the questionnaire (which is highly unlikely). Data analysis shows the mean score of this group to be 31 (of a possible 35 points), with a standard deviation of 3. The mean score is rather encouraging. Joan decides that the nurses in her state are fairly knowledgeable about legal issues. Excitedly, she reports the results to a friend. The friend says, "How can you be so confident about your results? There were only 100 nurses in the sample. I don't think you would find an average score of 31 if you tested all of the nurses in the state." Feeling somewhat deflated, Joan decides to determine how much confidence to place in the results. This is done by estimating the knowledge level of the total population of nurses in the state based on the test scores of a sample of 100 nurses. She decides that she wants to be 95% confident about her estimation when she goes back to talk to her friend again. First she determines the standard error of the mean ($s_{\bar{x}}$).

$$s_{\bar{x}} = \frac{3}{\sqrt{100}} = \frac{3}{10} = 0.3$$

Next, she inserts 0.3 into the formula for obtaining the 95% confidence interval (LL = lower limit, UL = upper limit).

$$LL = -1.96\,(\ )$$
$$UL = +1.96\,(\ )$$
$$LL = 31 - 1.96\,(0.3)$$
$$31 - 0.588 =$$
$$30.412$$
$$UL = 31 + 1.96\,(0.3) =$$
$$31 + 0.588 =$$
$$31.588$$

Joan then determines the 95% confidence interval to have a lower boundary of 30.41 and an upper boundary of 31.59. She was right after all. Her estimation of the knowledge of legal issues in nursing practice among the total population of nurses in her state indicates that their knowledge levels would be quite close to the mean of her sample of 100 nurses. She can be 95% confident that if she had selected another sample of 100 nurses from the mailing list, the mean score would be between 30.41 and 31.59. Another way to state this is that she is 95% confident the interval of 30.41 to 31.59 contains the population mean. If she wanted to be 99% confident of her estimate, she would replace 1.96 in the formula with the figure 2.58.

$$LL = 31 - 2.58\,(0.3) =$$
$$31 - 0.774 =$$
$$30.226$$
$$UL = 31 + 2.58\,(0.3) =$$
$$31 + 0.774 =$$
$$31.774$$

Joan is now 99% confident that the mean of the population lies between 30.23 and 31.77. With this statistical ammunition, she can again approach her friend and see if she is any more successful in convincing this friend that nurses in her state are fairly knowledgeable about legal issues in nursing practice.

Imagine you were asked to be a subject in a weight loss study. The researcher tells you that you will lose significantly ($p < .05$) more weight on this new diet than you did on the one you had previously tried. Wouldn't you also want to know how *much* weight you would lose? If the researcher said, "I am 95% sure that you will lose between 10 pounds and 15 pounds in 6 weeks," she would be giving you a confidence interval.

For some reason, confidence intervals have not been reported very often in nursing studies. As a matter of fact, Gaskin and Happell (2014) reported that confidence intervals were reported in only 28 % of the papers that were reviewed from a sample of 10 nursing journals with the highest 5-year impact factors from the publication year of 2011.

Generally, only significance levels are reported for hypothesis-testing studies. However, nurse researchers should be aware of the value of reporting confidence intervals in their research reports as well. Confidence intervals serve the purpose of informing clinicians or other researchers about the degree to which a particular strategy has influenced a study outcome (O'Mathuna & Fineout-Overhold, 2015).

A review of research journals provided examples of how some nurse researchers are reporting confidence intervals. Huis et al. (2013) reported a confidence interval of 95% for hand hygiene compliance when they compared the effects of a state-of-the-art strategy alone with team and leaders-directed strategies to promote hand hygiene and reduce hospital-acquired infections. A confidence interval (95%) was also reported by Fincher, Ward, Dawkins, Magee, and Wilson (2009) in their study of patients with Parkinson disease. They found visualization through videophone sessions to be more effective than telephone sessions in counseling these patients about their medications and self-management activities. In another study (Marshall, Cowell, Campbell, & McNaughton, 2010), cancer screening rates were compared between women with diabetes and those without diabetes. Again, a 95% confidence interval was reported in this study. Women with diabetes were less likely to receive cervical screening when compared to women in the general population.

Testing Hypotheses

As previously mentioned, the testing of hypotheses is very important to nurse researchers. Steps in testing hypotheses include the following:

1. State the study hypothesis (generally, a directional research hypothesis).
2. Choose the appropriate statistical test.
3. Decide on the level of significance (alpha level).
4. Decide if a one-tailed or two-tailed test will be used.
5. Calculate the test statistic, using the research data.
6. Compare the calculated value to the critical value for that particular statistical test.
7. Reject or fail to reject the null hypothesis.
8. Determine support or lack of support for the research hypothesis.

The Study Hypothesis

A researcher should take great pains in formulating the hypothesis (or hypotheses if more than one hypothesis) for a study. The hypothesis should be based on the theoretical/conceptual framework of the study; therefore, the hypothesis should generally be a directional research hypothesis that predicts the results of the study.

In quantitative research, the research hypothesis is the primary interest to the investigator, but the research hypothesis is not tested statistically. The null hypothesis (H_0) is the one that is tested using statistical analysis. The null hypothesis states that *no difference* exists between the populations from which the samples were chosen, or *no correlation* exists between variables in the population. Because the researcher expects to find a difference or a correlation, why is the null hypothesis necessary? Statistical measures are "set up" to test the null hypothesis. Remember, *all inferential statistical tests are based on the assumption that no difference or relationship (correlation) exists*. However, if small differences or low correlations are found, chance is considered to be the reason for this finding and the *null hypothesis is not rejected*. The null hypothesis is accepted. If the results of the analysis show that the difference or correlation is too large (or too significant) to be the result of chance, the null hypothesis is rejected. Of course, rejection of the null hypothesis provides support for the research hypothesis. Researchers are never able to say that they "proved" their research hypotheses. It is possible for them to say, however, with a specified degree of certainty, how likely it is that the null hypothesis is false.

The null hypothesis is frequently depicted using the following symbols:

$$H_0 : \mu_A = \mu_B$$

The symbols are those used for population parameters. Remember that statistical inference uses data from samples to draw conclusions about populations. The null hypothesis in the preceding formula indicates that there is no difference in the two populations from which the samples were drawn. Even if the two samples were drawn from the same population, for statistical purposes, the samples are assumed to have come from two separate populations concerning the variable of interest. For example, suppose a group of patients were divided into two treatment groups by a random assignment procedure.

The null hypothesis assumes these two groups have been selected from one hypothetical population. Although this idea is somewhat difficult to understand or to visualize, the concept is used in all of the inferential statistical tests that examine differences between groups. If the null hypothesis is rejected, the statistical decision is made that the two samples came from two hypothetical populations that were different on the variable being measured. If the null hypothesis is not rejected, the statistical decision is made that the two samples came from the same hypothetical population in respect to the variable being studied.

The correct words to use when discussing the results of testing the null hypothesis are *to reject* or *fail to reject*. *Retain* is also an acceptable word to use when the null hypothesis is not rejected. Although you will also see the word accept used in the literature, technically you never accept the null hypothesis. As Elzey (1974) noted, "We can only 'not reject' the hypothesis that there is no difference. We are not justified in concluding that there is no difference" (pp. 36–37).

When discussing the research hypothesis, it is correct to say that the hypothesis was supported or not supported. You do not reject the research hypothesis because it was never actually tested. These points may seem minor and overly fussy, but if you learn to use the correct terminology in the beginning of your research career, you will not have to change bad habits later, and your readers will have more faith in your conclusions.

Choosing a Statistical Test

Being able to choose an appropriate statistical test to use in analyzing your data and knowing the rationale for this choice are more important than being able to calculate the statistic. Currently, nearly all of the actual numerical calculations are done by computer. Although it is important to be familiar with the theoretical principles behind formulas used in the various tests, there is no need to memorize these formulas. When students take a statistics course, frequently they are so concerned with being able to perform mathematical calculations that they lose sight of the purposes of the various statistical tests and of how the choice of a particular test is made.

Basically, there are two types of inferential procedures: those that search for differences in sets of data and those that search for correlations between sets of data. Are you trying to determine if there is a significant difference between groups (i.e., between the experimental and control groups) or do you want to know if there is a significant correlation between variables within one group (levels of pain reported and number of requests for pain medication by open heart surgery patients)?

The choice of a statistical test is based primarily on the hypothesis(es) for the study or the research question(s). The hypothesis will indicate, for example, that the pain level of one group of subjects is going to be measured before and after some specific nursing intervention to relieve pain. The study design based on this hypothesis (one group, pretest and posttest) tells you that you will have two sets of dependent data. The data are considered dependent or related because the same subjects are measured both times. If the level of measurement of the dependent variable (pain) is interval or ratio, the most appropriate statistical test is a paired *t* test. The *t* test will be discussed later in this chapter.

Here are some of the questions that need to be answered when choosing the appropriate inferential procedure:

1. Are you comparing groups or sets of scores? Are you correlating variables?
2. What is the level of measurement of the variables (nominal, ordinal, or interval/ratio)?
3. How large are the groups (sample size)?
4. How many groups or sets of scores are being compared?
5. Are the observations or scores dependent or independent?
6. How many observations are available for each group?

Level of Significance

After analyzing data from a study, the decision must be made whether to reject or fail to reject the null hypothesis. The researcher wants to know how likely it is that a wrong decision has been made when two groups are said to be different or when an independent variable is said to cause the change in the dependent variable. To make this decision, the researcher must decide how certain or how accurate the decision must be. In other words, how willing is the researcher to be wrong when declaring that one group really is different from the other group on the variable being measured? The **level of significance** can be defined as the probability of rejecting a null hypothesis when it is true, and it should not be rejected. The level of significance is the researcher-determined chance that the difference or relationship that is found would be the result of random chance (or undetected sampling error), and the researcher has mistakenly said that the difference is related to the treatment variable.

The level of significance, represented by the Greek letter alpha (α), is an extremely important concept in inferential statistics. No matter what statistical test is used, a decision must be made about whether or not the specified level of significance was reached and, therefore, whether or not to reject the null hypothesis.

The letter p and the symbol α are used to symbolize the probability level that is set. The most common level of significance that is found in nursing studies is $p = .05$ [notice that no leading zero (0) is needed before the decimal point]. Traditionally, scientists have set this value as a decision point for testing the null hypothesis. A significance level of .05 means that the researcher is willing to risk being wrong 5% of the time, or 5 times out of 100, when rejecting the null hypothesis. If the decision needs to be much more accurate, such as deciding if a drug is effective or not, the level of significance might be set at .01 or even at .001. With a .01 level of significance, the researcher stands the risk of being wrong 1 time out of 100 when rejecting the null hypothesis. At the .001 level of significance, the risk of error is 1 time out of 1000.

An argument is occasionally made for setting a less stringent level of significance, such as .10. In research where no great harm would come from rejecting a true null hypothesis, a .10 level of significance might be acceptable. Again, nursing has accepted the .05 level as the standard in most studies. Note the researcher must decide how accurate the decision needs to be concerning the hypothesis.

It is important not to confuse level of significance with clinical significance or clinical importance. Although findings that are statistically significant are more likely to be clinically significant than findings that are not statistically significant, the two do not always go hand in hand. Findings that are statistically significant may not be clinically significant. The reverse situation is also possible.

One-Tailed and Two-Tailed Tests

A research hypothesis may be stated in the directional form (the degree of difference or type of correlation is predicted) or the nondirectional form (a difference or correlation is predicted, but the degree of difference or type of correlation is not indicated). Directional research hypotheses should be based on a sound conceptual or theoretical framework. In other words, the rationale for the prediction contained in a directional research hypothesis should be quite clear.

If the researcher has stated a directional research hypothesis, it is appropriate to use a one-tailed test of significance. When a **one-tailed test of significance** is selected, differences or correlations are sought in only one tail of the theoretical sampling distribution (either the right or the left tail). The word *tail* is used to indicate the values on each end of the distribution. A **two-tailed test of significance** is used to determine significant values in both ends of the sampling distribution. The nondirectional research hypothesis, therefore, calls for a two-tailed statistical test.

The type of research hypothesis that is chosen will determine the significance level needed to reject the null hypothesis. It is much easier to reject the null hypothesis when a one-tailed test rather than a two-tailed test is used. The entire area of rejection of the null hypothesis is in one tail, rather than being split

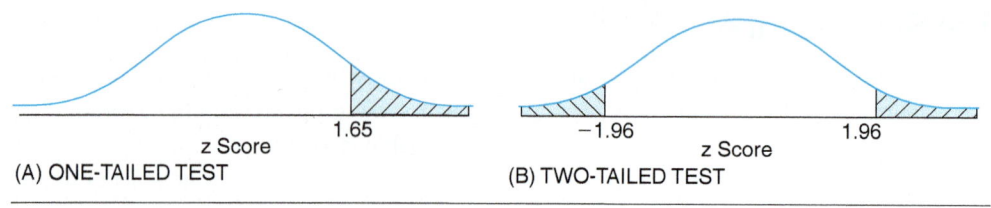

Figure 16–1 Significant values for one-tailed and two-tailed tests at α = .05

between the two tails, as would be necessary if a two-tailed test were used. If a two-tailed test is used, and the .05 level of significance has been chosen, the .05 must be divided into .025 in each tail of the distribution. For a one-tailed test, the region of rejection is all in one end of the distribution, and the entire .05 is sought in one tail. A z-score of 1.65 is significant at the .05 level for a one-tailed test. A z-score of 1.96 is necessary for significance at the .05 level for a two-tailed test. Figure 16–1 shows the area of significant values for a one-tailed and a two-tailed test when the probability level is set at .05.

To illustrate the use of a one-tailed test, consider the following example. The framework for a study indicates that play is an effective means of introducing children to unfamiliar environments or unfamiliar equipment. This is the hypothesis for the study: "Four-year-old children who have played with physical examination equipment, including a stethoscope and a tongue blade, before a physical examination are more cooperative during the examination than children who have had no such previous play experience." This hypothesis would allow the researcher to expect higher cooperation scores for the experimental group who had had experience with physical examination equipment than for the control group. The entire .05 probability level will be sought in the right tail or the positive end of the distribution. Suppose the mean co-operation score of the experimental group was higher than the mean score of the control group. If a z-score of 1.65 or higher was obtained for the difference between the means of the experimental and control groups, the researcher would conclude that the children in the experimental group were significantly more cooperative than the children in the control group.

Nursing research that is based on a conceptual or theoretical framework allows the prediction of the results. One-tailed tests, therefore, are appropriate for studies based on a sound study framework.

Calculating the Test Statistic

Although this step in hypothesis testing may seem like the most difficult, these days you rarely have to do any hand calculations. Numerous statistical software programs are available. Of course, a nurse researcher may want to take advantage of a statistician.

Comparing Calculated Value and Critical Value

Critical values may be determined by consulting tables found in the backs of statistics textbooks. However, today computer printouts generally provide critical values with which to compare the statistical results. A critical value is a scientific cutoff point. It denotes the value in a theoretical distribution at which all obtained sample values that are equal to or beyond that point in the distribution are said to be statistically significant. Critical values are found in the tails of a distribution. All values beyond the critical value are said to lie in the **critical region** or **region of rejection**. The critical value is determined by the level of significance chosen and the degrees of freedom. If the computed value of a statistic is less than the critical value, the null hypothesis is not rejected; if the computed value is equal to or greater than the critical value, the null hypothesis is rejected.

The interpretation of a statistical test depends on the degrees of freedom (df). **Degrees of freedom** relate to the number of values that are free to vary. Although the degrees of freedom indicate the number of values that can vary, the concern is really focused on the number of values that are *not* free to vary. Procedures to calculate the degrees of freedom for a particular statistical test are usually included in the description of that test. Degrees of freedom are generally denoted by the letters df and a number (e.g., $df = 2$). The concept of degrees of freedom is somewhat complex. A simplified example may help you gain a basic understanding of this concept. Suppose you were told to pick a number between 1 and 10. You would have 10 degrees of freedom because you could pick any of 10 numbers. Now imagine you are told to pick three numbers that add up to 10. After you have picked the first two numbers, the third number is not free to vary. For example, if you chose the numbers 3 and 5, the third number must be 2 to arrive at a sum of 10. You were, thus, allowed 2 degrees of freedom in this calculation.

Support for the Study Hypothesis

If a directional research hypothesis has been formulated for a study, support for this hypothesis is based on whether or not the null hypothesis is rejected. In nearly every study, the goal of the researcher is to reject the null hypothesis. Occasionally, the null hypothesis is actually a statement of the researcher's expectation. For example, in a study to determine if an inexpensive educational program was as effective as an expensive program, the researcher's prediction or expectation might be that there would be no difference in the effectiveness of these two programs. Again, as previously mentioned, the researcher generally hopes to be able to reject the null hypothesis.

After examining the obtained p value, if it is less than the level of significance that was set for the study (generally, $p = .05$), the researcher rejects the null hypothesis. Conversely, if the p value is greater than the set level of significance, the researcher must fail to reject the null hypothesis. Therefore, a researcher would reject the null hypothesis if the obtained value was .03, and would fail to reject the null hypothesis if the obtained value was .30, for example.

Factors Affecting Choice of Statistical Measures

There are different kinds of issues that affect the researcher's choice of the best statistical test for a particular study. These relate to the level of data being examined (nominal, ordinal, interval, or ratio); the different assumptions (such as sample size) that various tests may require; the ability of a test to detect a difference or correlation (power); and the consequences of errors (type I and type II) from the study.

Parametric and Nonparametric Statistical Tests

First, we will discuss the two different broad categories of inferential statistics, parametric and nonparametric, and those issues that affect which category is the appropriate choice for a study. As the term implies, **parametric tests** are concerned with population parameters, and these tests make assumptions about the population from which a sample was drawn. **Nonparametric tests** are less stringent in the requirements for their use and do not make assumptions about the population from which a sample is selected. The assumptions of parametric statistical tests include the following: (a) the level of measurement of the data is interval or ratio, (b) data are taken from populations that are normally distributed on the variable being measured, and (c) data are taken from populations that have equal variances on the variable being measured.

One major difference in the measures associated with parametric tests (compared to nonparametric tests) is that parametric tests use the mean as part of the calculation. The mean is a more accurate representation when a distribution is normal. Nonparametric tests tend to use either the median or the mode as part of the calculation, neither of which requires a normal distribution. Because nonparametric tests make no assumptions about the distribution of the population, they are often called distribution-free statistics. Nonparametric statistical tests may be used with nominal and ordinal data, and when sample sizes are small.

A growing body of research suggests that violations of the assumptions of parametric tests do not adversely affect statistical decisions. The parametric tests are quite robust, which means these tests are still reliable even if one of the assumptions of the test has been violated. Some researchers, therefore, routinely use parametric tests if data meet the requirement of being at the interval or ratio level of measurement.

Because it appears that nonparametric tests have fewer restrictions, you may ask why these types of tests are not used when analyzing all data. The answer lies in the power of the tests. If the assumptions of parametric tests are met, these types of statistical tests are more powerful than nonparametric tests. However, if the assumptions are violated, it is possible that a nonparametric test might be more powerful and generate results that more closely approximate reality.

Power of a Statistical Test

The **power of a statistical test** is defined as the ability of the test to reject a null hypothesis when it is false. In other words, the more powerful a test, the more likely it will detect a significant difference between groups or a significant correlation between variables in one group. The power of a statistical test depends on the sample size and the level of significance that is chosen. The larger the sample chosen, the more power the statistical test will have. The larger the *p* value selected, the greater the power. A *p* value of .10 would increase power when compared to a *p* value of .05. A *p* value of .05 would increase power when compared to a *p* value of .01.

Also, a test will be more powerful if a one-tailed test rather than a two-tailed test is used.

Type I and Type II Errors

Four possible decisions may be made concerning the null hypothesis. Two of the decisions are correct ones. If the null hypothesis is actually false and you reject it, you have made a correct decision. If the null hypothesis is actually true and you fail to reject it (retain the null), you have made a correct decision. However, two mistakes can be made: type I and type II errors. If the null hypothesis is actually true and you reject it, you have made a **type I error**. If the null hypothesis is actually false, and you fail to reject it, you have made a **type II error**.

Figure 16–2 depicts these four decisions. Because sample data are used to make a decision about a population, you never know for sure if you have made the correct decision.

As the probability of a type I error increases, the probability of a type II error decreases and vice versa. The level of significance (a) set for a study determines the probability of a type I, or alpha, error. For example,

		ACTUAL SITUATION IN POPULATION Null Hypothesis	
		True	False
Statistical Decision	Null Rejected	Type I Error	No Error
	Null *Not* Rejected	No Error	Type II Error

Figure 16–2 Type I and type II errors in hypothesis testing

if the level of significance for a study is set at .05, the probability of a type I error is .05 or 5%. The probability of a type II, or beta, error (b) can be controlled by using power analysis.

Type I errors in research findings usually result in unnecessary changes being instituted, whereas type II errors result in failure to institute needed changes. Both of these errors may be serious. In general, however, researchers are more concerned with a type I error than a type II error. A type I error seems to be more embarrassing to the researcher because something, such as an intervention, is said to work when it actually does not work. For example, a significant difference might be said to exist between the reactions to an intervention by the experimental group compared to the control group when, in fact, the difference was related to chance.

Statistical Tests Used in Nursing Research

Three of the most common statistical tests used in nursing research are the *t* test, analysis of variance, and chi-square, and are discussed next.

t Test

The ***t* test** is a parametric test that examines the difference between the mean values of some variable in two groups. It is one of the most popular statistical tests. The *t* test is appropriate for samples of nearly any size, but is particularly useful with small sample sizes (fewer than 30). Because the test compares means, interval or ratio data are required. Also, because the *t* test is a parametric test, the sample data are assumed to have been selected from populations that are normally distributed and have equal variances on the variable being measured.

Another name for the *t* test is the *Student t test*. This name was derived from the pseudonym used by the originator of the test, William Gosset. Gosset worked for a brewery in Dublin, Ireland. To maintain brewing secrets, a company policy prohibited publications by employees. Gosset chose to publish his mathematical formulas secretly under the pseudonym of Student.

The *t* test uses a *t* distribution. Actually, there is a set of *t* distributions, one for each different degree of freedom. As the number of degrees of freedom decreases, the shape of the distribution flattens from that of the normal curve. The more the number of degrees of freedom increases, the more the distribution shape resembles the normal curve.

There are two forms of the *t* test. One form is used with independent samples, and the other is used with dependent samples. An independent sample is one in which there is no association or connection between the scores of the groups that are being observed (e.g., an experimental group and a control group are compared). The test for independent samples is called an independent *t* test or independent samples *t* test or unrelated samples *t* test.

Independent *t* Test

An independent *t* test was used to analyze data from a study concerning the effectiveness of an audiotape educational program for the postoperative home care of patients following a coronary artery bypass graft (Hoseini, Soltani, Beygi, & Zarifsanaee, 2013). The data for the independent *t* tests were collected before and 6 weeks following the interventions. The researchers compared levels of depression between participants who received routine home care training (n = 35) and participants who received the audiotaped educational program in addition to routine training (n = 35). Six weeks following the interventions, the group with the audiotaped program demonstrated significantly lower depression scores than the routine training group (p < .0001). A closer look at the means of the scores indicated that audiotaped program group scores were reduced, while the scores of the routine home care training group had increased.

The **dependent *t* test**, also called *paired t test* or *correlated samples t test*, is used when scores or values are associated or have some connection. For example, anxiety scores of mothers and daughters might be compared. If each mother is matched with her daughter on some variable such as age or weight, the sets of values are dependent data. Dependent data are also obtained when the same subjects are measured before and after they receive an experimental treatment.

> ## Dependent *t* Test
>
> Stacey et al. (2015) studied the impact of training registered nurses' perceived confidence to use symptom protocols for remotely supported patients undergoing cancer treatment. The nurses' posttest scores (n = 90) were compared with their pretest scores. One-tailed, paired *t* tests (dependent *t* tests) demonstrated improved self-confidence to assess, triage, and guide patients in self-care for cancer treatment related symptoms and use protocols to facilitate symptom management ($p < .01$) after completion of the workshop.

Separate formulas are used to calculate the independent *t* test and the dependent *t* test. These can be found in statistics textbooks. The *t* value obtained is compared with the critical value associated with the *t* distribution appropriate for the data (based on the degrees of freedom). If the *t* value that is obtained is greater than the critical value, the null hypothesis is rejected, and the mean scores or values for the groups are considered to be significantly different.

Analysis of Variance

The *t* test is a very useful technique to determine the significance of the difference between two means. However, many studies compare more than two groups. For example, a researcher might want to compare the effectiveness of four different methods of teaching clients how to give insulin injections (four levels of the independent variable). The dependent variable might be the number of correct insulin injections that patients are able to perform in a given time period. If four groups were being compared, six separate *t* tests would have to be computed. Suppose Groups A, B, C, and D were being compared. The following pairs would result: A and B, A and C, A and D, B and C, B and D, and C and D (for a total of six comparisons).

Whenever the researcher wishes to compare the difference(s) among more than two means, the appropriate statistical test is the **an**alysis **o**f **va**riance (ANOVA; pronounced un-nóv-uh). ANOVA enables the researcher to analyze the difference between several means at one time.

ANOVA is a parametric statistical test and, therefore, is based on the assumption that data are interval or ratio level, and the data have been selected from populations that are normally distributed and have equal variances on the variable being measured.

ANOVA uses the *F* distribution, named after Sir Ronald Fisher. As is true with the *t* distribution, there is more than one *F* distribution. Each *F* distribution is based on the degrees of freedom. There are several different types of ANOVA procedures: one-way ANOVA, two-way ANOVA, and repeated measures ANOVA. The one-way ANOVA is discussed here.

As the name of the statistic indicates, analysis of variance examines the variance in data obtained. Two types of variation are examined: variation between the means of the groups and variation of individual scores within each of the groups. These two types of variation are called "mean square between" groups and "mean square within" groups. These terms are symbolized by MS_B and MS_W.

You may wonder why the difference between the means of the groups does not provide enough information to make a decision about the difference between the groups. It has been determined that the variability of the scores or values in the population affects the mean. By examining only the differences among the means of the samples, the researcher might falsely conclude that a true difference exists between the populations represented by the sample data when, in actuality, this seeming difference occurred because there is a great deal of variability within the samples. To avoid rejecting a true null hypothesis, the ANOVA examines two types of variability: the variability between the groups and the variability within each of the groups. The means of each of the groups are compared to the grand mean of all of the groups combined. Then each value within a group is compared to the mean value for that particular group. These two estimates of population variation are then compared by dividing the "between" estimate by the "within" estimate. An F ratio is obtained. This F ratio is symbolized by:

$$F = \frac{MS_B}{MS_W} \quad \begin{array}{l}\text{(Between group variance)} \\ \text{(Within group variance)}\end{array}$$

If the null hypothesis is true, these two measures of variability should be very similar, and the result of the division will be a value less than 1. If the null hypothesis is false, a value greater than 1 will be found. The larger the F value, the greater is the variation or difference between the groups as compared to the variation within the groups. The significance of the F value or F ratio is determined by consulting an F table in a statistics textbook to ascertain the critical value for F. If a computer program is used to analyze the data (which is nearly always the case today), the computer printout will usually provide the obtained value and the critical value.

If the difference or variation between the groups is significantly greater than the difference within the groups, the null hypothesis is rejected. In contrast, if the between-groups variation is not significantly greater than the within-groups variation, the null hypothesis is not rejected.

If the F value is significant, the researcher knows there is a significant difference between the means of at least two of the groups. The F statistic, however, does not tell exactly where the difference occurs. Other statistical procedures are necessary. You might think that the appropriate statistic to calculate would be t tests between all of the various pairs of groups. This technique will result in an increased likelihood of a type I error. The more comparisons that are made, the more likely it is that one of the comparisons will be significant, by chance. For example, if 20 t tests were run and the level of significance was set at .05, the researcher could expect to find statistical significance in at least one of these tests even if there was no true difference between the means of any of the groups that were being compared. Several multiple comparison tests may be used that decrease the probability of making a type I error, including the Duncan, Newman-Keuls (also called the Student-Newman-Keuls or S-N-K), Tukey B, and Scheffé tests.

Analysis of Variance (ANOVA)

The effects of implementing quiet times in a medical-surgical intensive care unit on levels of light, noise, and nurses' stress were studied by Riemer, Mates, Ryan, and Schleder (2015). The study consisted of 124 observations of 22 clinical nurses who worked in the intensive care unit. The lights were dimmed and quiet time was implemented from 2:00 pm to 4:00 pm. Measurements of nurses' stress levels, unit noise, and unit light were collected at 30 minutes before, 30 minutes, 1 hour, and 2 hours after implementation of the quiet time. ANOVA and comparisons of the means of the measurements over time indicated that both light levels and nurses' stress levels were significantly decreased after quiet time ($p < .001$).

Chi-Square

Statistical tests that were previously discussed, the t test and ANOVA, are appropriate for interval data. The **chi-square test** is a *nonparametric inferential* technique appropriate for comparing sets of data that are

Table 16–2 Smoking Behavior of Psychiatric and Medical-Surgical Nurses

	Smokers		Nonsmokers		Total
	50		50		
Psychiatric nurses	60		40		100
	50		50		
Medical-surgical nurses	40		60		100
Total	100		100		200

in the form of frequencies or percentages (nominal data). The chi-square statistic (χ^2) is probably the most commonly used statistic with nominal data.

Using the chi-square technique, the researcher compares the frequencies that are obtained or observed in categories with the frequencies that would be expected to occur if the null hypothesis is true. Observed frequencies are compared to expected frequencies. If the observed frequencies are quite different from the expected frequencies at a specified level of significance (such as .05), the null hypothesis is rejected.

The chi-square distribution is the theoretical sampling distribution used when the chi-square statistic is calculated. Actually, there is a set of chi-square distributions. The shape of each of these distributions is governed by the degrees of freedom. To consult a chi-square table, you need to know the degrees of freedom, just as you do when examining a t-distribution table or an F-distribution table.

Although the chi-square distribution may be used for several purposes, probably the most common use is with the chi-square test for independence, also called the chi-square test for contingency tables. Contingency tables are those tables used to illustrate data that are presented in frequencies. The chi-square test for contingency tables is used to analyze the data that are displayed in contingency tables. The observed and expected frequencies in each cell of the table are compared.

Examine the data in Table 16–2. The research problem of the study was to determine whether psychiatric nurses are more or less likely to smoke than medical-surgical nurses. The sample has 100 psychiatric nurses and 100 medical-surgical nurses. The data show that half of the total sample, 100 subjects are smokers, and 100 subjects are nonsmokers. The data also show that 60 psychiatric nurses smoke, and 40 psychiatric nurses do not smoke. The figures are reversed for the medical-surgical nurses. The number 50 displayed in the upper-right corner of each cell in the table is the number of smokers and nonsmokers that would be expected in each group if these two variables were not related.

The chi-square distribution will be used to determine if the observed values might have occurred by chance. If many samples, each containing 100 psychiatric nurses and 100 medical-surgical nurses, were chosen from the population, how many times would this size difference between groups occur by chance? To make this decision, the obtained value is compared to the critical value. In this case, the obtained value for χ^2 is 8.00, and the critical value is 3.84. The null hypothesis, therefore, would be rejected, and the researcher would conclude that this large a difference would occur by chance less than 5 times out of 100. Therefore, the conclusion is made that there is a significant difference in the smoking behavior of the two groups. Psychiatric nurses are more likely to smoke than medical-surgical nurses.

Because the chi-square test that was used is called the chi-square test of independence, another way to state the results is that smoking behavior *depends* on the type of nurse (psychiatric versus medical-surgical) you are. The null hypothesis says that smoking behavior and type of nurse are independent, or not related, and, therefore, there will be no difference between the observed frequencies and the expected frequencies in the cells of the table. Rejection of the null hypothesis indicates that these two variables are dependent or related. Smoking behavior and type of nurse (psychiatric versus medical-surgical) are related.

Chi-Square Test

Heidari and Norouzadeh (2015) examined nursing students' views of clinical nursing education. Chi-square was used to determine the differences between male and female nursing students. Male participants ranked all aspects of clinical education higher than female participants. Examples of measured domains evaluated through chi-square included (a) learning objectives (male 79.75, female 56.17, $p = .001$), (b) instructor (male 75.82, female 61.35, $p = .046$), clinical environment (male 79.09, female 54.29, $p = .0001$), and evaluation and supervision (male 79.15, female, 59.60, $p = .005$).

Testing the Significance of Correlation Coefficients

A correlation coefficient presents the degree to which the values of one variable (X) are related to the values of another variable (Y). The closer the correlation coefficient is to +1.00 or –1.00, the greater is the relationship between these two variables. Although the size of the correlation coefficient gives some indication of the degree to which two variables are related, an inferential statistical procedure is necessary to determine if this correlation coefficient is the result of chance (sampling error) or whether there is a true relationship between these variables in the population.

In testing the significance of a correlation coefficient, the researcher wants to determine if the obtained r, based on sample data, came from a population of pairs of values for which the actual correlation is 0. The null hypothesis states that there is 0 correlation between these two variables in the population. If the correlation coefficient that is obtained from the sample data is too high to have come from a population in which the correlation is actually 0, the null hypothesis is rejected, and the conclusion is made that the two variables are correlated at a level that is significantly higher than 0.

If a correlation of .80 is obtained between two variables, the variables are quite probably actually related. However, if a correlation coefficient such as .15 or .20 is obtained, this value possibly occurred as a result of sampling error or chance.

To determine if a correlation coefficient is significant, a t test can be calculated or a table of significant values consulted. The degrees of freedom for the Pearson product-moment correlation are equal to the number of subjects minus 2 (n – 2). When the sample contains a large number of subjects, the size of the correlation coefficient may be quite small and still be significant. For example, with 20 degrees of freedom (22 subjects), an $r = .42$ is significant at the .05 level. If the degrees of freedom are increased to 80 (82 subjects), a correlation of $r = .22$ is significant at the .05 level. When interpreting the significance of correlation coefficients, it is important to examine the sample size. Comparisons can be found in tables in the backs of statistics books or determined by examining a computer printout of the data.

Rather than using an inferential procedure to determine the statistical significance of a correlation coefficient, a more accurate interpretation of a correlation coefficient is obtained by squaring the coefficient (r^2), thereby determining the percentage of variance shared by the two variables. The r^2 for the first example, $r = .42$, would be .18 ($.42 \infty .42 = .1764$). This means that these two variables share a common variance or overlap of 18%. If you knew the value of one variable, you would possess 18% of the knowledge you needed to be able to predict the value of the other variable. A correlation coefficient of .42 may not sound very significant to you now, even though it might have been determined to be statistically significant. Remember, when a correlation coefficient is determined to be statistically significant, it only means that it is significantly different from 0. It does not take a very large correlation for it to be larger than 0. It is hoped that this information will help you understand why some small correlations that are reported in research articles are said to be statistically significant. Occasionally, you will see correlation coefficients as small as .15 or even .09 reported in the literature, and they will be starred (*) as being significant at the .05 level or even doubled starred (**) for the .01 level. Don't let these stars (******) fool you. Look at the actual size of the correlation coefficient.

Advanced Statistical Tests

Many advanced statistical tests are available for the researcher who wishes to study more than two variables in one study. One frequently used inferential procedure is multiple regression. **Multiple regression** is the procedure used when the researcher wishes to determine the influence of more than one independent variable on the dependent variable. For example, a researcher might want to determine what factors would most accurately predict a woman's decision to perform breast self-examination. A number of factors might be examined, such as history of breast cancer in the family, fear of cancer, and type of teaching received concerning the performance of breast self-examination.

Multiple Regression

Liebermann, Muller, Weigl, and Wegge (2015) used multiple regression to analyze those factors related to nurses remaining in the same job until they retire. Respondents were classified into three age groups: (a) younger than 30 years, (b) 30–50 years, and (c) older than 50 years. Findings indicated that work-time control, role clarity, and colleague support were positively related to the expectation to remain in the same job, but the relative importance of these variables differed by age group. All of these variables were mediated by the respondent's "vitality" or individual energy capacity.

Another frequently used test is the **analysis of covariance** (ANCOVA). ANCOVA is a powerful statistical test used when the researcher wishes to control statistically for some variable that may have an influence on the dependent variable. This test can also be used to make two groups statistically equal on some variable for which they are quite different before the experimental treatment is administered. For example, suppose a researcher wishes to determine if the anxiety levels of open-heart surgery patients will be lower postoperatively in the group that receives explicit pictorial information about postoperative procedures compared to the group that receives only verbal information. It is self-evident that the anxiety levels of patients preoperatively will influence their postoperative anxiety levels, regardless of the intervention that they receive. Therefore, the researcher needs to measure the preoperative anxiety levels of both groups. Even if subjects are randomly assigned to the experimental and control groups, the average anxiety levels of one group, just by chance, might be higher than the other group. ANCOVA enables the researcher to make the two groups statistically similar. You might consider it like a golf game where an average player is given a handicap to allow him or her to have a chance of winning against a great player. Improvement is the criterion.

Analysis of Covariance (ANCOVA)

Steinhardt et al. (2015) examined the effects of diabetes self-management education that incorporated resilience in African American adults with type 2 diabetes. The researchers assessed baseline knowledge, lab values, physical measures, and psychological well-being at baseline and six months later. Analysis of covariance (ANCOVA) was used to determine the effects of the diabetes education intervention controlling for these baseline measures. ANCOVA indicated that the experimental group had greater knowledge of diabetes ($p < .01$), improved fasting blood sugar ($p < .05$), and higher HDL cholesterol ($p < .01$) than the control group that did not receive the educational intervention.

Two other advanced statistical tests about which you may read in research reports are canonical correlation and multivariate analysis of variance. **Canonical correlation** examines the correlation between two or more independent variables and two or more dependent variables. **Multivariate analysis of variance** (MANOVA) examines the difference between the mean scores of two or more groups on two or more dependent variables that are examined at the same time.

Researchers may examine the results of several research studies simultaneously, using statistical measures. **Meta-analysis** is a technique that combines the results of several quantitative studies that have been conducted on the same topic. The results of a large number of different studies are combined and statistically analyzed as if only one study had been conducted with one large group of subjects. An effect size is presented for a treatment or intervention. The **effect size** indicates how useful a treatment or intervention was in several studies as indicated by the difference between data from control groups and experimental groups. The effect size may be reported as small, medium, or large, or the actual effect size may be reported (e.g., .23, .44). Anderson (2003) wrote that meta-analysis uses statistical methods to derive quantitative implications of many different studies about a common problem or question. She called for researchers to provide all of the needed information in their research articles that would allow their studies to be included in a meta-analysis. For example, the exact p value should be reported (rather than just reporting that the results were significant or not significant). In an editorial in the *Western Journal of Nursing Research*, Conn (2009) reported that the literature contains many small studies with insufficient statistical power because of small sample sizes. She asserted that meta-analysis provides a means of examining patterns across many small related studies.

Meta-Analysis

Urquhart, Currell, Harlow, and Callow (2015) did a meta-analysis on research related to the effectiveness of home uterine monitoring in pregnant women to prevent preterm birth. The authors identified 15 randomized clinical trials (6008 women), but determined that only 13 of these met the established criteria to contribute to the analysis. The result of this analysis using the higher quality clinical trials was that the use of home uterine monitoring had no effect on preterm birth. There was no difference in perinatal death. The authors concluded that home uterine monitoring did not impact major maternal and/or perinatal outcomes.

A fairly new meta term is appearing in the literature. **Metasynthesis** is a technique used in summarizing reports of qualitative research studies; it combines the results of several qualitative studies that cover the same topic. Beck (2009) called for qualitative researchers to synthesize their findings in order to promote qualitative research as a reliable source of evidence for evidence-based practice.

Metasynthesis

Daker-White et al. (2015) conducted a metasynthesis of qualitative research related to patient safety in primary care. Meta-ethnography was used to summarize the groups of findings found in the initial studies. These authors examined 48 studies and identified five subsets: patient's perspectives about safety, staff perspectives about safety, medication safety, systems issues, and the primary/acute care interface. Both clinical guidelines and electronic health records were presented as being both detrimental and beneficial to patient safety. The major threats to patient safety related to the larger healthcare system.

Critiquing Inferential Statistics in Research Reports

Readers are quite often intimidated by the statistics of a research report. The inferential statistics are even more intimidating than the descriptive statistics to many consumers of research. Although a thorough background in statistics is necessary to understand each and every statistical test discussed in research reports, a minimal understanding of inferential statistics is sufficient for the reader to understand the majority of the study results. Many of the same inferential statistics (e.g., t tests, ANOVA) are reported in a large number of research articles. Box 16–1 presents some guidelines for critiquing inferential statistics.

Box 16–1 Guidelines for Critiquing Inferential Statistics

1. Are inferential statistics presented in the research report?
2. If inferential statistics are presented, is enough information presented for the reader to determine whether or not the appropriate tests were used?
3. Is the reader provided with the calculated value of the inferential statistic, the degrees of freedom, and the level of significance that was obtained?
4. Were parametric or nonparametric tests used when the other type of measure would have been more appropriate?
5. Are the chosen tests appropriate considering the level of measurement of the variables, the number of groups that were tested, the size of the sample, and so on?
6. Are inferential statistics presented for each hypothesis that was stated in the study?
7. Are the results of inferential tests clearly and thoroughly discussed?
8. Are the results presented both in the text and in the tables?

First, the reader searches the report for any inferential statistics used in data analysis. Every time you see a p value listed, you know an inferential statistical test was used. Then a determination must be made if there is enough information to make a decision about the appropriateness of each test that was used. For example, the research report should include the level of measurement of the variables, number of groups that were tested, and sample size.

The reader should be provided with the value of the statistical test that was obtained, the degrees of freedom, and the significance level reached when each hypothesis was tested. The actual p value should be listed, not just that the p value was significant or not significant. The reader should be able to determine if each of the researcher's hypotheses was or was not supported. Therefore, every research report should clearly present the results of hypothesis testing. These results should be presented both in the text of the report and in tables.

Summary

The two broad purposes of inferential statistics are to estimate population parameters from sample data and to test hypotheses. The second purpose has been of more interest to nurse researchers.

When a sample is chosen to represent a population, there is some likelihood that the sample will not accurately reflect the population. The phenomenon in which sample values tend to be normally distributed around the population value is known as the central limit theorem. A frequency distribution based on an infinite number of samples is called a sampling distribution. Theoretical sampling distributions are used to estimate population characteristics. The standard deviation of the sampling distribution of the mean is called the standard error of the mean $s_{\bar{x}}$.

A confidence interval is a range of values that, with a specified degree of probability, is thought to contain the population value. The researcher might establish a 95% confidence interval or a 99% confidence interval, for example.

Steps in hypothesis testing include (a) stating the study hypothesis, (b) choosing an appropriate statistical test, (c) deciding on the level of significance, (d) deciding if a one-tailed or a two-tailed test will be used, (e) calculating the test statistic, (f) comparing the calculated value to the critical value, (g) rejecting or failing to reject the null hypothesis, and (h) determining support or lack of support for the research hypothesis.

Although the study hypothesis (generally a directional research hypothesis) is of primary interest to an investigator, the null hypothesis (H_0) is the one subjected to statistical analysis.

Some of the questions that need to be answered when choosing a statistical procedure include the following: Are you comparing groups? Are you correlating variables? What is the level of measurement of the variables? How large are the groups? How many groups are being compared? Are the observations dependent or independent? How many observations are available on each group?

The level of significance, also called alpha (α), is defined as the probability of rejecting a null hypothesis when it is true. The most common level of significance used is .05. This means that the researcher is willing to risk being wrong 5% of the time or 5 times out of 100 when rejecting the null hypothesis. More stringent levels of significance are .01 and .001.

If the researcher has stated a directional research hypothesis, it is appropriate to use a one-tailed test of significance. If a one-tailed test of significance is employed, values will be sought in only one tail of the theoretical sampling distribution. A two-tailed test of significance is used to determine significant values in both ends of the sampling distribution.

A critical value is a cutoff point that denotes the place in a theoretical distribution at which all obtained values from a sample that are equal to or beyond that point are said to be statistically significant. Values beyond the critical value are said to lie in the critical region or region of rejection. If the computed value of a statistic is equal to or greater than the critical value, the null hypothesis is rejected.

The interpretation of a statistical test depends on the degrees of freedom (df). Degrees of freedom concern the number of values that are free to vary.

If the null hypothesis is actually true and it is rejected, a type I error is made. If the null hypothesis is actually false and is not rejected, a type II error is made. The level of significance set for the study determines the probability of a type I error. Power analysis will help prevent a type II error.

Inferential statistical tests can be classified as parametric and nonparametric. Parametric tests require interval or ratio data and assume the sample data have been taken from populations that are normally distributed and have equal variances. Nonparametric tests can be used with nominal and ordinal data and make no assumptions about the distribution of the population. Nonparametric tests are sometimes called distribution-free statistics. The power of a statistical test is the ability of the test to reject a null hypothesis when it is false. The power of a test depends on the sample size and the level of significance chosen. The t test is a parametric test that examines the difference between the means of two groups. The t test uses the t distribution. One form of the test is used with independent samples and is called the independent t test or *independent samples t test* or *unrelated t test*. The dependent t test, also called paired t test or *correlated samples t test*, is used when scores or values are associated.

Analysis of variance (ANOVA) is used to compare the difference among more than two means. The ANOVA is a parametric test that uses the F distribution. The chi-square test is a nonparametric inferential technique that is appropriate for comparing sets of data that are in the form of frequencies or percentages. The frequencies that are obtained or observed are compared to the expected frequencies. The chi-square distribution is the theoretical sampling distribution used when the chi-square (χ^2) statistic is calculated.

An inferential procedure is necessary to determine if a correlation coefficient is statistically significant. The researcher may determine the significance of a correlation coefficient using a t test or by consulting a table of significant values.

Advanced statistical tests include multiple regression, analysis of covariance (ANCOVA), canonical correlation, and multivariate analysis of variance (MANOVA). Meta-analysis combines the results of several similar studies that gathered quantitative or numerical data. An effect size indicates how useful a treatment or intervention was in several studies as indicated by the difference between data from the control and experimental groups. Metasynthesis combines the results of several similar studies that involve qualitative inquiries.

Self-Test

1. Statistical significance means that the study findings:
   A. are important to the nursing profession.
   B. apply to a large target population.
   C. have proven the study hypothesis.
   D. are not likely to be the result of sampling error.
2. If study findings are statistically significant, this implies that the:
   A. null hypothesis should be rejected.
   B. research hypothesis should be rejected.
   C. null hypothesis should not be rejected.
   D. research hypothesis should not be rejected.
3. Parametric statistical tests would be appropriate for which type of data?
   A. pulse rates
   B. religious affiliation
   C. blood type
   D. patients' identification numbers
4. Which is true concerning nonparametric statistical tests? They:
   A. should never be used with interval/ratio data.
   B. estimate population parameters.
   C. are generally used with large samples.
   D. none of the above
5. A research hypothesis states that "Male appendectomy patients ask for more pain medication on the first postoperative day than female appendectomy patients." When the data are analyzed, the mean number of requests for pain medication is 3.5 for males and 2.3 for females. The p value is calculated to be .04. What decision should be made about the findings of this study?
   A. Male appendectomy patients asked for significantly more pain medication on the first postoperative day than did female appendectomy patients.
   B. Female appendectomy patients needed less pain medication on the first postoperative day than did male appendectomy patients.
   C. There was no statistically significant difference in male and female patients' requests for pain medication on the first postoperative day after an appendectomy.
   D. No determination can be made about the difference in male and female appendectomy patients' requests for pain medication on the first postoperative day.
6. A researcher is trying to determine if the type of educational preparation is associated with the level of professional commitment. The mean scores on the Commitment to the Nursing Profession instrument are obtained for 30 diploma school graduates, 30 associate degree graduates, and 30 baccalaureate graduates. The probability level associated with the obtained F value is .03. What is the level of measurement of the dependent variable?
   A. nominal
   B. ordinal
   C. interval/ratio
   D. percentage

7. A researcher is trying to determine if the type of educational preparation is associated with the level of professional commitment. The mean scores on the Commitment to the Nursing Profession instrument are obtained for 30 diploma school graduates, 30 associate degree graduates, and 30 baccalaureate graduates. The probability level associated with the obtained F value is .03. How many sets of scores are being compared?
    A. one
    B. two
    C. three
    D. four
8. A researcher is trying to determine if the type of educational preparation is associated with the level of professional commitment. The mean scores on the Commitment to the Nursing Profession instrument are obtained for 30 diploma school graduates, 30 associate degree graduates, and 30 baccalaureate graduates. The probability level associated with the obtained F value is .03. What inferential statistic was calculated?
    A. dependent t test
    B. analysis of variance
    C. independent t test
    D. chi-square test
9. A researcher is trying to determine if the type of educational preparation is associated with the level of professional commitment. The mean scores on the Commitment to the Nursing Profession instrument are obtained for 30 diploma school graduates, 30 associate degree graduates, and 30 baccalaureate graduates. The probability level associated with the obtained F value is .03. Which decision concerning scores on the Commitment to the Nursing Profession instrument is correct, based on the probability level of .03 that was obtained when the data were analyzed?
    A. No significant difference was found among diploma, associate degree, and baccalaureate graduates' scores.
    B. A significant difference was found among diploma, associate degree, and baccalaureate graduates' scores.
    C. No decision can be made as to whether a significant difference was found among diploma, associate degree, and baccalaureate graduates' scores.
    D. A significant difference was found between diploma and associate degree scores
10. A researcher is trying to determine if the type of educational preparation is associated with the level of professional commitment. The mean scores on the Commitment to the Nursing Profession instrument are obtained for 30 diploma school graduates, 30 associate degree graduates, and 30 baccalaureate graduates. The probability level associated with the obtained F value is .03. A computer printout reveals $t = -2.5$; $df = 40$; $p = .03$. Given that the researcher selected an α 0f .05, the researcher would:
    A. reject the null hypothesis.
    B. fail to reject the null hypothesis.
    C. conclude that an error in calculation had been made.
    D. conclude that an error in analysis was made because this information does not relate to the t-test.

See answers to Self-Test in the Answer Section at the back of the book.

References

Anderson, E. H. (2003). Facilitating meta-analysis in nursing [Guest editorial]. *Nursing Research, 52,* 1. doi:10.1097/00006199-200301000-00001

Beck, C. T. (2009). Metasynthesis: A goldmine for evidence-based practice. *AORN Journal, 90,* 701–702; 705–710. doi:10.1016/j.aorn.2009.06.025

Conn, V. S., Hafdahl, A. R., & Brown, L. M. (2009). Meta-analysis of quality-of-life outcomes from physical activity interventions. *Nursing*

Research, 58, 175–183. doi:10.1097/NNR.0b013e318199b53a

Daker-White, G., Hays, R., McSharry, J., Giles, S., Cheraghi-Sohi, S., Rhodes, P., & Sanders, C. (2015). Blame the patient, blame the doctor or blame the system? A meta-synthesis of qualitative studies of patient safety in primary care. *PLoS ONE 10*(8): e0128329. doi:10.1371/journal.pone.0128329

Elzey, F. (1974). *A first reader in statistics* (2nd ed.). Monterey, CA: Brooks/Cole.

Fincher, L., Ward, C., Dawkins, V., Magee, V., & Wilson, P. (2009). Using telehealth to educate Parkinson's disease patients about complicated medication regimens. *Gerontological Nursing, 35,* 16–24. doi:10.3928/00989134-20090201-10

Gaskin, C. J., & Happell, B. (2014). Power, effects, confidence, and significance: An investigation of statistical practices in nursing research. *International Journal of Nursing Studies, 51,* 795–806. doi:10.1016/j.ijnurstu.2013.09.014

Heidari, M. R., & Norouzadeh, R. (2015). Nursing students' perspectives on clinical education. *Advances in Medical Education & Professionalism, 3*(1), 39–43. PMCID: PMC4291507

Hoseini, S., Soltani, F., Beygi, M. B., & Zarifsanaee, N. (2013). The effect of educational audiotape programme on anxiety and depression in patients undergoing coronary artery bypass graft. *Clinical Nursing, 22,* 1613–1619. doi:10.1111/jocn.12125

Huis, A., Hulscher, M., Adang, E., Grol, R., van Achterberg, T., & Schoonhoven, L. (2013). Cost-effectiveness of a team and leaders-directed strategy to improve nurses' adherence to hand hygiene guidelines: A cluster of randomized trial. *International Journal of Nursing Studies, 50,* 518–526. doi:10.1016/j.ijnurstu.2012.11.016

Liebermann, S. C., Müller, A., Weigl, M., & Wegge, J. (2015) Antecedents of the expectation of remaining in nursing until retirement age. *Advanced Nursing, 71*(7), 1624–1638. doi:10.1111/jan.12634

Marshall, J. G., Cowell, J. M., Campbell, E. S., & McNaughton, D. B. (2010). Regional variations in cancer screening rates found in women with diabetes. *Nursing Research, 59,* 34–41. doi:10.1097/NNR.0b013e3181c3bd07

O'Mathuna, D. P., & Fineout-Overholt, E. (2015). Critically appraising quantitative evidence for clinical decision making. In B. M. Melnyk & E. Fineout-Overholt (Eds.), *Evidence-Based Practice in Nursing & Healthcare: A Guide to Best Practice* (3rd ed.). China: Wolters Kluwer Health.

Riemer, H. C., Mates, J., Ryan, L. & Schleder, B. J. (2015). Decreased stress levels in nurses: A benefit of quiet time. *American Journal of Critical Care, 24,* 396–402. doi:10.4037/ajcc2015706

Shott, S. (1990). *Statistics for health care professionals.* Philadelphia: W. B. Saunders.

Spatz, C., & Johnston, J. (1984). *Basic statistics: Tales of distribution* (3rd ed.). Monterey, CA: Brooks/Cole.

Steinhardt, M. A., Brown, S. A., Dubois, S. K., Harrison, L., Lehrer, H. M., & Jaggars, S. S. A resilience intervention in African-American adults with type 2 diabetes. *American Journal of Health Behavior, 39,* 507–518. doi.org/10.5993/AJHB.39.4.7

Urquhart, C., Currell, R., Harlow, F., & Callow, L. (2015). Home uterine monitoring for detecting preterm labour. *Cochrane Database of Systematic Reviews* 2015, Issue 1. Art. No.: CD006172. doi:10.1002/14651858.CD006172.pub3

Chapter 17
Presentation and Discussion of Study Findings

Rose Nieswiadomy, PhD, RN, and Verdell Marsh, PhD, RN

Objectives

On completion of this chapter, you will be prepared to:

1. Summarize the parts of a presentation of findings.
2. Explain the discussion of findings, study hypotheses, and statistical and clinical significance.
3. Describe the purpose of conclusions, implications, and recommendations for research studies.

Introduction

We have reached the final steps in the research process. However, these final steps are very important. We might say, the best has been saved for last. The findings, discussion of findings, conclusions, implications, and recommendations help pull together all of the pieces of a research study. They indicate not only what has been learned from this particular study, but also point out what needs to be done in the future related to this area of research.

The presentation of these final sections of a study may be placed under various headings in the research report. In theses and dissertations, you will probably find each of these sections under a separate heading. There is a great deal of variation in research journal articles. All of these elements of a report may be found under a section titled "Discussion of Findings" or there may be a section on "Findings" and another section for "Discussion." Many qualitative study reports contain a section titled "Discussion." Some articles may have a section titled "Results and Conclusions." Regardless of the division of the material under various headings, each research report should contain the elements mentioned: findings, discussion of findings, conclusions, implications, and recommendations. Each area is discussed individually here.

Presentation of Findings of the Study

Most research reports present the findings in both a narrative form and in tables. There is some disagreement about the function of the table in relation to the narrative presentation. Some people want to see all of the results in both places. Other individuals contend that results presented in tables should not be reported in their entirety in the text and that only highlights or important items from the table should be presented in the narrative. According to the publication manual of the American Psychological Association (2010), if the text discusses every item in the table, the table is unnecessary.

Findings of the Study

The findings of a quantitative study are the results presented in the form of empirical data or facts. Have you ever seen reruns of the old TV show *Dragnet*? Sergeant Friday would say, "Just the facts, ma'am." This holds true for the findings of a research study. This is not the place for the researcher to express opinions or reactions to the data.

Findings are written in the past tense, of course, because data are being reported that have already been gathered and analyzed before the writing of the report. A note of caution: *Data are plural.* The word *data* frequently is used incorrectly as a singular noun rather than a plural noun. *Datum*, the singular noun, is rarely used because the information that is gathered nearly always involves more than one piece of information.

The findings come from the analysis of the data obtained in the study. Descriptive statistics are always used to describe the sample and to present the findings. Inferential statistics are always used to present the findings in studies in which hypotheses were tested.

Ethical Issues in Presenting Research Findings

The researcher has the responsibility to ensure no subjects can be identified. The names of subjects should never be reported. Generally, in quantitative studies, only group data are presented. In qualitative studies, narratives by individual participants are common. Therefore, protecting subjects from being identified in a qualitative report is very important.

If data are collected in an agency, the name of this agency should never be mentioned unless permission has been obtained. The agency should be described in very general terms such as "a large public teaching hospital in the northeastern United States."

Narrative Presentation of Findings

The findings of a study should be clearly and concisely presented in the text. In qualitative studies, narrative presentations predominate. These narrations generally contain direct quotes from participants. The researcher may then present a summary of the findings by discussing patterns and themes found in the data. Do the themes appear to capture the meaning found in the participants' own words?

In quantitative studies where hypotheses are tested, the narrative presentation should present data that support or fail to support each study hypothesis. Certain information should always be included in the text when discussing the study hypothesis(es). The statistical test that was used, the test results, degrees of freedom, and the probability value should be listed. Here are two common methods of reporting the same information:

$$t(30) = 2.75; \quad p = .01$$
$$t = 2.75; \quad df = 30; \quad p = .01$$

In the past, the probability value was frequently reported with a "less than" symbol in front of it ($p = < .05$) to indicate that the actual probability level was less than the given figure. Today, with the use of computers, the exact probability value should be reported. The computer printout will usually provide the probability value to four or more decimal places. The probability value is then listed in a research report as two decimal places. So, if the probability level was .0212, it probably would be reported as .02 and not as < .05, as was common in years past.

In qualitative research studies, hypotheses are not tested. Therefore, inferential statistics are not included in these reports.

Tables

Tables are a means of organizing data so they may be more easily understood and interpreted. The discussion of the table should be as clear as possible in the text. Some of the responsibility, however, for understanding the table is left with the reader. If a table is being used to present the results of hypothesis testing, the results should be placed in the table or a footnote added that provides the test results, degrees of freedom, and probability level. This information would be presented in the format described under the narrative type of presentation. For example, the following might be found under a table:

$$x^2 = 13.39; \ df = 5; \ p = .02$$

Here are some general guidelines concerning tables:

1. Tables should appear as soon as possible in the report after they have been referred to in the text.
2. Information presented in tables should also be discussed in the narrative of the report.
3. Titles should be clear, concise, and contain the variables that are presented in the data. The name of the statistical test should not be used. For example, the following would be an inappropriate title: *T Test for Difference in Anxiety Levels of Cardiac Patients*. An appropriate title might be: *Guided Relaxation and Anxiety Levels of Cardiac Patients*.
4. All data entries should be rounded to the same number of decimal places (one or two decimal places is common).
5. The decimal points, if present, should be lined up under each other in the data columns.
6. If data are not available for a section of the table, a dash (—) should be entered, rather than leaving a blank space, to make it clear that no data have accidentally been left off the table.

Some tables contain rows, some contain columns, and some contain both rows and columns. The vertical entries in a table are referred to as columns, and the horizontal entries are called rows. **Cells** are the boxes that are formed where rows and columns intersect.

Figures

The word *figure* is the term used to indicate any type of visual presentation other than a table. Figures include graphs, diagrams, line drawings, and photographs. Figures may help enliven a narrative presentation and should be considered as a valuable means of displaying research results. These methods are particularly useful in presenting demographic data about subjects.

Discussion of Findings and Significance

The discussion of the findings is a much more subjective section of a research report than the presentation of the findings. The discussion section of a study report allows the researcher to make interpretations of the findings. The findings are interpreted in light of the theoretical framework and within the context of the literature review. No literature sources should be cited in the discussion of the findings section that were not referred to in the review of the literature section of the report. When new literature sources are cited, it appears as if the investigator went back to the library or the internet after the data were collected to search for a source or sources that would be in agreement with the study findings.

In the discussion of the findings, the researcher discusses aspects of the results that are in agreement and those that are not in agreement with previous research and theoretical explanations. The researcher also reports study limitations. Study limitations are uncontrolled variables that may affect study results and limit the generalizability of the findings.

Limitations

Chang et al. (2015) examined the aspects of professional commitment on the retention of professional nurses. One finding was that continuance commitment contributes to retaining nurses in the nursing profession.

A study limitation mentioned was the use of a simple random sampling process, which did not provide a representation of the unique characteristics of each of the units studied.

Although study limitations should be discussed, this is not the time to focus on every fault of the study. A beginning researcher frequently lists all of the weaknesses and problems of the study and appears to ask the reader to disregard the findings of the present study when they are not in agreement with the theoretical framework or past research results. Experienced investigators are able to interpret findings within the context of the strengths and the weaknesses of their studies.

Discussion of Study Hypotheses

Nurses need to have a basic understanding of hypothesis testing prior to reading an article that contains a hypothesis. Delaney (2010) published an informative article in the *British Journal of Cardiac Nursing* about the importance of understanding statistical hypothesis testing. She pointed out that hypothesis testing involves a systematic and well-defined process that enables the researcher to make assumptions about a population based on data from a sample.

The most important aspect of the findings in studies where hypotheses have been formulated is the presentation of inferential statistics used to test the hypotheses. The null hypothesis is subjected to statistical analysis, and the results allow the researcher to reject or fail to reject the null hypothesis. Another way to describe failure to reject the null hypothesis is to "accept the null hypothesis." However, if the null hypothesis is rejected, support is provided for the research or hypothesis. Remember, the research hypothesis predicts study results based on the theoretical framework or on previous research studies.

The results of hypothesis testing fall into one of three categories: (a) the null hypothesis is not rejected; (b) the null hypothesis is rejected, and the research hypothesis is supported; and (c) the null hypothesis is rejected, and the results are in the opposite direction from the prediction of the research hypothesis.

When the study results are congruent with the study prediction found in the research hypothesis, the researcher is overjoyed, and the task of describing the results of the study is relatively easy. The explanation for the findings will have already been discussed in the section on the theoretical framework or in the review of the literature section where previous research results were presented. Although the researcher should never say that the results "proved" the study hypothesis, the findings of a study provide empirical support for the hypothesis, and the investigator asserts with a degree of certainty (probability level) that the results were not related to chance. When significant results are found, the researcher will feel like celebrating and may begin to think about publishing the results.

When the null hypothesis is not rejected, the researcher may become discouraged and start trying to determine what went wrong. Beginning researchers are particularly prone to start picking apart their studies when the null hypothesis is not rejected. They discuss the small sample size and the inadequate instrument and all the other limitations that can be identified. It is not uncommon for a graduate student who is writing a thesis to become upset after discovering nonsignificant study results. Researchers must be objective when considering negative results (those not in agreement with the prediction). Negative results may be as important as positive results. They just are not as exciting for the researcher.

Some researchers think the only studies that are published are those in which the findings are in agreement with the study predictions. Many of the published research studies *do* report positive findings. In fact, you will find that most of the study results you examine report positive findings. However, a recent review of the research journals revealed that studies are being published in which nonsignificant results were found. As previously mentioned, negative results may be as important as positive results.

Although the discovery of nonsignificant results is disheartening, the discovery of results that are in the opposite direction of the study prediction is even more disappointing and puzzling. These types of results do not support the study's theoretical framework. These results may also be incongruent with previous research results. For an investigator faced with this dilemma, the best thing that can be done is to try to make some sense out of the findings and give some tentative explanations for the results. Recommendations may then be made for further research based on these explanations.

Statistical and Clinical Significance

It is very important to distinguish between statistical and clinical significance. Statistical significance means that the null hypothesis has been rejected and that the differences found between groups on the variable of interest, or the correlations found between two variables, are not likely to be a chance occurrence. The differences or correlations are probably real. These real differences or correlations, however, may not be clinically important. Clinical significance means that the findings can be useful in the clinical setting with patients. The researcher's greatest desire is that study findings are both statistically and clinically significant.

Statistical and Clinical Significance

A study examined the differences in patient outcomes of discharge planning rounds held at the bedside compared to the conference room (Wrobleski, Joswiak, Dunn, Maxon, & Holland, 2014). Hospital length of stay between the two groups of patients was significantly different ($p = .02$). The patients in the conference room discharge planning rounds stayed on an average of 8.0 days; those patients in the bedside discharge planning rounds stayed an average of 5.4 days. Both a statistically and a clinically significant difference (three-day difference) were determined.

The significance of a correlation coefficient depends on the sample size. As the sample size increases, the smaller the correlation needs to be to reach significance. For example, with a sample size of 15, a correlation coefficient of .48 is needed to be statistically significant at the .05 level. With a sample of 100 subjects, a correlation of .19 is statistically significant at the .05 level. Remember, a statistically significant correlation means only that you are reasonably sure the actual correlation between these two variables in the population from which the sample was obtained is greater than zero. It does not take a very large correlation to be greater than 0.

Sometimes the difference between the scores of two groups (experimental and control) on the dependent variable are so large that the statistical and clinical significance are quite apparent. However, there are instances where no statistical significance is found, but the researcher believes the findings have some clinical significance. Sometime the researcher will find an intervention to have no significant effect for the experimental group, as a whole, but will find the intervention to be effective for a certain subgroup within the experimental group.

Conclusions, Implications, and Recommendations

The study conclusions are the researcher's attempt to show what knowledge has been gained by the study and are an attempt to generalize the findings. In writing conclusions, the researcher returns to the study problem, purpose, hypothesis, and theoretical framework. Was the study problem addressed adequately? The research purpose met? The research hypothesis supported? The theoretical framework supported? The researcher should leave no doubt in the reader's mind about what the study has demonstrated in these areas. Conversely, it is probably wise to be somewhat conservative in drawing conclusions from the findings.

Conclusions

In formulating conclusions, the researcher must consider the sample size and the population from which the sample was drawn. An example of a study conclusion that was generalized beyond the findings of the study is found in Jones's (1981) report published in *Nursing Research*. Self-reported theft behavior among 33 nurses in one hospital in the northeast was examined. These nurses were asked if they ever took anything home from the hospital (supplies, etc.). Based on their responses, the investigator reported that theft behavior was prevalent among this group of nurses. One of the researchers' conclusions was, that employee theft among nursing personnel was rampant and was a serious issue that required attention. Do you agree that this is an example of overgeneralization? A sample size of 33 nurses in one hospital does not warrant the use of the word *widespread*. Although this study is 35 years old, we have mentioned it in each edition of this textbook because the conclusion is so awful.

Whereas the findings of a study are concrete and tied into the specific data of the study, the conclusions are more abstract and are presented in more general terms. Conclusions are *not* just a restatement of the findings. It is somewhat common to find a conclusion in a student's initial research report that states, "There is a significant relationship between anxiety and test scores among nursing students." This is a finding and not a conclusion. The conclusions should go beyond the findings. For example, a study finding might be, "There is a significant increase in the exercise performance of a group of senior citizens who have used mental practice to increase their exercise performance." A conclusion based on this finding would be, "Mental practice appears to be an effective means of increasing exercise performance in the elderly." You may think that these two statements are quite similar, but examine them more closely and you will see that the conclusion goes beyond the finding. The finding addresses the difference in exercise performance of one group of people from the pretest to the posttest. A conclusion is an attempt to generalize the result to other senior citizens and to other points in time. The word *appear* may worry you. You have been taught in nursing to avoid words that could have subjective meanings. You would never chart "It appears that the patient is bleeding." That statement probably makes you cringe. However, the word *appears* is an acceptable term for a study conclusion. Conclusions are tentative. We never prove our findings when we conduct research with human beings, which is usually the case in nursing research. We can say only "mental practice appears to increase exercise performance in the elderly."

The purpose of scientific quantitative research, as you may recall, is to be able to generalize results to the broad population, not just to the study sample. In some types of research, such as phenomenological studies, nurses may be more interested in the responses of individuals than in those of groups.

However, in the traditional scientific method the interest is in populations rather than in samples or in individuals. The generalization of findings, therefore, is of great interest to quantitative study investigators.

Generalizations are risky business. The study design and sampling procedures must always be considered. If the senior citizens in the previous example had consisted of 10 volunteers who said before the study that they enjoyed exercising, there would be no basis for making the conclusion that mental practice was the reason for the increase in exercise performance. There would be too many threats to the validity of the study because of the design used and the sampling technique. You would have no way of knowing if the group changed because of the treatment or other factors, such as the Hawthorne effect. Because the subjects were volunteers who said that they enjoyed exercising, they may have been more motivated to increase their exercise performance.

Implications

Both quantitative and qualitative researchers should present the implications of their studies. This section of the research report gives the researcher an opportunity to be creative. Imagine you have the power to change the way certain courses are taught in your curriculum or certain procedures are carried out in the hospital where you work. Based on the findings and conclusions of your study, what changes would you suggest?

The implications of a study contain the *should* or what needs to happen next. "Nurse educators should . . ." or "it would be appropriate for nurse clinicians to . . ." are the types of statements found in the implications section of a research report. Based on the study, what changes, if any, should be considered?

A study implication might be that no change is needed, or that more research is called for to further verify the study results, or that changes need to be made based on the study conclusions. Although it is possible that no change is deemed necessary and that nurses should continue with their current practices, it is more common to see implications that call for more research in the subject area or for certain changes to be made based on the conclusions of the study.

For every conclusion of a study, there should be at least one implication. Implications can be addressed to any or all of the following: clinicians, educators, researchers, administrators, or theorists.

Consider this conclusion: "Guided relaxation is an effective means of controlling anxiety in patients about to undergo a proctoscopic examination." An implication of this conclusion might be "Nurses might want to consider using guided relaxation techniques with patients about to undergo proctoscopic examinations." Another implication might be that nurse educators teach nursing students about the usefulness of guided relaxation techniques in their nursing practice. Although these implications may seem to be quite simple and derived from common sense, the implications of a study may be very challenging to write at times.

Recommendations

It has often been said that every research study raises more questions than it answers. The last section of every research report should contain recommendations for further research. Both quantitative and qualitative researchers should make recommendations for future research, based on their studies. This section may propose replication of the study or a new study in which the present study limitations are considered. The researcher might also suggest some logical extension of the present study.

Replication of the Research Study

Replication of a study involves carrying out a study similar to one that has previously been done. Only minor changes are made from the previous study, such as using a different type of sample or setting. Partial replication studies are probably more common than exact replications. If an instrument is changed or a new tool is added, it is probably more accurate to call this type of study a partial replication study.

Nurses have appeared to be reluctant to replicate the studies of other investigators. Polit and Beck (2010) contended that often replication of studies is not viewed as valuable and with graduate students sometimes discouraged. Knowledge is augmented through replication of studies, not simply by testing new theories, instruments, or constructs (Polit and Beck, 2010). They asserted that "in both qualitative and quantitative research, intentional replication only makes sense when there are strong, thoughtful studies that yield evidence worth repeating" (p. 1454).

As a result of nurses' reluctance to replicate studies, many isolated pieces of nursing research exist. Researchers must become convinced of the value of replication. The body of nursing knowledge needs to be based on research findings. Hypotheses must be tested over and over on different samples and in different settings to build confidence in research results.

Replication studies are very appropriate for beginning researchers. This type of research is an excellent means of gaining research experience. Experienced researchers must also be willing to conduct replications to verify or repudiate previous research results. Unfortunately, few replication studies are found in the nursing literature.

Consideration of Study Limitations in Future Research

When recommending future research studies, the limitations of the present study should be considered. Some of the most common recommendations that are made concerning limitations are (a) alteration in the sample (different age group or educational level of the subjects), (b) alteration in the instrument (either a change in an existing instrument or use of another instrument), (c) control of variables (taking only a certain age group in the sample or selecting a random sample instead of using a convenience sample), and (d) change in methodology (providing 6 weeks of the experimental treatment instead of 4 weeks or using structured observations to collect data from respondents rather than using self-report measures).

Extensions of the Research Study

Recommendations concerning extension of the research study should answer the question, "What comes next?" After completing a study, the investigator should be in a good position to determine the next step that needs to be taken to examine the subject area under consideration. It is important to distinguish extensions of the study from the common recommendations often found in research studies. These common recommendations suggest a larger sample, or a different setting, or more reliability studies on the instrument. Although the limitations of a study need to be discussed, this is not the most important function of the recommendations section. In this section of the report, the researcher has the opportunity to make suggestions for future research based on the findings of this particular study, the findings of previous research, and the current state of the theoretical framework used in the study. This is a great challenge.

Recommendations for Future Research

A study was conducted to examine how often and long nurses were involved in the mobility of older patients in acute care settings and to determine who initiated the mobilization of these patients (Doherty-King, Yoon, Pecanac, Brown, & Mahoney, 2013). The study used a time and motion design for observations of 15 Registered Nurses for two to three 8-hour periods and chart reviews to collect characteristics data for 47 patients. Thirty-two percent of these patients had no mobility activity by an RN. The mean duration of walking was 1.8 minutes and 1.5 minutes for standing. Patients initiated all of the ambulation activity. The authors of this study recommended that future research be conducted to study mechanisms to encourage patients to become self-advocates in promoting ambulation during their hospitalization stay. The researchers further suggested examining how best to engage nurses in mobility activities of older patients.

Critiquing the Presentation of Study Findings

When presenting the findings of a study, the investigator must be very objective. None of the investigator's personal opinions should be included. However, in discussing the study results, the researcher has an opportunity to interject some subjective interpretation of the data. For example, the researcher might mention some environmental factor that was thought to affect the study results. In one study, a group of subjects were trying to improve the time needed to complete a run around a track. Subjects had been taught the use of guided imagery to help them run faster. During the time the subjects were running on the track, a dust storm came up. The researcher proposed that this might have been the reason for the nonsignificant study findings.

The discussion section of a research report should discuss the findings of each hypothesis that was tested or each research question that was answered. The findings should be interpreted in light of the study framework and previous literature on the topic. If the study hypotheses were not supported, the researcher should present an argument about why these findings may have occurred. If these findings were thought to be related to the limitations of the study, the researcher should acknowledge these limitations and make suggestions for how these problems could be corrected in future studies. The study conclusions should be presented; implications for nursing practice, nursing education, and nursing research should be indicated; and recommendations for replication or extension of the study should be suggested. Box 17–1 presents some guidelines for critiquing the presentation and discussion of study findings.

Box 17–1 Guidelines for Critiquing the Presentation of Study Findings

1. Is the information concerning the study findings presented clearly and concisely?
2. Are the findings presented objectively?
3. In qualitative studies, are the participants' subjective narrations clear and do the themes derived from these narratives capture the meaning of the data?
4. In quantitative studies, is each study hypothesis or research question addressed separately?
5. Are the findings described in relation to the study framework?
6. Are the findings compared to those of other studies discussed in the literature review section of the report?
7. Does the investigator discuss the limitations that may have influenced the findings of the study?
8. Is clinical significance discussed, and is statistical significance discussed in a quantitative study where inferential statistics are presented?
9. Are study conclusions clearly stated?
10. In quantitative study reports, are generalizations made that are based on the data and take into consideration the sample size and sampling method, or does it appear the investigator has overgeneralized the findings of the study?
11. Are implications suggested for nursing practice, nursing education, and/or nursing research?
12. Are recommendations made for future research studies? If so, do these recommendations take into consideration the limitations of the present study?

Summary

Each research report should contain the findings, discussion of findings, conclusions, implications, and recommendations for future research. These elements of a research report may be found under various types of headings.

The findings of a study are the presentation of the results in the form of empirical data. Methods of presenting findings include narrative presentations, tables, and figures.

The findings of a study should be clearly and concisely presented in the narrative text of the study report. The results of hypothesis testing should contain the statistical test used, the test results, the degrees of freedom, and the obtained probability level.

Tables are a means of organizing data to make study findings more easily understood and interpreted. Tables should never appear in a report unless they have been discussed in the text; they should appear as soon as possible after they have been referred to. The vertical entries in a table are the columns; the horizontal entries are called rows. Cells are the boxes formed where rows and columns intersect.

The word *figure* is the term used to indicate any visual presentation of data, other than a table. Figures include graphs, diagrams, line drawings, and photographs.

The discussion of findings is a more subjective section of a research report than the presentation of findings. The researcher interprets the findings in light of the theoretical framework and in the context of the literature review. The researcher also discusses any problems that may have occurred while conducting the study.

An important aspect of the findings of a study is the discussion of the hypothesis testing results. Results fall into one of three categories: (a) the null hypothesis is not rejected, and, therefore, the research hypothesis is not supported; (b) the null hypothesis is rejected, and the research hypothesis is supported; and (c) the null hypothesis is rejected, and the results are in the opposite direction from the prediction of the research hypothesis.

It is important to distinguish between statistical and clinical significance. Statistical significance means that the null hypothesis has been rejected and the study findings are probably not related to chance. Clinical significance means that the findings may be useful in the clinical setting.

The study conclusions are the researcher's attempt to generalize the findings. Conclusions are based on the findings and take into consideration the study problem, purpose, hypothesis, and theoretical framework. The population, sample, and sampling method must also be considered when trying to generalize study results.

The implications of a study contain the "shoulds" that result from the study. Appropriate changes are recommended that should be carried out by nurses in any of the following roles: clinician, educator, researcher, administrator, and theorist.

Recommendations for further research should be contained in each research report. This section of the report should propose replication of the study or a new study in which the present study limitations are considered. The researcher might also suggest some extensions to the present study.

When presenting research results, the rights of subjects must be protected. Names of subjects should never be reported, and, generally, only group data are presented.

Self-Test

1. Guidelines for the use of tables in research studies include which of the following?
   A. A table should appear in a research report after the narrative discussion of the table.
   B. If data are missing, a blank space should appear in the table to indicate missing data.
   C. Titles should include the name of the statistical test used to analyze the data.
   D. Information presented in a table does not need to be in the research report narrative.

2. Which type of study would generate direct quotes from the participants?
   A. statistical studies
   B. descriptive studies
   C. quantitative studies
   D. qualitative studies

3. The researcher has provided a comprehensive narrative of every item associated with the findings in the study. What should be said about planning for the accompanying table?
   A. Include only highlights or important items from the narrative in the table.
   B. There is no need for a table.
   C. There is a need to complete the table and delete the narrative of the findings.
   D. Include everything from the narrative of the findings in the table

4. Which of the following statements is true concerning statistical and clinical significance?
   A. Statistical significance is necessary for clinical significance.
   B. Findings may be both statistically and clinically nonsignificant.
   C. If findings are said to be clinically significant, they must also be statistically significant.
   D. Findings must be either statistically significant or clinically significant.

5. What can be said about the theory-based hypothesis when the findings of the study support the research intervention?
   A. The null hypothesis was rejected.
   B. The null hypothesis was not rejected.
   C. The research hypothesis was rejected.
   D. The research hypothesis failed to predict the outcome.

6. There is a statistically nonsignificant difference and a clinically significant difference in the variable of interest between the experimental and the control group members? What does this mean?
   A. The null hypothesis was rejected and it occurred by chance among the groups.
   B. The research hypothesis was supported with a clinically important difference.
   C. The null hypothesis was accepted with a clinically important difference between the groups.
   D. The research hypothesis was not supported and the findings are not clinically important.

7. The conclusions of a study are based on the:
   A. findings of the study.
   B. review of the literature.
   C. implications of the study.
   D. recommendations for future research.

8. Consider the following conclusion: "There is a positive relationship between children's anxiety levels and their failure to cooperate with physical examinations." Determine an appropriate implication derived from this conclusion.
   A. Nurses should try to assess the anxiety levels of children before physical examinations.
   B. Nurses must discover why high anxiety levels cause children to be uncooperative during physical examinations.
   C. Physical examinations should be conducted infrequently with small children.
   D. A parent should be instructed to remain in the room with the child during a physical examination.

9. The recommendations of a study might contain which of the following?
   A. a discussion of the study findings
   B. suggestions for extension of the study
   C. comparisons of results with previous research findings
   D. a means of implementing the study findings

See answers to Self-Test in the Answer Section at the back of the book.

References

American Psychological Association. (2010). *Publication manual of the American Psychological Association* (6th ed.). Washington, DC: Author.

Chang, H.-Y., Shyu, Y.-I., L., Wong, M.-K., Friesner, D. Chu, T-L., & Teng, C.-I. (2015). Which aspects of professional commitment can effectively retain nurses in the nursing profession? *Nursing Scholarship 47*, 468–476. doi:10.111/nu.12152

Doherty-King, B., Yoon, J. Y., Pecanac, K. J., Brown, R., & Mahoney, J. (2013). Frequency and duration of nursing care related to older patient mobility. [Special issue on basic nursing care]. *Nursing Scholarship 46*, 20–27. doi:10.1111/jnu.12047

Jones, J. (1981). Attitudinal correlates of employee theft of drugs and hospital supplies among nursing personnel. *Nursing Research, 30*, 349–351. doi:10.1097/00006199-198111000-00013

Polit, D. F. & Beck, C. F. (2010). Generalization in quantitative and qualitative research: Myths and strategies. *International Journal of Nursing Studies 47*, 1451–58. doi:10.1016/j.ijnurstu.2010.06.004

Valdovinos, N. C., Reddin, C., Bernard, C., Shafer, B., & Tanabe, P. (2009). The use of topical anesthesia during intravenous catheter insertion in adults: A comparison of pain scores using LMX-4 versus placebo. *Emergency Nursing, 35*, 299–304. doi:10.1016/j.jen.2008.08.005

Wrobleski, D. M., Joswiak, E. M., Dunn, D. F., Maxson, P. M., & Holland, D. E. (2014). Discharge planning rounds to the bedside: A patient- and family-centered approach. *MEDSURG Nursing, 23*(2), 111–116. http://www.medsurgnursing.net/cgi-bin/WebObjects/MSNJournal.woa

PART VI Research Findings and Nursing Practice

Chapter 18
Communication and Utilization of Nursing Research

Rose Nieswiadomy, PhD, RN, and Verdell Marsh, PhD, RN

 Objectives

On completion of this chapter, you will be prepared to:

1. Describe the means of communicating nursing research findings.
2. Summarize issues related to research utilization.

Introduction

Your research project is completed, and you have been asked to present your study results at a national research conference. Does this sound like delusions of grandeur? Maybe so, but it is hoped that some day you will present the results of a study you have conducted. Once a researcher has completed a study, plans should be made to communicate or disseminate the results. In fact, these plans should be made before the beginning of the project. A research project is really not completed unless the findings have been communicated to others.

Although the communication of research findings is frequently considered to be the last formal step in the research process, it is only the beginning of the most important phase of research—the utilization of research findings. Utilization of research findings is the final step of the research process. Nurse researchers need to exert as much effort in implementing research findings as they do in conducting research in the first place. This chapter discusses various means of communicating nursing research findings and promoting their utilization.

Communication of Nursing Research Findings

Researchers can communicate the results of their studies in two major ways: They can talk about them or write about them. A nurse researcher might begin by presenting study results to peers. Next, this researcher might attend a research conference at which study results are discussed in an oral presentation or in a poster session. As a next step, study results might be published in a journal article. If funding has been received for a research project, the researcher probably will be required to submit a written report of the study to the funding agency. Finally, many nurses are pursuing advanced degrees and will present their research results associated with their theses and dissertations.

Although researchers have the prime responsibility of communicating the findings of their studies, other nurses and nursing organizations also bear the responsibility of seeing that research findings are distributed inside the nursing profession, to other healthcare professionals, and even to the general public.

Preparing a Research Report

A **research report** is a written or oral summary of a study. No research project is complete until the final report has been written. Even when an oral presentation is planned, the research report should be written out in its entirety.

Writing is not easy (Kotz, Cals, Tugwell, & Knottnerus, 2013). Kotz et al. state that many novice researchers may struggle with writing scientific papers. Researchers often learn the skill of writing by doing it and receiving feedback on their drafts from more experienced writers, such as their instructors. Of course, that takes time.

Effective writing is the result of planning and organization before writing begins. Good writing should be clear, accurate, and concise. Technical or scientific writing is not meant to be humorous or entertaining, but it also should not be dull. The results of a study should be presented in an interesting and informative manner.

The research report should be presented in the order of the research process, beginning with the problem of the study and ending with conclusions, implications, and recommendations for future studies. The major part of the research report is written in the past tense because the study has already occurred. Hypotheses and conclusions are written in the present tense, and the implications and recommendations are directed toward the future.

Presenting Research Results at Professional Conferences

Many nurse researchers give first consideration to nursing journals as a publication medium for their research results. However, the time delay for publication of a report in a journal may be two years or longer. This process has been speeding up in recent years, because journal editors now allow manuscripts to be submitted online. However, presentations of research findings at local, regional, and national conferences provide more rapid distribution of study results. Nurses should present their research results at nursing conferences as well as at interdisciplinary conferences.

The two ways to disseminate research results at professional conferences are oral presentations and poster presentations. Traditionally, oral presentations have been used most frequently, but in the last 15 to 20 years, poster presentations have increased in popularity.

Nurses have many opportunities to present their study results at research conferences and seminars. Nursing organizations such as the American Nurses Association and Sigma Theta Tau International Honor Society of Nursing sponsor research seminars. Many nursing schools, regional nursing associations, and most recently, large medical centers also sponsor research conferences. Some organizations make special provisions for presentations by students.

Potential participants are contacted through a **call for abstracts**, which request a summary of a study that the researcher wishes to present at a conference. These requests are published in professional journals and distributed to educational institutions, healthcare agencies, and potential participants whose names have been obtained through the mailing lists of professional organizations. Notices of research conferences are generally distributed 6 to 12 months before the event.

Each conference or seminar will provide special guidelines for presenters and deadlines for submission of abstracts. The required length of the abstract varies from 50 to 1000 words, but many have a 200-to-300-word limit. Abstracts should contain the purpose, research question(s) or hypothesis(es), design, methodology, major findings, and conclusions. If the research is still in progress, the last two items are not required. Abstracts will be evaluated, and participants will be notified about the selection decisions.

Generally, those individuals selected to be presenters at conferences receive no pay and are required to cover their own travel expenses. Sometimes the conference registration fee is waived or reduced for participants. A commitment to nursing research is a prime motivator for participants. Of course, personal recognition and career advancement are also rewards.

Presenting a Research Paper

The oral presentation of a research report is usually referred to as a paper presentation. The word *paper* is used because the report of the study has been written out on paper and is referred to or read by the investigator during the presentation. Guidelines for paper presentations are found in the literature (Davis, M., Davis, & Dunagan, 2012; Leng, 2012).

If the principal investigator is unable to attend the conference, a co-investigator or another person familiar with the study presents the paper. A written report of the study will be necessary if the proceedings of the conference are to be published.

Presenting research results at a conference has advantages over publishing the findings in a journal article. First, the investigator has the opportunity to present findings that are recent. Because of the time lag in publishing, research presented in journals may be outdated when it is printed. Some journals have attempted to reduce this lag time by offering published-ahead-of-print or advanced-released articles on their websites, at which the electronic publication of accepted papers occurs before the printed publication. Second, the researcher will have the opportunity to interact with people who are interested in studying the same or similar phenomena.

Although many presentations are read directly from the research paper, more interest is created when an outline is used and the presenter communicates with the audience informally. The use of audiovisual aids, such as slides and PowerPoint displays, greatly enhances a presentation. Audiences generally appreciate written handouts in the form of abstracts or summaries of the study.

A presenter is usually allotted 15 to 30 minutes. At some conferences, additional time is allocated for questions. At other conferences, the presenter may have to allow time for questions if questions are desired. Even when no time remains for questions, presenters are usually willing to respond to questions during break times or after the conferences.

The format of the oral presentation is similar to that of a journal article or other written presentations of the study, in that the steps of the research process are usually presented in chronological order. The main difference lies in the condensation of the material to fit the time constraints of the conference. Some presenters prefer to attract the attention of the audience by reporting the findings first, proceeding with the other parts of the study, then returning to discuss the findings in more detail later in the presentation. The review of the literature is usually not discussed in detail; only pertinent studies are mentioned.

Typically, conference organizers distribute evaluation sheets so the audience can rate each presenter. The presenter should try to read the evaluations with an open mind. Although 99 of 100 comments may be favorable, the presenter probably will react most strongly to that 1 unfavorable comment. A colleague was devastated when reading a comment given to her after a presentation. The comment read, "You forgot to take the price tag off your dress sleeve." She was able to laugh about it later but was thoroughly embarrassed at the time.

Presenting a Research Poster

A popular way to present research results is through poster presentations. This visual method of presentation may be seen by a large number of people in a short time period.

Because of time constraints, a research conference participant can attend only a few oral presentations in a 1- or 2-day research conference. However, it is possible to view a fairly large number of posters in just an hour or two. Research poster sessions are an excellent way for beginning researchers to present their research findings. This type of presentation does not seem as scary as the idea of standing up in front of an audience and discussing a study orally.

Occasionally, educational institutions and clinical agencies hold research conferences in which the only method of presentation is through posters. If posters are placed in a hallway in a clinical setting, patients, their visitors, and the nursing staff can view the materials at their leisure. At a poster session, the presenters usually remain with their posters and interact with the viewers. In fact, Hand (2010) asserted that a poster should be a springboard for discussion. Needless to say, poster sessions are an excellent source of research information, particularly for beginning researchers.

Many sources in the nursing literature discuss the process of constructing a poster, including Durkin, 2011, and Hand, 2010. Careful consideration should be given to the construction of posters (Durkin, 2011). The size of the posters varies according to different research conference requirements. Many conferences are held in hotels, and the size of the assigned rooms may dictate the number and size of the posters. Technical help may be sought from a graphic artist, or researchers may design and construct their own posters. The poster should not appear as if it had been thrown together at the last minute or constructed by a young child. The initial view of the poster is important. Attractive color combinations should be used. Some examples of eye-catching posters have included contrasting colors between the fonts and background, such as black on tan, white on blue, or white on black (Ecoff & Stichler, 2015). Size, thickness, and color of the poster board may be determined after visiting an art store.

It is better not to place too much material on a poster. A cluttered poster distracts the viewers or, worse yet, causes them to pass by the poster because they think it will take too long to decipher the meaning of all of the material. Ecoff and Stichler (2015) have called for the material to be arranged purposefully and with appeal to the eye. The major titles on the poster should be in large letters, at least 1 inch high. Viewers need to be able to see these letters from about 3 feet away. Typed material should be prepared with large letters. Computer software programs have this capability, but letters also can be prepared freehand, with the use of a stencil or vinyl adhesive letters. Posters should contain the research question(s), hypothesis(es), a description of the sample, the methods, the findings, and major conclusions. Diagrams, graphs, and tables are an effective means of presenting certain aspects of the study, such as the findings.

If a poster is displayed on a table, some type of support is needed to make the poster stand erect. Commercial products may be purchased or a support can be built out of materials such as plastic foam blocks or wooden wall moldings. When posters must be transported long distances, such as by airplane, care should be taken that the poster does not get dirty or bent.

Publishing a Journal Article

The growth of the nursing profession depends on the ability of its members to build and share a body of knowledge. According to Northam, Yarbrough, Haas, and Duke (2010), nurses "have an obligation to the profession and to society to share their knowledge and experience through publishing" (p. 36).

Nursing research is the method of building knowledge, and publications are the major outlet for sharing this knowledge.

The preparation of an article for a journal is a service to the profession and a means of obtaining recognition as an author. Nurse authors usually do not receive any compensation. Some journals provide authors with complimentary copies of the journal issue in which the article appears, while others send reprints of the article to the author.

The process of manuscript submission has been speeded up, as mentioned before. Many journals allow submission either by email attachments or directly to a website. *Nursing Research* requests that authors submit their manuscripts to a web-based editorial manager system at their website.

Galley proofs show how the article will appear in typeset form. When the author receives the galleys (about 2 months before the publication date), these pages must be proofread for errors. The length of time from submission of a manuscript to the decision about acceptance varies. In the study by Northam et al. (2010), this time period varied from 4 months to more than 20 months. When an author receives an acceptance letter from a journal, an approximate date or month of publication is usually included. The time period from acceptance to publication is called "lag time." The nurse editors in Freda and Kearney's (2005) survey reported a mean lag time of 6 months for the 90 journals they surveyed, with a range of 1 to 18 months. In January 2009, the editors of the *Journal of Nursing Education* reported a 17-to-24-month backlog in manuscripts awaiting publication and a desire to reduce the backlog to 6 to 9 months (Tanner & Bellack, 2009). Later in 2014, Brandon and McGath stated that one of the long-term goals for the editors of the *Advances in Neonatal Care* was to reduce the length of time from submission to publication for all their manuscripts.

One of the reasons for the lag times is because many manuscripts have to be revised. Patricia Yoder-Wise, editor-in-chief of the *Journal of Continuing Education in Nursing*, discussed manuscript resubmissions in a March 2009 editorial (Yoder-Wise, 2009). She reported that requests for manuscript resubmissions approximated 75%.

The *Journal of Nursing Education* has introduced "online advanced releases" as an attempt to speed up the availability of articles to readers. These articles, which have been peer-reviewed and accepted for publication, are posted online a few weeks before final proofing has been done. Online versions will be accessed through subscriptions only once the final version is available in print. Other journals, including *Advances in Nursing Science* and *Research in Gerontological Nursing*, have this same feature. Anyone can access the abstracts that accompany these articles, but a subscription to the journal is necessary to read the entire article.

The acceptance rate for manuscripts seems to vary with the number of manuscript submissions. The The *Journal of Nursing Education* reported an acceptance rate of 20% from 473 manuscript submissions for 2009 compared to 42% from 279 manuscript submissions in 2005 (Bellack, 2010). Authors may want to become familiar with the acceptance rates of the journals of interest before they submit their manuscripts.

The results of several surveys of nursing journal editors have been published since 1990. These include: Swanson, McCloskey, and Bodensteiner (1991); Freda and Kearney (2005); and Northam et al. (2010). The number of nursing journals continues to grow. The survey by Freda and Kearney (2005) examined the roles and practices of nurse editors of 71 journals published in the United States and 19 journals published in other countries. The survey by Northam et al. (2010) covered 230 English-language nursing journals. In addition to journals published in the United States, there are also web-based links to journals in countries such as Australia, Brazil, Canada, England, Japan, the Netherlands, New Zealand, Scotland, and South Africa.

PREPARING THE ARTICLE Because of space constraints, journal articles provide somewhat brief coverage of research reports. The length of journal articles varies a great deal, but most editors prefer manuscripts of 10 to 15 typed pages. The sections of the article and the format vary according to the journal. Most articles contain an introduction, review of literature, methods, findings, and discussion. It is important for the researcher to examine the target journal carefully for style and format.

SELECTING A JOURNAL Selecting an appropriate journal for an article is an important decision. With each passing year, more nursing and allied health journals are coming into existence. Before 1978, *Nursing Research* was the only journal devoted to the publication of nursing research studies. Since that time, more research-focused journals have become available: *Applied Nursing Research, Biological Research for Nursing, Clinical Nursing Research, Research and Theory for Nursing Practice, Research in Gerontological Nursing, Research in Nursing and Health, Western Journal of Nursing Research*, and *Worldviews on Evidence-Based Nursing*. Additionally, journals such as *Advances in Nursing Science* and the *Journal of Nursing Scholarship* devote a large percentage of space to coverage of research studies. Many other journals, including journals that focus on clinical issues, contain research reports.

The choice of a journal may be made before or after a manuscript is prepared. If the manuscript is written first, the author then seeks a journal that is appropriate for the proposed article. Another option is to determine the journal most appropriate for the content of the article then prepare the manuscript according to the guidelines of that particular journal and the needs of that journal's readers.

The selection of a journal may be based on its impact factor. The **impact factor** (IF) is a number used to evaluate the influence of a particular journal. The higher the impact factor number, the more influence the journal is thought to have on the scientific community. Impact factors are listed in the *Journal Citation Reports* published by Thomson Reuters. You may be able to gain access to the entire database through your library. In the 2010 survey by Northam et al. of nursing journal editors, 50 of the 63 editors did not report an impact factor, and several indicated their journal had not been rated.

The IF rating is based on how frequently the articles in a particular journal are cited. The 2-year impact factor is calculated by dividing the number of citations in a given year by the number of articles published in that journal during the previous 2 years. For example, to determine a specific journal's impact factor for 2016, first identify the number of citations from 2014 and 2015 journal issues that are also found in the 2016 literature. If 100 articles were published in the 2014 and 2015 issues, and 75 citations of these articles appeared in the 2016 literature, the impact would be 0.75 (75/100 = .75). The impact factor would actually be reported in early 2017 after all of the 2016 literature had been examined. On February 16, 2016, the website for *Nursing Research* listed an impact factor of 1.356, whereas the *Journal of Professional Nursing* listed an impact factor of 0.945. The 1.36 impact factor indicates that articles published 1 or 2 years ago in *Nursing Research* have been cited, on average, 1.36 times. For the sake of a comparison, a review of the *Journal of the American Medical Association's* website on February 19, 2016, provided an IF of 35.29 for 2014 and 2015.

As you begin to publish more articles throughout your career, you will be able to determine your h-index. This score is a ranking generated from the number of articles in which authors have cited your publications in comparison to your actual number of publications. For example, if you published seven articles and you were cited seven or more times, your h-index score would be 7. The higher your h-index is; the greater impact it is thought that you have contributed to your field. You will be able to find your h-index from such web databases as Web of Science, Scopus, or Google Scholar (Kearney, 2015).

The nurse author should not forget magazines designed for the general public. Although the format would need to be simple and the content presented in easily understood terms, nurses will reach a wide section of healthcare consumers by publishing study results in appropriate lay magazines.

Choosing Between Refereed and Nonrefereed Journals

The author may choose to publish in a refereed or nonrefereed journal. Generally speaking, a **refereed journal** is one in which subject experts chosen by the journal's editorial staff evaluate manuscripts. A **nonrefereed journal** uses editorial staff members or consultants who are not necessarily content experts to review manuscripts. The issue of publication in refereed versus nonrefereed journals seems to be almost moot. In Freda and Kearney's 2005 report of the policies of 90 journals, all of the nurse editors indicated that peer review was in place at their journals. In both refereed and nonrefereed journals, the journal editor makes the final decision about the publication of an article.

Panels of expert colleagues evaluate each manuscript submitted to refereed journals. The nurse editors who responded to the Freda and Kearney (2005) survey reported that the median size of the review panels for their journals was 40. These nurse editors indicated several ways of providing recognition for their reviewers. Ninety-one percent of the nurse editors of the journals reported that reviewers' names were listed each year. Six of the journals (representing 7%) provided an honorarium, while another 25% provided free journal subscriptions to their reviewers.

The review of manuscripts by professional colleagues who are content or methodological experts is called **peer review**. The gold standard of publishing scientific papers is the peer-review process (Oermann & Hays, 2016). Oman (2009) said peer reviewers share in the process with authors and editors toward writing and vetting pioneering, original, and valid contributions to nursing science.

This process allows journal editors to obtain objective opinions about a manuscript from experts in the field. Peer review is usually an unpaid contribution to the nursing profession by some of its accomplished members. Journals usually list their reviewers for the past year in their December issue or in next year's January issue. The March-April 2015 issue of *Heart & Lung* listed 422 reviewers for 2014.

In a **blind review**, the reviewers are not aware of the author's identity before the manuscript is evaluated. This process is very important to a writer with a limited publication record. An unknown writer would have an equal chance with a well-known author. Blinded peer review was reported by 98% of the journals in Freda and Kearney's (2005) survey of nurse editors.

Some journals use an open review process. In an open review, the reviewers sign their comments associated with the review. Open reviews enable the reader to examine the original manuscript and see the reviewers' comments. An example of a posted open review relates to an article titled *Meta-Analysis of Fitness Outcomes From Motivational Physical Activity Interventions* by Chase and Conn (2013). This review can be found at the manuscript review website for the *Nursing Research* journal.

Applied Nursing Research uses a unique approach to manuscript review. Each manuscript submitted to this journal is sent to two teams of reviewers who have individuals with expertise in the content area or the research methods presented in the manuscript. Each team member individually writes a review of the manuscript, and then the two reviewer teams write a joint review.

SENDING QUERY LETTERS Before submitting an article to a journal, it may be wise for the author to first determine the journal's interest in the manuscript. A **query letter** contains an outline of a manuscript and important information about the manuscript that is sent to an editor to determine interest in publication. The letter should be addressed to the editor by name. It is never wise to address a query letter to "The Editor of . . ." or to "Dear Sir or Madam." Many journals allow query letters to be submitted via email.

The advantage of a query letter is that the writer does not waste time submitting a manuscript where a similar article is already in line for publication (Moos, 2010) or for which the content of the proposed manuscript is not appropriate for the targeted journal. In the survey conducted by Northam et al. (2010), 24 editors (38%) rated query letters as somewhat important, and 10 (16%) rated them as very important. Although query letters may be sent to several journals simultaneously, a manuscript should be sent to only *one* journal at a time. Most journals require a signed statement that the manuscript is not being considered by any other journal.

REASONS FOR MANUSCRIPT REJECTION Researchers have examined why manuscripts are rejected. Swanson et al.'s (1991) survey revealed that the highest-ranked reason for rejection of manuscripts by editors of nursing journals was that the manuscript was poorly written. A poorly written manuscript continued to be the highest-ranked reason for rejection reported in McConnell's (2000) survey of English-language journals published outside the United States. It appears that nurse authors must work on their writing skills, because a poorly written manuscript was, again, the most common reason for rejection of manuscripts (35.8%), according to a survey of 63 nursing journal editors published in the January–February 2010 issue of *Nurse Educator* (Northam et al., 2010).

Other reasons reported by Northam et al. (2010) were that the topic was not relevant to the focus of the journal (32.8%), or the manuscript had methodology problems (16.4%). Additionally, seven editors indicated that manuscripts were "too short and superficial."

If an article is rejected outright, the reasons for the rejection will be indicated. Rejection of an article does not necessarily mean that it is not a good article (Oermann & Hays, 2016). There is a lot of competition for the limited space in the nursing and allied health journals. Editors do not want to discourage authors. In fact, the editor of the journal who rejects a manuscript may make suggestions for submission to another journal.

Preparing Research Reports for Funding Agencies

Research projects cost money, and researchers frequently seek funding sources. Many organizations provide funds for nursing research. Some public organizations that might be approached for support are the National Institute of Nursing Research, National Institute of Mental Health, Veterans Health Administration, and the U.S. Public Health Service.

Although public sources have provided most of the funding for nursing research, nurses are increasingly seeking funds from private foundations. Some of these private foundations are AARP, Robert Wood Johnson, John Hartford, Kellogg, Alcoa, and Lilly. Voluntary health organizations such as the American Cancer Society and the American Heart Association have supported nursing research. Businesses and corporations such as Apple was formerly called Apple Computer, this name was changed 10 years ago. . . Now it is formally "Apple, Inc." and Del Monte Foods have provided funds for nurse researchers. Charitable organizations, including churches and sororities, as well as individual philanthropists, may be approached for funding. Intramural funding is available in many universities and healthcare agencies. Finally, various groups within the nursing profession, such as Sigma Theta Tau International Honor Society of Nursing (STTI) and the American Nurses Foundation (ANF), make funds available for research. According to the ANF website, this organization has provided over $3 million dollars to more than 1000 nurse researchers since 1955.

If funding is received for a study, the researcher is nearly always expected to provide a final report at the completion of the project. This report may be a brief summary or a lengthy report.

Preparing Theses and Dissertations

Theses and dissertations are an important means of communication for research studies conducted to fulfill educational requirements. Because these documents serve a dual purpose of communicating research findings and providing educators with evidence of the students' ability to perform scholarly work, theses and dissertations are usually lengthy documents that may contain 100 pages or more, divided into several chapters. Dissertations contain more in-depth investigations than theses and provide new knowledge for the profession. Theses are concerned usually with testing existing theory, whereas dissertations focus on refining existing theories or generating new theories.

Utilization of Nursing Research Findings

Recall the first goal for conducting nursing research was to promote an evidence-based nursing practice. It is no longer acceptable for nurses to base their actions on tradition or authority in this day of evidence-based practice. Nurses should be able to justify the decisions they make and the care they give. For nursing research to be useful to the profession, study findings must be implemented in nursing practice. The utilization of research findings in nursing practice means going beyond the somewhat artificial research setting to the real world of nursing. Despite efforts to promote an evidence-based practice, there are still gaps between nursing research and nursing practice (Chau, Lopez, & Thompson, 2008; Kajermo et al., 2008; Yava et al., 2009).

Additional Barriers to Nursing Research Utilization

Barriers to the utilization of research evidence have been mentioned elsewhere in this book; however, a focus on the dissemination of the research findings is relevant to the topic in this chapter. For example, researchers have reported that the dissemination of research findings has been inadequate and the findings of research studies are often not translated into practice.

Inadequate Dissemination of Research Findings

Inadequate dissemination of nursing research findings involves two areas. First, most nursing research studies are rarely published or presented at research meetings or workshops. Second, published or presented studies are often not written or orally presented at a level at which the practicing nurse can understand the findings.

Many references in the literature attest to the unhappiness with the dissemination of nursing research findings among practicing nurses (Hutchinson & Johnston, 2004; Kajermo et al., 1998; Retsas, 2000). Swedish nurses in the 1998 study by Kajermo et al. ranked the lack of availability of research findings as the greatest barrier to the use of these findings. Fifty-one percent of Australian nurses in Hutchinson and Johnston's (2004) study reported that research reports were not readily available.

Practicing nurses have complained about their inability to understand articles in the research journals. The language is technical, and the articles are often lengthy. Research reports are frequently written for researchers rather than clinicians. To help reduce this barrier, Yoder et al. (2014) have suggested that doctorally prepared nurses should develop and teach nurses in the practice setting how to read research literature and understand statistical findings.

In Funk et al.'s (1991b) seminal study, respondents suggested that research should be reported in journals that are read most frequently by clinicians and these reports should be more readable and contain clinical implications. Nurse researchers tend to present their research findings in very formal research meetings and in research publications. Researchers in academic settings are sometimes rewarded (e.g., promotions, salary raises, tenure) more for publications in prestigious research journals than for publications in practice journals.

Nurses need to make an effort to publish in the popular clinical journals. This remark does not mean that nurse researchers should not publish in scholarly journals, but that they have an obligation also to disseminate the findings in a manner understandable to the nurse in practice; this usually means publishing findings in practice journals. Nurses need to make an effort to publish in the popular clinical journals.

Betz, Smith, Melnyk, and Olbrysh (2015) have suggested that researchers should consider the dissemination of evidence through digitalization media, such as podcasts, videocasts, webinars, and social media. We define a podcast as either digital audio or video, intended by its creator to be downloaded to a personal electronic device. Podcasts are often part of a series, either related parts or with a larger theme. A podcast is defined as a "digital audio or video file or recording, usually part of a themed series, that can be downloaded from a website to a media player or computer" (*Online Etymology Dictionary* [n.d.]). An advantage of using this media is the ability to download information into smart devices, giving easy access to information. Although Betz et al. (2015) believe that the use of digitalization may help to enhance the translation of research findings into practice, future research is needed to determine the feasibility and effectiveness of this type of dissemination of research.

FINDINGS ARE NOT READY FOR USE IN PRACTICE In an editorial in *Nursing Research*, Downs (1981) asserted, "Research is not something that can be brewed over night and ingested the next morning" (p. 322). She warned against the "premature consumption" of research findings. She stated that this practice might be "hazardous to someone's health" (p. 322).

Blegen (2005), in an editorial in *Nursing Research*, asserted that no research exists on which to develop protocols for many nursing practice problems. She further asserted that some nursing practice problems have a few studies on the topic, but some of these studies contain serious threats to validity, which makes use of their findings questionable. Duffy (2004), in contrast, contended that since the mid-1980s, qualified nurse researchers have completed, presented, and published many studies. She asserted that an available knowledge base is waiting to be used in the development of evidence-based practice.

No study findings should be implemented if the study has not been replicated in several clinical settings, with similar results being found. Norwood (2010) has emphasized the need for replication of nursing studies to ensure that the findings are powerful; Norwood has contended that a strong evidence-based practice usually requires replication studies. Replication of nursing studies ensures findings are powerful and strengthens evidence-based practice.

Bridging the Gap between Research and Practice

In the past few years, the nursing literature has shifted some of the emphasis from research utilization (RU) to evidence-based practice (EBP). Although these terms sometimes are used interchangeably, distinctions can be made between these two concepts (Yoder et al., 2014).

Burns and Grove (2009) have described RU as "the process of synthesizing, disseminating, and using research-generated knowledge to make an impact on or a change in the existing practices in society" (p. 720). EBP is viewed as broader in scope than RU. Burns and Grove asserted that EBP is the "conscientious integration of best research evidence with clinical expertise and patient values and needs in the delivery of quality, cost-effective health care" (p. 699). Thus, EBP encompasses evidence that is based not only on scientific findings, but also expert clinical opinions, and patient and family preferences.

Many nursing research utilization projects have been described in the literature, beginning in the 1970s. Two widely known projects that have fostered research utilization are the Western Council on Higher Education for Nursing (WCHEN) Regional Program for Nursing Research Development project conducted in the early 1970s and the Conduct and Utilization of Research in Nursing (CURN) project conducted later that same decade. Both projects received funding from the Division of Nursing of the Western Interstate Commission for Higher Education.

WCHEN PROJECT In the research utilization aspect of the WCHEN project, nurses from various settings attended 3-day workshops in which they were taught how to use the change process to bring about research utilization. The nurses came in pairs from the same geographic location but worked in different settings. For example, a school nurse and a community health nurse who came from a rural community developed a plan together to provide nursing interventions for elementary school students who had high rates of absenteeism (Elliott, 1977). Although the WCHEN project was considered successful, one major problem encountered was the lack of reliable nursing studies that were appropriate for implementation in nursing practice.

CURN PROJECT The most well-known nursing research utilization project is the CURN project, a 5-year project sponsored by the Michigan Nurses Association. The two major goals of this project were to stimulate the conduct of research in clinical settings and to increase the use of research findings in the daily practice of nurses. As a result of this project, nursing innovations (protocols) were developed for nine practice problems. The titles of the nine published volumes are:

- *Mutual Goal Setting in Patient Care*
- *Closed Urinary Drainage Systems*
- *Distress Reduction through Sensory Preparation*
- *Pain*
- *Intravenous Cannula Change*
- *Preventing Decubitus Ulcers*
- *Preoperative Sensory Preparation to Promote Recovery*
- *Reducing Diarrhea in Tube-Fed Patients*
- *Structured Preoperative Teaching*

ROGERS'S INNOVATION-DIFFUSION MODEL   Rogers's (1995) innovation-diffusion model contains five stages: knowledge, persuasion, decision, implementation, and confirmation.

In the knowledge stage, the nurse becomes aware of a research-based nursing intervention. This knowledge can be obtained through such sources as conferences, journal articles, and from talks with colleagues. In the persuasion stage, the nurse forms a positive or negative attitude toward the intervention. This attitude can be based on the intervention's advantage, compatibility, complexity, trialability, and observability. After an attitude is formed, the decision stage is reached. In this stage, the nurse decides whether or not to adopt the new intervention. The decision should be based on the research evidence that has been gathered. The implementation phase is reached when the nurse actually puts into practice the intervention or uses the knowledge indirectly, such as by discussing the findings with colleagues or citing the findings at a conference or in one of his or her own publications. An intervention may be introduced exactly as it was described in research studies, or there might be some adaptation for the particular healthcare setting where the intervention is being introduced.

Finally, in the confirmation stage, the intervention is evaluated for its effectiveness. The decision is then made whether or not to continue using the intervention. Validation concerns the overall examination of the strengths and weaknesses of a study. The nurse consumer must question every step of the research process that was carried out. A traditional research critique is done. If a biased sample was used, or operational definitions were not provided, or invalid statistical procedures were used, the findings would be questionable for application in practice. If the study design and procedures were determined to be valid, nurse consumers should also search for findings and conclusions that might be valid in their clinical settings.

If the nurse determines that the study is valid, then a comparative evaluation should be done. What variables would affect the decision to change practice based on research findings? Would it be possible to implement the findings in the nurse's practice? The nurse would want to know how similar the research setting was to her or his own setting and how similar the study sample was to patients/clients with whom the nurse works. Finally, in doing a comparative evaluation, the nurse must determine the feasibility of implementing the findings based on the constraints of the particular practice setting. Are there any legal or ethical risks to the involved clients, nurses, or institution? Are the resources (time, money, equipment) available?

Once the nurse has examined the feasibility, the decision about application is made. The nurse may decide against application or make a cognitive or direct application of the findings. Cognitive application means the nurse is not yet ready to apply the findings in practice but will use the information to enhance her or his knowledge base and may consider moving to a direct application in the future. Direct application of research findings means the nurse chooses to test out the findings in practice.

The Stetler Model of Research Utilization and the Iowa Model for Evidence-Based Practice to Promote Quality of Care, described in another chapter of this book, are two conventional process-driven models that have been used to implement evidence-based research findings in clinical settings. Only after all of the steps described above are completed is the evidence-based project ready for implementation. Of course, evaluation of the project must follow.

Many research utilization studies and projects have been discussed in recent literature. One project is presented below.

Research Utilization Study

The Iowa Model of Evidence-Based Practice to Promote Quality Care was used in a collaborative project of a clinical nurse specialist (CNS), health science librarian, and a nurse (Krom, Batten, & Bautista, 2010). Their aim was to heighten staff nurses' awareness of the evidence-based practice (EBP) process. They developed an EBP educational program for staff nurses. The CNS was considered an expert advisor for knowledge transformation because of clinical expertise, advanced educational preparation, and exposure to graduate-level research. The librarian was deemed capable of meeting the nurses' information needs. A staff nurse was considered the appropriate person to ask clinical questions and to find and critique relevant literature. The collaborators concluded that the project had increased staff nurse exposure to, and knowledge of, EBP principles and techniques.

Summary

A research report is a written or spoken communication of the findings of a study. The report should be presented in the order of the research process. Research reports may be presented as oral presentations, poster presentations, journal articles, written reports for funding agencies, and in theses and dissertations.

Research conferences are sponsored by many nursing organizations. Participants are contacted through a call for abstracts, which is a request for summaries of research studies that researchers wish to present.

An oral presentation of a research report at a conference is referred to as a *paper presentation*. The researcher may also present research results in the form of a poster.

Research is generally published in journal articles. Refereed journals use subject experts to review manuscripts. Nonrefereed journals use editorial staff members or consultants to review manuscripts. Impact factor is a journal rating based on the number of article citations from that journal in a given year compared to the actual number of articles published in that journal in the past, usually a 2-year period.

During the peer review process, professional colleagues who have content and methodological expertise in the study area review the manuscript. Journals frequently use a blind review process in which no authors' names are included on the manuscripts. In an open review, reviewers sign their names to their reviews.

Before submitting an article, a letter of inquiry, called a query letter, should be sent to determine the editor's interest in reviewing a certain manuscript. Unlike a query letter, a manuscript must never be sent to more than one journal at a time.

About 2 months before an article is published, the author will receive the galleys. Galley proofs contain the article as it will appear in typeset form.

If funding is received for a study, the researcher is usually expected to provide a final report at the completion of the project. This report may be either a brief summary or a lengthy report.

Theses and dissertations are a means of communicating results of research studies that are conducted in conjunction with educational requirements. These documents are generally quite long and divided into several chapters.

Common barriers to the utilization of evidence-based nursing research findings that relate to the dissemination and the implementation of findings are an inadequate means of disseminating nursing research findings and study findings that are not ready for use in nursing practice.

Two widely known nursing research utilization projects are the Western Council on Higher Education for Nursing (WCHEN) Regional Program for Nursing Research Development project conducted in the early 1970s and the Conduct and Utilization of Research in Nursing (CURN) project conducted in the late 1970s. Three models that have been very influential in the utilization of research findings in nursing are Rogers's innovation-diffusion model, Stetler's model for research utilization, and the Iowa model for evidence-based practice.

Self-Test

Select the letter before the *best* answer.
1. What communication medium is most likely to reach the largest percentage of nurses?
   A. dissertation
   B. journal article
   C. conference oral presentation
   D. poster
2. The communication medium for research findings that is probably most appropriate for a beginning researcher is:
   A. a journal article.
   B. an oral presentation at a conference.
   C. a research paper.
   D. a poster presentation.
3. Which statement concerning journal articles is true?
   A. Revisions generally are not needed in manuscripts that are submitted to journals.
   B. It is a good idea to send a query letter before submitting the manuscript.
   C. There is a general agreement among nursing journals about research article formats.
   D. Journals do not accept manuscripts from beginning researchers.
4. Support for nursing research has been furnished primarily by:
   A. public sources.
   B. private foundations.
   C. businesses.
   D. individual philanthropists.
5. Which statement is true?
   A. Most nurses have adequate knowledge of nursing research findings.
   B. Many nursing research findings are never published.
   C. Inadequate research skills of nurses is the most cited reason for lack of utilization of research findings.
   D. Most nursing research findings are ready for use in practice.
6. In the implementation stage of the Rogers's Innovation-Diffusion Model, the nurse:
   A. becomes aware of a research-based nursing intervention.
   B. uses, discusses, or cites the intervention.
   C. develops a positive or negative attitude about the intervention.
   D. evaluates the effectiveness of the intervention.

See answers to Self-Test in the Answer Section at the back of the book.

References

Bellack, J. P. (2010). Get ready, get set, write. *Nursing Education, 49,* 63–64. doi:10.3928/01484384-20100119-01

Betz, C. L., Smith, K. N., Melnyk, B. M., & Olbrysh, R. T. (2015). Disseminating evidence through publications, presentations, health policy briefs, and the media. In B. Melnyk & Finout-Overhold, E. (Eds.), *Evidence-Based practice in nursing & health care* (3rd ed., pp. 391–431). Philadelphia: Wolters Kluwer | Lippincott Williams & Wilkins.

Blegen, M. A. (2005). Research thrust changing? At risk [Editorial]. *Nursing Research, 54,* 1. http://journals.lww.com/nursingresearchonline/Citation/2005/01000/Research_Thrust_Changing__At_Risk.1.aspx

Burns, N., & Grove, S. K. (2009). *The practice of nursing research: Appraisal, synthesis, and generation of evidence* (6th ed.). St. Louis, MO: Saunders Elsevier.

Brandon, D., & McGrath, J. M. (2014). Provision of and response to manuscript reviews. *Advances in Neonatal Care, 14*(3), 137–138. doi:10.1097/ANC.0000000000000097

Chase, J. A., & Conn, V. S. (2013). Meta-analysis of fitness outcomes from motivational physical activity interventions. *Nursing Research, 62*(5), 294–304. doi:10.1097/NNR.0b013e3182a0395c

Chau, J. P., Lopez, V., & Thompson, D. R. (2008). A survey of Hong Kong nurses' perceptions of barriers to and facilitators of research utilization. *Research in Nursing & Health, 31,* 640–649. doi:10.1002/nur.20289

Davis, M., Davis, K. J., & Dunagan, M. (2012). *Scientific papers and presentations.* London: Academic Press.

Downs, F. (1981). Soap [Editorial]. *Nursing Research, 30,* 322. http://journals.lww.com/nursingresearchonline/pages/default.aspx

Duffy, M. E. (2004). Resources for building a research utilization program. *Clinical Nurse Specialist, 18,* 279–281. http://journals.lww.com/cns-journal/pages/default.aspx

Durkin, G. (2011). Promoting professional development through poster presentations. *Nurses in Staff Development, 27*(3), E1-3. doi:10.1097/NND.0b013e318217b437 [doi]

Ecoff, L., & Stichler, J. F. (2015). Disseminating project outcomes in a scholarly poster. *HERD, 8*(4), 131–138. doi:10.1177/1937586715583463 [doi]

Elliott, J. E. (1977). Research programs and projects of WCHEN. *Nursing Research, 26,* 277–280. http://journals.lww.com/nursingresearchonline/pages/default.aspx

Freda, M. C., & Kearney, M. (2005). An international survey of nurse editors' roles and practices. *Nursing Scholarship, 37,* 87–94. doi:10.1111/j.1547-5069.2005.00006.x

Funk, S. G., Champagne, M. T., Wiese, R. A., & Tornquist, E. M. (1991b). Barriers to using research findings in practice: The clinician's perspective. *Applied Nursing Research, 4,* 90–95. http://www.appliednursingresearch.org/

Hand, H. (2010). Reflections on preparing a poster for an RCN conference. *Nurse Researcher, 17,* 52–59. http://dx.doi.org/10.7748/nr2010.01.17.2.52.c7462

Heart & Lung's 2014 reviewer list. (2015, March-April). *Heart and Lung, 44*(2), 179–181. http://www.heartandlung.org/

Hutchinson, A. M., & Johnston, L. (2004). Bridging the divide: A survey of nurses' opinions regarding barriers to, and facilitators of, research utilization in the practice setting. *Clinical Nursing, 13,* 304–315. doi:10.1046/j.1365-2702.2003.00865.x

Kajermo, K. N., Nordström, G., Krusebrant, Å., & Björvell, H. (1998). Barriers to and facilitators of research utilization as perceived by a group of registered nurses in Sweden. *Advanced Nursing, 27,* 798–807. doi:10.1046/j.1365-2648.1998.00614.x

Kajermo, K. N., Undén, J., Gardulf, A., Eriksson, L. E., Orton, M.-L., Arnetz, B. B., & Nordström, G. H. (2008). Predictors of nurses' perceptions of barriers to research utilization. *Nursing Management, 16,* 305–314. doi:10.1111/j.1365-2834.2007.00770x

Kearney, M. H. (2015). Distinguishing impact from productivity. *Research in Nursing & Health, 38*(6), 417–419. doi: 10.1002/nur.21698

Kotz, D., Cals, J. W., Tugwell, P., & Knottnerus, J. A. (2013). Introducing a new series on effective writing and publishing of scientific papers. *Clinical Epidemiology, 66*(4), 359–360. doi: 10.1016/j.jclinepi.2013.01.001

Krom, Z. R., Batten, J., & Bautista, C. (2010). A unique collaborative nursing evidence-based practice initiative using the Iowa model. *Clinical Nurse Specialist, 24,* 54–59. doi:10.1097/NUR.0b013e3181cf5537

Leng, S. (2012). Style: What it is and why it matters. In G. M. Hall (Ed.), *How to write a paper* (pp. 133–140). John Wiley & Sons. doi:10.1002/9781118488713.ch19

McConnell, E. A. (1995). Journal and publishing characteristics for 42 nursing publications out side the United States. *Image: Journal of Nursing Scholarship, 27,* 225–229. doi:10.1111/j.1547-5069.1995.tb00863.x

McConnell, E. A. (2000). Nursing publications outside the United States. *Nursing Scholarship, 32,* 87–92. doi:10.1111/j.1547-5069.2000.00087.x

Moos, D. (2010). Writing for publication: An interview with the editors. *Perianesthesia Nursing, 25,* 46–49. doi:10.1016/j.jopan.2009.11.004

Northam, S., Yarbrough, S., Haas, B., & Duke, G. (2010). Journal editor survey information to help authors publish. *Nurse Educator, 35,* 29–36. doi:10.1097/NNE.0b013e3181c42149

Norwood, S. L. (2010). *Research essentials: Foundations for evidence based practice.* Upper Saddle River, NJ: Pearson.

Oermann, M. H., & Hays, J. C. (2016). *Writing for publication in nursing.* Springer.

Oman, K. (2009). Peer review: The art of supporting colleagues and advancing our profession. [Editorial]. *Emergency Nursing, 35,* 278. doi:10.1016/j.jen.2009.05.011 Online Etymology Dictionary. (n.d.). Podcast. http://dictionary.reference.com/browse/podcast

Retsas, A. (2000). Barriers to using research evidence in nursing practice. *Advanced Nursing, 31,* 599–606. doi:10.1046/j.1365-2648.2000.01315.x

Rogers, E. M. (1995). *Diffusion of innovations* (4th ed.). New York: Free Press.

Swanson, E. A., McCloskey, J. C., & Bodensteiner, A. (1991). Publishing opportunities for nurses: A comparison of 92 U.S. journals. *Image: Journal of Nursing Scholarship, 23,* 33–38. doi:10.1111/j.1547-5069.1991.tb00632.x

Tanner, C. A., & Bellack, J. P. (2009). The new wave of nursing education scholarship [Editorial]. *Nursing Education, 48,* 3–4. doi:10.3928/01484834-20090101-04

Yava, A., Tosun, N., Çiçek, H., Yavan, T., Terakye, G., & Hatipoglu, S. (2009). Nurses' perceptions of the barriers to and the facilitators of research utilization in Turkey. *Applied Nursing Research, 22,* 166–175. doi:10.1016/j.apnr.2007.11.003

Yoder, L. H., Kirkley, D., McFall, D. C., Kirksey, K. M., StalBaum, A. L., & Sellers, D. (2014). CE: Original research: Staff nurses' use of research to facilitate evidence-based practice. *American Journal of Nursing, 114*(9), 26–37. doi:10.1097/01.NAJ.0000453753.00894.29

Yoder-Wise, P. S. (2009). Manuscript resubmissions: The dialog of changes [Editorial]. *Continuing Education in Nursing, 40,* 99–100. doi:10.3928/00220124-20090301-07

Chapter 19
Nursing Research and Healthcare Economics

Rose Nieswiadomy, PhD, RN; Michael L. Nieswiadomy, PhD;
and Charles McConnel, PhD

 Objectives

On completion of this chapter, you will be prepared to:

1. Explain economic terms that have an impact on nursing.
2. Determine the cost-effectiveness of nursing care based on the results of selected nursing research studies.
3. Summarize the impact of governmental agencies and related organizations on nurses and the cost of healthcare.

Nursing is a very admired profession. Since 1999, nurses have been included in the Gallup Poll that measures the general public's trust of various professionals in the United States. Nurses have been chosen as the most trusted professionals every year, except for 2001, when firefighters were selected. The most recent (December 19, 2016) poll again rated nurses far above all other professions in honesty and ethics.

As nurses, we have an obligation to live up to the trust that has been placed in us. We must continually demonstrate our knowledge and abilities in the healthcare arena. As members of the largest group of healthcare professionals, we should have a great deal of influence on healthcare. However, because it is difficult to measure the value of all that nurses contribute to the business of patient care, we need to understand some basic concepts about economics as they pertain to the nursing and healthcare profession.

With prospective payment systems determining the amount of reimbursements that hospitals receive, nursing care services are being closely examined. It is not difficult to determine that hospitals could cut costs by curtailing nursing services, but they will be reluctant to do so if nursing care can be demonstrated to be cost-effective or cost saving.

Before proceeding with a discussion of how nursing contributes to the provision of services (care), it is necessary to point out that the economist's explanations rely on models that are composed of theoretical parts that only represent a characterization of a complex real world. For instance, the theoretical term *demand* does not mean forceful insistence but the set of preferences or desire of a buyer of a good, service, or factor of production. The reader is called upon to use economic models and terminology as a way to organize the discussion, hopefully toward understanding real-world relationships and events.

Healthcare Economics and Nursing

Nurses are an economic factor, along with physicians and other staff, in the production of healthcare services. Nurses must become more aware of healthcare economics as the healthcare industry becomes increasingly cost conscious. In order for nurses to demonstrate their value in providing healthcare services (what we call *production*), they must attempt to quantify their productive value in pecuniary terms. **Pecuniary terms** means a monetary value must be placed on care. Of course, only a portion of the services that professional nurses provide can be quantified in pecuniary terms (Dall, Chen, Seifert, Maddox, & Hogan, 2009). To begin this valuation process we estimate the monetary value of nursing care services. This section provides some of the insight needed to understand healthcare economics as it relates to nurses.

Understanding Market Forces Affecting Nurses

In order to understand economic issues affecting nursing, we must first understand the market forces that affect nurses. As in any market, two primary forces affect the number of nurses hired and the wage rate paid: the demand for and supply of nursing skills.

Let's start the discussion of the demand for nurses by first examining a medical service provider's (we will call this entity a *firm*) demand for labor. A firm (for example a hospital, urgent care facility, or clinic) produces a good or service (e.g., treating patients), with what economists model as a **production function**, indicating the output (e.g., a patient recovers from surgery) that can be produced with a given set of inputs (e.g., physician, nursing and physical therapist care). In economic terms, because the demand for labor is *derived* from the demand for the product (or service) that the firm produces and sells, we say that firms have a **derived demand** for labor. For example, a hospital hires nurses because its customers (i.e., patients) want to purchase medical care. Since 81% of hospitals are not-for-profit hospitals (American Hospital Association, 2015) it is important to note that many hospitals only need revenues to sufficiently cover costs. A smaller percentage of hospitals attempt to maximize profits. But even not-for-profit hospitals, because they must live within their budgets, must make decisions that are similar to the ones made by for-profit hospitals.

To determine the optimal number of nurses to hire, the hospital determines the *profit maximizing* number of staff to hire by comparing the marginal expense with the marginal benefit. The **marginal expense (cost)** of a worker is the additional cost of hiring one more worker. Usually, the marginal expense of hiring an additional worker is the market-determined wage rate [e.g., $34.14 was the mean hourly wage for a RN in the U.S. in 2015 (U.S. Bureau of Labor Statistics, 2016)]. An exception can occur when a large buyer of an input, such as the only hospital in town, sets the wage for nurses; this is called a **monopsony**. Generally, this wage will be lower and fewer nurses will be hired than in a competitive market. The **marginal benefit** of a worker is the product of two components: (a) the **marginal product** of labor—the additional output produced by an additional worker, and (b) the **marginal revenue**—the additional revenue generated by selling an additional unit of output. This concept addresses how much additional work will be accomplished by an additional worker, and how much revenue can be gained through that worker's efforts.

The law of **diminishing marginal returns** says that as more of a variable input (like labor) is hired (given that the amount of capital is fixed), the marginal product (or output) of a worker declines. Primarily due to this diminishing marginal product, the demand for labor curve is downward sloping. Once the hospital has determined the marginal benefit, it must compare this to the marginal expense of hiring another nurse. The hospital should hire additional nurses as long as the marginal benefit is greater than the wage rate (i.e., the marginal expense). The optimal number of nurses to hire is reached when the marginal benefit of the last nurse hired equals the marginal expense. The hospital must also decide how much of other inputs (e.g., computers, CT scanners) to use. The process to determine the optimal combination of all inputs is somewhat complex and is in the domain of financial managers and accountants. Essentially, the marginal benefits must be compared to the marginal expenses for each input and ideally these ratios should be equal to one another. This is referred to as making sure that each input gives the firm the same "bang for the buck."

Determining the Value of Nursing

A hospital (or other medical facility) has many similarities, along with some significant differences, with other kinds of businesses. A hospital provides healthcare services and has a derived demand for many inputs such as doctors, nurses, equipment, and office staff. In this way, a hospital is similar to many companies. However, a hospital administrator's task is very complex because it is much more difficult to measure the output of a hospital. Consequently, it is very difficult to measure the value (i.e., the marginal benefit) of a nurse. For example, it is easy for a paper mill to see how many feet of paper have been produced. But it is much more difficult to measure the output of a nurse's job because the output is ultimately measured in terms of the patient's health, something inherently difficult to measure. Herein lies the crux of the problem for the nursing profession: How do nurses demonstrate the value of their services? Although nurses pride themselves on being compassionate caregivers, in terms of economics, they are an input jointly used (with other staff and equipment) in providing healthcare, and we recognize that the demand for their productive services is *derived*. Nurses must be able to demonstrate the value of services for which they are paid or risk losing hospital nursing positions.

Part of the problem with determining the value of nursing care is that hospitals traditionally have not billed separately for nursing services. The cost of nursing services are generally undifferentiated and bundled within a total hospital bill. Recently, healthcare economists and nursing experts have begun to grapple with the issue of "costing out" nursing care.

In the current system, hospitals can make more profit in the short run if they increase the workload of nurses. However, this strategy is likely to lead to long-term losses if the quality of care is significantly reduced. The hospitals will lose future customers as their reputations are tarnished. Even worse, hospitals may expose themselves to legal liabilities for harm caused to their patients. Thus, hospitals need to carefully examine the value of nursing care in balance with other inputs. Nurses need to play a pivotal role in this valuation process.

The Dall Study

The Dall et al. (2009) study provides an excellent example of how to quantify the economic value (i.e., cost savings) of professional nursing. This study provides many interesting ideas for developing a cost-effectiveness study for nursing. The researchers examined the relationship between registered nurse staffing levels and nursing-sensitive patient outcomes (NSOs) in acute care hospitals. They synthesized findings from the literature and from hospital discharge data. These researchers examined patient risk for urinary tract infections, hospital-acquired pneumonia, pressure ulcer, upper gastrointestinal bleeding, sepsis, shock/cardiac failure, pulmonary failure, central nervous system complications, deep vein thrombosis, postoperative infection, adverse drug events, and patient falls. They also looked at in-hospital mortality (failure to rescue).

Estimates of the total societal costs were made by adding together values from three categories of economic costs associated with NSOs: (a) medical costs, (b) patient's lost income due to increased length of stay, and (c) family lost income due to mortality of a member.

For the first category, medical costs, they assumed each inpatient day that is avoided generates cost savings of approximately $1,522 per patient day (the 2005 national average cost per inpatient day in community hospitals). This is a real savings to a hospital, especially as the federal government and private insurers increasingly refuse to pay for nosocomial complications (complications arising in a hospital).

For the second cost category, they assumed each additional day of stay causes a person to lose income. The researchers used U.S. Bureau of Labor Statistics data on average earnings and labor force participation rates by age and gender to estimate the lost productive value to society of patients being delayed in returning to the workforce. A speedier return to the workforce results in a cost saving to the patient.

For the third cost category, they assumed families of the deceased lose the lifetime stream of the deceased's income. They used standard economic assumptions on the growth in a worker's earnings and discounted these earnings to present value (the value in today's dollars of future losses). They multiplied the reduction in the probability of death (due to an increase in nurse staffing levels) times the lifetime earnings to obtain the expected cost savings.

The second and third cost categories are costs to the patient (and thus to society), but not necessarily to the hospital. However, as mentioned above, hospitals may bear the liability in lawsuits. Thus, hospitals need to be keenly aware of these costs.

The Dall et al. (2009) study results indicated that as nursing staffing levels increase, patient risk of nosocomial complications and hospital length of stay decrease. After combining the three cost saving categories, they estimated that adding 133,000 full-time equivalent (FTE) RNs to the acute care hospital workforce in the United States would save 5900 lives per year. When medical savings and increased productivity were considered, the economic value to society of each additional RN was $57,700. They noted that this is only a partial estimate of the value of an additional nurse. Furthermore, their estimates consider only the marginal value. Because of diminishing marginal returns, the average value of a nurse is higher than the marginal value. Thus, the average value of a nurse is higher than $57,700.

Nursing Research Cost-Effectiveness Studies

Only a few studies can be found in the literature that demonstrate the cost-effectiveness of nursing care or the substitutability of specialized nursing services for other professional services. The results of some of these studies are presented here in chronological order. The areas studied include: home care of early birth-weight infants, a nurse-practitioner-managed healthcare unit in a factory, home nursing visits of newborns, a nurse case management program for patients experiencing syncope, an admission nurse program, a perinatal program, a collaborative nurse practitioner (NP) care management model on pharmaceutical usage, with a focus on antibiotics, nurse-led education for management of chronic heart failure, nursing intervention for elderly self-medication, shifting care from doctors to nurses, and infection rates for different dressing types for tunneled central venous catheters and the cost of infections for cancer patients in Canada, and several telephone nursing programs.

The study by Brooten et al. (1986) clearly demonstrates the cost-effectiveness of nursing care. This study examined early hospital discharge and home follow-up care of very-low-birth-weight infants. The researchers found that follow-up care by a nurse specialist was safe and cost-effective. This type of care potentially reduces hospital care costs, decreases iatrogenic (meaning caused by a healthcare professional) illnesses and hospital-acquired infections, and enhances parent-infant interactions.

Ferguson (1996) discussed the cost-effectiveness of a nurse practitioner–managed healthcare unit (HCU) that was implemented in a meat packing/rendering plant in the northern United States. During the first 5 years (1988–1992), a net savings of more than $1.3 million was realized in the cost of workers' compensation alone.

The cost-effectiveness of providing home nursing visits after newborn discharge was studied by Paul, Phillips, Widome, and Hollenbeak (2004). Nurse visits to newborns were made 1 to 2 days after their hospital discharge to determine if these visits would reduce the incidence of rehospitalization for jaundice and dehydration. These visits were found to reduce rehospitalization within the first 10 days of life from 2.8% of 2641 newborns who were not seen by a nurse to only 0.6% of the 326 infants who received a home visit by a nurse. The home visits were significantly less costly than visits to the emergency department.

Bourdeaux et al. (2005) studied the use of a nurse case management program with patients experiencing syncope. The program was implemented at a large urban teaching hospital. The experimental (case management) group had 359 patients, and the control (no case management) group had 331 patients. Length of stay was reduced by 0.15 days over the 12 months of the case management program for diagnosis-related group (DRG) 141 (syncope and collapse with comorbidities). The decrease in direct cost was $376 per patient. Length of stay was decreased by 0.28 days for DRG 142 (syncope and collapse without comorbidities), with a cost savings of $292 per patient.

The staff of one Pennsylvania hospital created an admission nurse position (Hlipala, Meyer, Wallace, & Zaremba, 2005). This nurse initiates and completes the patient's health history and assessment and promotes consumer satisfaction. A time study revealed that 30 to 60 minutes less staff nurse time was needed for new admissions. The annual cost savings, based on the salary of staff nurses, was between $100,000 and $201,296. Also, $64,000 annually was saved in overtime pay. Overtime pay related to admissions was found to be 93% less than prior to implementation of the admission nurse's services.

Perinatal outcomes were evaluated based on a nurse-driven quality improvement program (Jallo, Bray, Padden, & Levin, 2009). Preterm birth, which is birth before 37 weeks' gestation, is an acute and complex problem. A nursing team, composed of a perinatal clinical nurse specialist and several experienced obstetrical nurses, joined a large managed care organization (MCO) to develop and implement a program, Partners in Pregnancy (PnP), for pregnant women enrolled in the MCO. Four quarters of data from the pre-PnP program were compared to four quarters of data after the program was implemented. Neonatal Intensive Care Unit (NICU) length of stay (LOS) and cost data were compared. The preprogram LOS was 13.8 days, whereas the postprogram LOS was 11.6 days. The NICU payment per admission was reduced from $14,482 to $11,310.

A study was conducted to evaluate the economic impact of a collaborative nurse practitioner (NP) care management model on pharmaceutical usage, with a focus on antibiotics (Chen, McNeese-Smith, Cowan, Upenieks, & Afifi, 2009). The researchers used pharmaceutical claims data of 1200 subjects who participated in the Multidisciplinary, Physician, and Nurse Practitioner Study from 2000 to 2004. The NP-led intervention group was associated with a significant reduction in overall drug cost, drug days, antibiotic cost, and antibiotic days per hospitalization episode. The researchers presented the advantages of "dedicating NPs in acute care settings to achieve quality care and contain inpatient drug costs" (p. 166).

Fergenbaum, Bermingham, Krahn, Alter, and Demers (2015) recently conducted an extensive literature review on the management of chronic heart failure and established that nurse-led education and home care compared to "usual care" was a cost-effective alternative. By establishing that nurse-related care is both "more effective and less costly" compared to usual care, they provide the strongest evidence of the cost-effectiveness findings.

In an analysis of a home-based nurse coordinated medication program, Marek et al. (2014) found that nursing intervention was cost-effective when applied to the self-management of medications by elderly subjects.

One of the most interesting and provocative studies regarding the nursing profession is a systematic review by the Cochrane Database scholars on the question if nurses can be substituted for doctors in primary care (Laurant et al., 2005). The analysts examined the potential of shifting care from physicians to nurses by screening 4253 articles of which 25 articles met the inclusion criteria. Though not explicitly a cost-effectiveness study, the analysts did conclude that in general there were "no appreciable differences . . . between doctors and nurses in health outcomes for patients, process of care, resource utilization or cost," excluding the professional costs, of course.

Keeler et al. (2015a) studied the effect of three different nursing care strategies (transparent dressing, no dressing, or a gauze dressing) for tunneled central venous catheter (CVC) exit sites on catheter-related bloodstream infections (CRBSI) in adult Canadian blood and marrow cell transplant recipients. A sample of 432 records at a single center found no significant differences in CRBSI, number of organisms, gram stain of organisms, or days until the onset of an infection among the three dressing groups. Since the gauze dressing was considerably more expensive (in terms of nursing labor costs and supplies) than both the transparent dressing and the no-dressing strategy, the latter two strategies were most economical.

In a related study (Keeler et al., 2015b), patients with a CRBSI were paired for comparison to patient records not indicating CRBSI in the following domains: length of stay, laboratory tests, diagnostic tests, medications used, consultations to a specialty physician, catheter replacement costs, and length of stay in the intensive care unit. Patients with CRBSI stayed on average an extra 19.37 days in the hospital. The total estimated burden of CRBSI in Canadian blood and marrow transplant patients for the 2013 fiscal year was $44,816 per incident. Thus, there is a strong economic reason to adhere to best possible infection control practices.

Telephonic Nursing Studies

Nursing researchers are always searching for new and innovative practices. One such cost reducing and quality enhancing strategy is telenursing (TN)—the use of telephone follow-up as a demand management strategy. A seminal study of the merits of telenursing was reported by Greenberg (2000), who presents a fairly comprehensive discussion of the many facets of telenursing interventions based on a survey of experience of a pediatric outpatient clinic. Her study took place in a pediatric outpatient clinic setting in the southwestern United States. Results of 90 calls (25% of the calls for one month) were examined. The dollar savings for one month were estimated to be $2,360. This figure was determined by subtracting the money ($2,216) spent on actual outcomes from the money ($4,576) that would have been spent based on outcomes without TN, a savings of over 50%.

More recently a number of sophisticated studies have examined areas of care as diverse as the follow-up telephone experience of patients discharged after undergoing orthopedic surgery (Clari et al., 2015), nurse-led telephone follow-up after treatment for breast cancer (Kimman et al., 2010), and a follow-up intervention aimed at improving outcomes following hospital care for myocardial infarction (Hanssen, Nordrhaug, Eide, & Hanestad, 2007). Favorable patient outcomes that could be tied directly to telenursing were found in each of these studies. Throughout this selection of literature, analysts report finding telenursing not only a quality-enhancing method of follow-up for care and reassurance, but highly complementary to a favorable outcome in other more direct forms of prior medical care delivered in hospitals and clinics. This is especially true of the randomized tele-trial following orthopedic surgery (Clari et al., 2015), in which regression analysis was employed to isolate differences between intervention and controls in favorable outcomes. Telenursing was found to significantly reduce post-discharge health problems and reduce the drain on the community's health resources. Baker et al. (2011) examined the impact of the Health Buddy program, which integrates a telehealth tool with care management for chronically ill Medicare beneficiaries. They compared the program's impact on spending for patients of two clinics in the U.S. northwest, one group which received the program, and a matched control group. They found significant savings for patients who used the Health Buddy telehealth program of approximately 7.7% to 13.3% ($312 to $542) per person per quarter.

Cryer et al. (2012) examined the Hospital at Home concept. As part of the post-hospital care team, nurses provide critical support both in-home and by telephone by "monitoring for clinical changes via daily telehealth encounters" (p. 1238). Overall, this program, of which telenursing was a major component, reduced the costs associated with similar inpatients by 19%. In this program, the "telehealth unit consists of a blood pressure monitor, stethoscope, oximeter, glucometer and video connection allowing communication for assessment and teaching" (p. 1238).

Need For More Research Studies on Nursing Care

Research is the means of demonstrating the value of nurses in the healthcare arena. Numerous sources call for more research on the economic value of nurses.

Peter Buerhaus, member of the editorial board of *Nursing Economic$*, interviewed influential nurse and nursing advocate John Welton, who researches the economic value of nursing. Welton stated, "We need to establish a price for nursing care and measure the clinical as well as economic contribution of nurses to patient care on an individual basis similar to physician care" (Buerhaus, 2010, p. 50). Welton says that we need to measure the marginal benefit of nursing care (Buerhaus, 2010).

Chen et al. (2009) have called for future research that validates specific roles and functions of advanced nurse practitioners (ANPs) in regard to specific quality outcomes and cost-effectiveness measures. Bednarski (2009) reported that the American Association of Nephrology Nurses supports an evidence-based approach for delineating the value of nursing; Bednarski wrote that it is critical to connect nursing care with the outcomes of this care. Rausch and Bjorklund (2010) have called for more research in the use of bachelor's-prepared psychiatric nurses in the role of psychiatric liaison nurse in medical patient-care settings. Other experts call for research on how nursing intensity, academic preparation, licensure, certification, and other variables affect care cost and quality.

Melynk (2014) argues that there is a need for evidence-based nursing research to be impactful. It is not enough for the research to be published and read; it must have a "so what" factor that convinces practitioners to implement it. For example, the Creating Opportunities for Parent Empowerment (COPE) was not widely implemented until the findings of a full-scale clinical trial with 260 premature infants and their parents that showed that the preemies of parents who received COPE were discharged by an average of 4 days sooner than preemies of the attention control parents. This earlier discharge rate created a cost saving of nearly $5,000 per COPE infant. Using COPE in NICUs for 500,000 preemies could save the U.S. healthcare system $2.5 billion annually.

Goetz, Janney, and Ramsey (2011) note that nurses will be called upon to be more proactive in delivering quality care at a lower cost. They describe a program at Northwest Memorial Hospital in Chicago, Illinois, where the nursing leadership team reduced costs by more than $10 million over 4 years while outperforming national benchmarks on nurse-sensitive quality indicators. Central-line associated blood stream infections were reduced 79%, hospital-acquired pressure ulcers were reduced 66%, and patient falls were reduced 23%. They used spreadsheets to track outcomes against goals, monitored variances regularly, and made adjustments accordingly.

For years, hospital readmission has been an expensive problem for the Medicare system. In a recent nursing perspective article, Brooks (2015) provides an insightful assessment of the problem, reviews Medicare's strategy of designing and implementing a system of incentives (or disincentives) to reduce readmissions, and focuses on the essential role of the professional nurse in making the strategy successful. Financial penalties are aimed at reducing readmission for the medical conditions most responsive to improved post hospital care, such as pneumonia and heart failure. The strategy is intended to promote superior home care, principally by well-trained nurses, the effect of which will reduce medical complications that otherwise lead to readmission. The first phase of the strategy is to target acute myocardial infarction, heart failure, and pneumonia; followed by chronic obstructive disease, elective hip and knee arthroplasty; and, by 2017, coronary artery bypass graft discharges. The three diagnostic conditions in the first phase alone are targeted to save $8 billion over the following decade. The value added by the nursing profession in its essential role in the success of the readmission reduction strategy is readily identified and acknowledged.

It is evident that more research is needed on the economic value of nursing. After reading this chapter on nursing research and healthcare economics, it is hoped that you will be more interested in the economic impact of nursing and be willing to participate in research to evaluate the economic importance of nursing in the healthcare arena.

Impacts of Governmental Agencies and Related Organizations

The U. S. healthcare system is a complex structure of various types of organizational forms and occupational descriptions. Providers are motivated by a variety of interests, with services and products being offered on the part of private for-profit firms; federal, state and municipal health agencies and organizations; along with non-profit providers and voluntary agencies. These agencies are all interwoven into arguably the largest, most expensive, and complex system in the world—not to mention the most extensively regulated and subsidized. Nurses must have a thorough understanding of the U.S. healthcare system as it affects both patients and nurses.

The federal government is by far the most important entity with the greatest economic and regulatory impact on the structure and functioning of the healthcare enterprise. The one governmental agency that has the largest dollar impact on healthcare is the Centers for Medicare & Medicaid Services (CMS). CMS controls both Medicare, the government system that pays for a large part of the care for the elderly, kidney dialysis for the victims of end-stage kidney disease and many of the disabled, and Medicaid, a federal/state program nearly as large as Medicare that pays for medical care for many poor and indigent patients and elderly poor requiring nursing home services. The U.S. Department of Health and Human Services controls the 27 National Institutes of Health that annually fund around $30 billion in biomedical research (of which $140.5 million funds the National Institute of Nursing Research), as well as the Agency for Healthcare Research and Quality, which funds health services research including patient-centered outcomes research (PCOR) and comparative effectiveness projects. Another important entity the public relies on for information and protection from catastrophic disease events (such as flu epidemics) is the National Center for Health Statistics that houses the Centers for Disease Control and Prevention (CDC) with its national corps of disease surveillance officers and biomedical research specialists.

Affordable Care Act

Clearly the most significant and controversial event impacting virtually every aspect of the U.S. healthcare system was the enactment in 2010 of the Patient Protection and Affordable Care Act (PPACA) and its implementation in 2014. The simplest interpretation of the act is that it is a nation-wide health insurance program formed and funded with the intention of providing health insurance coverage for nearly all U.S. citizens. Some of its more important features are the subsidization of insurance premiums for many low-income individuals and families, creation of well-regulated healthcare markets in which health insurance can be purchased, and the prohibition of denying health insurance to individuals having preexisting conditions.

Among the many effects of the PPACA that will indirectly impact nurses is an expected increase in employment possibilities. For instance, the U. S. Bureau of Labor Statistics (2016) estimates that the demand for nurses will increase 16% between 2014 and 2024; Frogner and Spetz (2013) estimate that fully one-third of that increase will be due to implementation of the PPACA. Few of these positions will be in the hospital sector (Spetz, 2014).

Another aspect of the act is the official insistence on the implementation of evidence-based practice (or medicine) (EBP or EBM) throughout the range of practices, from prevention, cure, care, and rehabilitation. In essence, EBP ensures that the most recent empirically based assessments of procedures are considered and the most current knowledge regarding the disease or injury process is incorporated into the treatment of the patient (Stevens, 2013; Johnson, 2013). Evidence-based practice as a concept was originally introduced as an initiative by the Institute of Medicine (IOM) (2001) in its effort to address the quality deficiency chasm. EBP is incorporated into the PPACA, with particular reference to prevention, mental health, and public health innovations.

Regulatory Agencies

One of the most important regulatory agencies of the federal government impacting the healthcare economy is the U.S. Food and Drug Administration (FDA). Some idea of the scope of public health concerns over which the FDA has at least a modicum of regulatory interest can best be appreciated by examining its tabs on the FDA's Home Page: food, drugs, medical devices, radiation-emitting products, vaccines, blood & biologics, animal & veterinary, cosmetics, and tobacco products. While the agency is often criticized by those it regulates and by consumers who disagree with its decisions, there is plenty of evidence that the agency is seriously underfunded (Strom, Kimmel, & Hennessy, 2012). Some financial help is provided by drug companies who want to expedite the process of approval of new drugs but there is criticism of this by consumer advocacy groups who see this as a conflict of interest.

Public Health

Finally, attention must be given to two premier governmental organizations that publicly provide healthcare: 1) the U.S. Department of Veterans Affairs and 2) the U.S. Public Health Service Commissioned Corps that provides rapid response to public health emergencies and advancement of public health practices and science. Another facet of this agency is what the service calls its best kept secret, the 6500 nurse officers that staff it. Of the assignments that these corps nurses might receive, the most interesting are the Indian Health Service (IHS), Federal Bureau of Prisons (BOP), Department of Homeland Security (DHS), Food and Drug Administration (FDA), National Institutes of Health (NIH), and Health Resources and Services Administration (HRSA) (U.S. Department of Health and Human Services, 2015).

Of the $2.9 trillion annual expenditure on healthcare in the United States, 43% of that total was the government's support (Hartman et al., 2015). Outside the government proper are a number independent organizations, most of which are nonprofit and represent the public's interest in improving the health of the population, as well as others representing specific interests of professional organizations or controlling the accreditation process. These organizations include professional societies such as the American Nurses Association, the American Medical Association, and the Institute of Medicine (renamed in 2016 the Health and Medicine Division (of the National Academies of Sciences, Engineering, and Medicine)) that provides findings from internal research projects focusing on the quality and safety of the nation's healthcare system.

The Joint Commission is another independent organization with which any nurse employed by a hospital will become familiar. The Joint Commission is an independent, not-for-profit organization that accredits and certifies more than 20,500 healthcare organizations. All hospital personnel must be alert to the demanding requirements related to patient safety that are ultimately enforced by the Joint Commission. For a brief look, see the Joint Commission's website.

Summary

Nursing care is a challenge to quantify. However, it is necessary that nurses demonstrate their contributions to healthcare in monetary terms.

This chapter defines some economic terms that nurses need to understand. Pecuniary terms indicates that monetary values must be determined. A production function indicates the output that can be produced with a given set of inputs. A derived demand means the demand for labor is derived from the demand for the product (or service) that a firm produces and sells. The marginal expense of a worker is the additional cost of hiring one more worker. The term monopsony is used to indicate a large buyer of an input, such as the only hospital in town, which is then able to set the wages for nurses. The marginal benefit of a worker has two components: (a) the marginal product of labor—the additional output produced by an additional worker, and (b) the marginal revenue—the additional revenue generated by selling an additional unit of output. The law of diminishing marginal returns means as more of a variable input (like labor) is hired, and the amount of capital and other inputs are fixed, the marginal product of a worker declines.

Seminal studies set the parameters of the debate over just how valuable nursing services are and what we can expect in future research. Findings from existing nursing research studies have demonstrated the cost-effectiveness of nursing care. Brooten et al.'s (1986) study on the cost-effectiveness of interventions for very-low-birth-weight infants is a classic study that has been cited over 220 times in the healthcare literature.

Many nursing and healthcare experts are calling for more research that will help determine the economic value of nursing care. Nonetheless, the working papers division of the National Bureau of Economic Research does not list even one study that reports on the economic aspects of nursing, yet lists a number of studies on physicians and nursing homes. The Brookings Institution does little better. A more robust effort on advocacy and promotion of economic research on nurses and nursing services is definitely needed.

The federal government along with state and local governments play a significant role in the U.S. healthcare system and support 43% of the $2.9 trillion in annual healthcare spending in the United States. Some of the significant agencies are the Centers for Medicare and Medicaid Services, the National Institutes of Health, the Agency for Healthcare Research and Quality, the Food and Drug Administration, and the National Center for Health Statistics (particularly the Centers for Disease Control and Prevention). The implementation of the Patient Protection and Affordable Care Act (PPACA) in 2014 will have a significant impact on the U.S. healthcare system through increased insurance coverage and emphasis on evidence-based medicine (EBM). Nurses in particular will be affected as it is expected to increase the demand for nurses by 16% between 2014 and 2024.

Self-Test

1. The Gallup Poll has revealed that:
   A. nursing is the most highly rated profession in the United States.
   B. nursing is the second most highly rated profession in the United States.
   C. the rating of the nursing profession has increased in recent years.
   D. the rating of the nursing profession has decreased slightly in recent years.

2. The demand for nursing is:
   A. a derived demand.
   B. impossible to determine.
   C. not affected by demographic forces.
   D. not affected by technological advances.
3. Published studies involving the cost-effectiveness of nursing care:
   A. are numerous in the literature.
   B. generally reveal that nursing care is cost-effective.
   C. have decreased in number in recent years.
   D. demonstrate mixed results on the cost-effectiveness of nursing care.

Indicate True or False for the following statements:

_____ 4. The economic value of nursing care is easier to determine than that of the services provided by many other professions.

_____ 5. Nurses do not need to be very interested in the monetary worth of the care they provide.

_____ 6. A profit-maximizing firm should hire additional workers as long as the marginal benefit of an additional worker is greater than the marginal expense of the additional worker.

_____ 7. One of the factors of nursing cost-effectiveness examined in the Dall et al. (2009) study was hospital-acquired pneumonia.

_____ 8. The Patient Protection and Affordable Care Act (PPACA) places little emphasis on evidence based medicine.

See answers to Self-Test in the Answer Section at the back of the book.

References

American Hospital Association (2015). http://www.aha.org/research/rc/stat-studies/fast-facts.shtml

Baker, L. C., Johnson, S. J., Macaulay, D., & Birnbaum, H. (2011, September). Integrated telehealth and care management program for Medicare beneficiaries with chronic disease linked to savings. *Health Affairs, 30*, 91689–1697. doi:10.1377/hlthaff.2011.0216

Beaver, K.,Tysver-Robinson, D., Campbell, M., Twomey, M., Williamson, S., Hindley, A., Susnerwala S., Dunn, G., & Luket, K. (2009, Jan 14). Comparing hospital and telephone follow-up after treatment for breast cancer: Randomized equivalence trial. *BMJ*, 338:a3147. doi:10.1136/bmj.a3147

Bednarski, D. (2009). President Elect Message: The value of nursing. *Nephrology Nursing, 36*, 115–117. https://www.annanurse.org/

Bourdeaux, L., Matthews, L., Richards, N. L., San Agustin, G., Thomas, P., & Veltigian, S. (2005). Comparative study of case management program for patients with syncope. *Nursing Care Quality, 20*, 140–144. http://journals.lww.com/jncqjournal/pages/default.aspx

Brooks, J. A. (2015). Reducing hospital readmissions. *American Journal of Nursing, 115*(1), 62–65. doi: 10.1097/01.NAJ.0000459639.76280.ae

Brooten, D., Kumar, S., Brown, L. P., Butts, P., Finkler, S. A., Bakewell-Sachs, S., . . . Delivoria-Papadopoulos, M. (1986). A randomized clinical trial of early hospital discharge and home follow-up of very-low-birth-weight infants. *New England Journal of Medicine, 315*, 934–939. doi: 10.1056/NEJM198610093151505

Buerhaus, P. (2010). Health care payment reform: Implications for nurses. *Nursing Economic$, 26*, 49–54. http://www.nursingeconomics.net/cgi-bin/WebObjects/NECJournal.woa

Chen, C., McNeese-Smith, D., Cowan, M., Upenieks, V., & Afifi, A. (2009). Evaluation of a nurse practitioner-led care management model in reducing inpatient drug utilization and cost. *Nursing Economic$, 27*, 160–169. http://www.nursingeconomics.net/cgi-bin/WebObjects/NECJournal.woa

Clari, M., Frigerio, S., Ricceri, F., Pici, A., Alvaro, R., & Dimonte, V. (2015). Follow-up telephone calls to patients discharged after undergoing orthopaedic surgery: Double-blind, randomized controlled trial of efficacy. *Clinical Nursing, 19–20,* 2736–44. doi: 10.1111/jocn.12795

Cryer, L., Shannon, S. B., Van Amsterdam, M., & Leff, B. (2012). Costs for "hospital at home" patients were 19 percent lower, with equal or better outcomes compared to similar inpatients. *Health Affairs, 31*(6), 1237–32. doi: 10.1377/hlthaff.2011.1132

Dall, T. M., Chen, Y. J., Seifert, R. F., Maddox, P. J., & Hogan, P. F. (2009). The economic value of professional nursing. *Medical Care, 47,* 97–104. doi: 10.1097/MLR.0b013e3181844da8

Feldstein, Paul J. (2011). *Health care economics* (7th ed.). Albany, NY: Delmar Cengage Learning.

Fergenbaum J., Bermingham, S., Krahn, M., Alter, D., & Demers, C. (2015). Care in the home for the management of chronic heart failure: Systematic review and cost-effectiveness analysis. *Journal of Cardiovascular Nursing, 4* S1 S44-51. doi: 10.1097/JCN.0000000000000235

Ferguson, L. A. (1996). Enhancing health care to underserved populations. *American Association of Occupational Health Nurses, 44,* 332–335. http://www.aaohn.org/aaohn-aboutus-files.html

Frogner, B., & Spetz, J. (2013). *Affordable care of 2010: Creating job opportunities for racially and ethnically diverse populations.* Washington, DC: Joint Center for Political and Economic Studies.

Gallup. (2016). Americans Rate Healthcare Providers High on Honesty, Ethics. http://www.gallup.com/poll/200057/americans-rate-healthcare-providers-high-honesty-ethics.aspx

Goetz, K., Janney, M., & Ramsey, K., (2011, July-August). When nursing takes ownership of financial outcomes: Achieving exceptional financial performance through leadership, strategy, and execution, *Nursing Economic$, 29*(4), 173–182. http://www.nursingeconomics.net/cgi-bin/WebObjects/NECJournal.woa

Greenberg, M. E. (2000). Telephone nursing: Evidence of client and organizational benefits. *Nursing Economic$, 18,* 117–123. http://www.nursingeconomics.net/cgi-bin/WebObjects/NECJournal.woa

Hanssen, T. A., Nordrehaug, J. E., Eide, G. E., & Hanestad, B. R. (2007). Improving outcomes after myocardial infarction: A randomized controlled trial evaluating effects of a telephone follow-up intervention. *European Journal of Cardiovascular Prevention & Rehabilitation, 14,* 429–37. doi: 10.1097/HJR.0b013e32801da123

Hartman, M., Martin, A., Lassman, D., Catlin, A., & the National Health Expenditure Accounts Team (2015). National health spending in 2013: Growth slows, remains in step with the overall economy. *Health Affairs, 34*(1), 150–160. http://www.healthaffairs.org/

Hlipala, S. I., Meyer, K. A., Wallace, T. O., & Zaremba, J. A. (2005). Profile of an admission nurse. *Nursing Management, 36,* 44–47. http://journals.lww.com/nursingmanagement/pages/default.aspx

Institute of Medicine. (2001). Crossing the quality chasm: A new health system for the 21st century. Committee on Quality of Health Care in America, Institute of Medicine. Washington, DC: National Academies Press.

Jallo, N., Bray, K., Padden, M., & Levin, D. (2009). A nurse-driven quality improvement program to improve perinatal outcomes. *Perinatal and Neonatal Nursing, 23,* 241–250. doi: 10.1097/JPN.0b013e3181af85ec

Johnson, R. (2013). An introduction to evidence-based practice. https://www.fmhs.auckland.ac.nz/en/soph/about/our-departments/epidemiology-and-biostaistics/research/epiq/evidence-based-practice-and-cats.html

Keeler, M., Haas, B. K., Nieswiadomy, M., Northam, S., McConnel, C., & Savoie, L. (2015a, Summer). Analysis of costs and benefits of transparent, gauze, or no dressing for a tunneled central venous catheter in Canadian stem cell transplant recipients. *Canadian Oncology Nursing, 25*(3), 289–298. http://www.canadianoncologynursingjournal.com/index.php/conj/index

Keeler, M., Haas, B. K., Nieswiadomy, M., Northam, S., McConnel, C., & Savoie, L. (2015b, Summer). Tunnelled central venous catheter-related bloodstream infection in Canadian blood stem cell transplant recipients: Associated costs.

Canadian Oncology Nursing, 25(3), 311–318. http://canadianoncologynursingjournal.com/index.php/conj/index

Kimman, M. L., Bloebaum, M. M., Dirksen, C. D., Houben, R. M., Lambin, P., & Boersma, L. J. (2010). Patient satisfaction with nurse-led telephone follow-up after curative treatment for breast cancer. *BMC Cancer, 10,* 174–183. doi: 10.1186/1471-2407-10-174

Laurant, M., Reeves, D., Hermens, R., Braspenning, J., Grol, R. & Sibbald, B. (2005). Substitution of doctors by nurses in primary care, *Cochrane Database Systematic Review,* 18. doi: 10.1002/14651858.CD001271.pub2

Marek, K. D., Stetzer, F, Adams, S. J., Bub, L. D., Schlidt, A., & Colorafi, K. J. (2014). Cost analysis of a home-based nurse care coordination program. *American Geriatrics Society, 62,* 2369–76. doi: 10.1111/jgs.13162

Melnyk, B. M. (2014). Speeding the translation of research into evidence-based practice and conducting projects that impact healthcare quality, patient outcomes and costs: The "so what" outcome factors. *Worldviews on Evidence-Based Nursing, 11*(1), 1–4. doi: 10.1111/wvn.12025

Paul, I. M., Phillips, T. A., Widome, M. D., & Hollenbeak, C. S. (2004). Cost-effectiveness of postnatal home nursing visits for prevention of hospital care for jaundice and dehydration. *Pediatrics, 114,* 1015–1022. http://www.jpeds.com/

Rausch, D. L., & Bjorklund, P. (2010). Decreasing the costs of constant observation. *Nursing Administration, 40,* 75–81. doi: 10.1097/NNA.0b013e3181cb9f56

Spetz, J. (2014). How will health reform affect demand for RNs? *Nursing Economic$, 32*(1), 42–44. http://www.nursingeconomics.net/cgi-bin/Web Objects/ NEC Journal.woa

Stevens, K. R. (2013). The impact of evidence-based practice in nursing and the next big ideas. *Online Journal of Issues in Nursing, 18*(2): Manuscript 4. http://www.nursingworld.org/

Strom, B. L, Kimmel, S. E., & Hennessy, S. E. (Eds.) (2012). Pharmacoepidemiology (5th ed., p. 8). (p. 8). Hoboken, NJ: John Wiley & Sons.

U.S. Bureau of Labor Statistics (2015). Occupational outlook handbook.ooh/healthcare/registered-nurses.htm#tab-6

U.S. Bureau of Labor Statistics. (2015). May 2014 National occupational employment and wage estimates United States. http://www.bls.gov/oes/current/oes_nat.htm#29-0000

U.S. Department of Health and Human Services, 2015. Commissioned Corps of the U.S. Public Health Services. http://www.usphs.gov/profession/nurse/activities.aspx

U.S. House of Representatives. Compilation of patient protection and affordable care act. Office of the Legislative Counsel for the use of the U.S. House of Representatives, 111th Congress, as amended through May 1, 2010. http://housedocs.house.gov/energycommerce/ppacacon.pdf

Chapter 20
Critique of Research Reports

Rose Nieswiadomy, PhD, RN, and Catherine Bailey, PhD, RN

Objectives

On completion of this chapter, you will be prepared to:

1. Summarize the guidelines for critiquing a quantitative research report.
2. Summarize the guidelines for critiquing a qualitative research report.

Introduction

As all nurses and nursing students know, their practice should be based on evidence. Evidence-based practice (EBP) is probably one of the most prevalent terms found in the nursing literature in this first part of the 21st century. You have learned that research evidence is the most critical component of EBP. To use research evidence, you must be able to evaluate this evidence. Hence, nurses need critiquing skills. Stevens (2011) stated that the critical appraisal of research evidence for clinical decision making is one of the most valuable skills that a clinician can possess in the present healthcare setting. To be able to distinguish the differences between the best evidence and unreliable or biased evidence is a basic requirement for providing clinical interventions that will produce the intended outcomes.

As a reader of this book, you may take some consolation in knowing that you are not the only one who is *not* an expert in critiquing research articles. However, if you have made it all the way through this book, you have gained some knowledge that will help you critique published research articles.

You may believe that all research articles that are published contain reports based on good research. Unfortunately, this is not always true. Although the review process used by most nursing journals helps ensure the publication of valid research, some published studies contain serious flaws.

All studies have strong and weak points. The word *critique* is often equated with the word *criticism*. This is unfortunate because the purpose of a research critique is to assess the strengths as well as the weaknesses of a study. In the past, when our students have been given a critique assignment, we asked them to list the strengths of the study as well as the weaknesses. Sometimes, it seemed they enjoyed pointing out the weaknesses rather than the strengths. They would ask, "How did this study get published?" It is well to remember that the author of the published report had the courage and motivation to become involved in nursing research, whereas many other nurses have not. This is not to say that critiquers should be lenient in their evaluation of published research. It is important, however, that nursing research be conducted. Severe criticism of their work may dim the enthusiasm of some nurse researchers. This is especially true for those who are just beginning to become involved in nursing research. Keep in mind that it is much easier to evaluate the research of others than to conduct research yourself.

There are no right or wrong answers when evaluating research reports. Even experts may disagree about certain aspects of a particular study. In evaluating research, reviewers should be as objective as possible and present a sound rationale for their judgments. If you use the Google search engine and type in "critical research appraisal checklists," you will obtain many hits for various types of rationales and scoring systems for appraising studies.

Critiquing research articles is particularly helpful to the beginning researcher because the critiquing process aids in the development of research skills. As the reader assesses the parts of a published study, ideas come to mind for the development of future research projects or for improvements in studies that have already been conducted or those that are in progress.

The research critique involves a thorough examination of all the parts of the study. Generally, the best way to conduct a critique is to read the entire study and make an initial evaluation of the report. Then, each part of the study should be subjected to an in-depth evaluation.

This chapter summarizes the material presented in other chapters on topics related to critiquing quantitative and qualitative study reports. The steps in critiquing qualitative studies are not as clear-cut and easily summarized as those of a quantitative study. Therefore, you may want to review other sources for critiquing certain aspects of qualitative study reports.

Some guidelines for evaluating research reports follow. These guidelines are certainly not an exhaustive list. Many other guidelines could be used and questions posed when reading research. As ideas come to mind while you are critiquing research reports, jot them down. In this way, you will be able to develop your own research critique assessment tool to use in the future.

Critiquing Quantitative Research Reports

Many nursing research textbooks contain information pertaining to the critique of quantitative studies. A number of published articles also contain guidelines for critiquing quantitative research reports (Fothergill & Lipp, 2014; Ingham-Broomfield, 2008; Kaplan, 2012).

When critiquing a quantitative study report, you generally begin with the abstract, placed either at the top of the article or along the left margin on the first page. The body of the article begins with an introductory section. A research article that discusses a quantitative study generally has four headings (there are variations): (a) "Literature Review," "Relevant Literature," or "Background," following the introduction; (b) "Methods"; (c) "Results"; and (d) "Discussion." Some articles contain additional headings for "Theoretical Framework" and "Conclusions." Even though the research article may contain only four or five headings, these sections should include all parts of the research study. For example, the methods section generally contains information about the study design, setting, population, sample, data-collection methods, and data-collection instruments.

Probably the most important part of a research article to focus on, after a cursory review of the entire article, is where the design is discussed. As mentioned, information on the design is usually found in the methods section. After you determine how the researcher actually carried out the study, you can go back and see if the other parts of the study are congruent. For example, if the design is described as a pretest-posttest control group design, two groups should be mentioned in the problem or purpose statement, in the hypothesis, and when the population and sample are discussed.

Researcher Qualifications

The first question to ask about quantitative research studies concerns the individuals who conducted the research and their qualifications regarding that particular study. Non-nurses conducted many nursing studies in past years. As nurses have become more qualified to conduct research, they are now conducting the majority of these studies.

A brief biographical sketch will assist the reader in evaluating the qualifications of the author(s). If this type of information is not provided, the academic credentials after the name, such as MSN or PhD, inform the reader of the educational background of the researcher. Generally, the researcher's current affiliation with a university or healthcare institution is listed, and a search of the university's website should also provide information about the researcher's scholarly interests. If the research has been funded by a reputable organization, such as the American Nurses Foundation, the reader of the report should have more confidence in the study results and conclusions.

Title

Clarity and conciseness are the major considerations in evaluating the title of a research article or report. The focus of the research should be apparent in the study title. It should contain the population and major variable(s). According to the *Publication Manual of the American Psychological Association* (2010, p. 23), the title should be no more than 12 words, whereas the Contributor Guidelines for the journal *Nurse Researcher* call for the title to be no more than 8 words. Extraneous words like "A Study of . . . ," "The Relationship Between . . . ," or "The Effects of . . . ," should be avoided. Nouns serve as the keywords in the title.

Abstract

Research reports, particularly those published in journals, frequently contain an abstract or summary of the study. Because the abstract may be the only section of the article that is read, the researcher should present the essential components of the study in the abstract. Abstracts typically are 150 to 250 words in length and they should describe the problem under investigation or purpose, the participants, essential features of the study method, basic findings, and conclusions and implications. Imbedding key words in an abstract enhances the reader's ability to access the report with the use of electronic searches.

Introduction

Although a research report is not meant to be a literary work of art, there is no reason to write the report in a dull and uninteresting fashion. The introduction should catch the interest of the reader and set the stage for the presentation of the research report. The best way to accomplish this is through a brief exploration of the study area. Background information on the problem and the significance of this problem to nursing needs to be addressed.

Identifying the Problem

The problem of the study should be clearly identified. Generally, there is a discussion, early in the research report, of the broad problem area of the study. In the abstract and at the end of the introductory section of the report, you will generally find a more specific statement of the problem. This may be in the form of a declarative problem statement, a purpose statement, or a research question. The problem statement, purpose statement, or research question should contain the population and major variable(s) and indicate that data may be gathered empirically (through the senses). The feasibility and significance of the study should be apparent. Sometimes, it may appear that a researcher has made the study focus too broad and tried to examine too many variables in one study. Although the problem, purpose, and research question are separate entities, many research reports identify only one of these aspects of the research process. In many published reports, the purpose of the study may be identified more clearly than the specific statement of the problem or research question. We prefer the research question as the best way to demonstrate what will be studied. Questions demand answers more than declarative statements.

Purpose

The author should leave no doubt in the reader's mind about the purpose of the study. The reason(s) for undertaking the study should have been clearly formulated before the research was begun, and the researcher should convey this information to the reader in the form of the study purpose. The broad purpose of the study may be made more specific in the form of objectives or goals. The purpose statement is usually found in the abstract and, again, at the end of the introductory section.

Review of the Literature

The literature review provides a context for the study (Kaplan, 2012). The literature review should flow logically and establish what is and what is not known about the problem (Kaplan, 2012). Generally, classic sources are presented, and current sources are discussed. Additionally, primary sources should be cited. If most of the references are from journals, you should have more confidence that primary sources were accessed. Key sources should be critically compared and appraised, rather than simply alluded to. Paraphrasing is preferred rather than the use of many direct quotations. A comprehensive literature review presents theory and research that both supports and opposes the expected study results. Finally, the review should conclude with a sentence or two that indicates how the present study will contribute to the existing body of knowledge in that subject area.

Theoretical/Conceptual Framework

In searching for the study framework in a research report, the reader may find a clearly identified section for the framework, or this information may be found in the introductory section or literature review section of the research article or report. If a framework is identified, ask if this is the most appropriate framework for the study. Is the framework based on a nursing theory or a theory from another discipline? With the great emphasis on theoretically based nursing research, nurse researchers are becoming aware of the need for a framework, but may not choose the most appropriate framework for the study. Support or lack of support for the framework, based on the findings, should be discussed at the end of the report.

Theoretical frameworks are not used for health services research, a branch of research which studies issues related to access to care, healthcare costs, and healthcare delivery (Kaplan, 2012). Additionally, clinical researchers who compare the effectiveness of drugs don't use theoretical frameworks.

Assumptions

All studies are based on assumptions. These assumptions may be of the universal type, such as "All human beings need to feel loved." Assumptions also come from theory and previous research. Finally, the researcher may make some commonsense assumptions that are necessary to proceed with the research. Such an assumption might be, "The respondents will answer the questions honestly." The reader should look for the researcher's explicit assumptions. Explicit assumptions are those asserted by the researcher and clearly identifiable by the reader.

The reader should also try to identify assumptions that the researcher appears to have made, but never stated specifically. These implicit assumptions are those made by the researcher, but not clearly identified in the research report. For example, if the study sought to determine if giving a back rub at bedtime would decrease patients' requests for sleeping medications, the researcher has made at least three either explicitly stated or unstated implicit assumptions: (a) Adequate sleep is necessary for patients, (b) Sleeping medications are not the most healthful type of sleep enhancer, and (c) One of the roles of nurses is to try to assist patients in obtaining adequate sleep.

Limitations

The reader should not have to search out the limitations of a study. Frequently, the first mention is found in the discussion section. The author will comment on the inappropriateness of the instrument or the small sample size. These limitations should be openly and honestly stated in the early part of a research report. The researcher should clearly identify those aspects of the research situation over which no control has been exercised. In experimental studies, internal and external threats to validity should be listed. As is the case with the assumptions of a study, many research reports do not contain a separate section on the study limitations. Because the researcher frequently acknowledges some of the study limitations in the discussion section, study limitations may be easier to identify than the assumptions on which the study was based. Additionally, readers frequently may be able to identify additional limitations of a study other than those acknowledged by the researcher.

Hypothesis(es)

Hypotheses should be clearly and concisely stated in a declarative sentence and in the present tense. Hypotheses should be based on theory or research findings. Directional research hypotheses, rather than null or nondirectional hypotheses, are the preferred type. The exception is those situations where there is no available research or theory that predicts the relationships among the variables being examined. The hypothesis should contain the population and the variables and reflect the problem statement, purpose, or research question. A hypothesis should be empirically testable and contain only one prediction. To be testable, it must be possible to gather empirical or objective data on the variables of interest. Single predictions are necessary in a hypothesis to avoid the partial support crisis that occurs when two predictions are made and only one is supported. An error sometimes detected in published hypotheses is the multiple predictions they contain.

Definition of Terms

A separate section on definition of terms may not be included in a journal article because of space constraints. Definitions of key terms in a research report are necessary, however, to make explicit what is being studied. Replication of a study is aided by clear definitions of terms. The key terms generally reflect the theoretical or conceptual framework for the study; therefore, some of the definitions of the terms may be derived from the section on the discussion of the study framework. Operational definitions are also necessary. These definitions indicate the observable, measurable phenomena associated with the study variables. Frequently, operational definitions are indicated in the discussion of the research instruments that were used to gather data.

Research Design

The research design should be clearly identified and adequately described. In experimental studies, the research consumer is concerned with the experimental treatment. Is the treatment adequately described and appropriate for the particular study? Is the method of assigning subjects to groups discussed? Means to control threats to internal and external validity should be included in the section on research design. In nonexperimental quantitative studies, the means of selecting study participants should be discussed. Any extraneous variables that have been controlled, such as age and educational background of the respondents, should be identified.

Setting

The setting for the research project needs to be described. Many agencies do not want to be identified in research reports. As a result, the description of the setting is usually general. The description might be "a small private psychiatric institution in the southeastern United States." The reader must then determine if the setting seems appropriate for the particular study.

Population and Sample

Generally, the study sample is easily identified when reading a research article. The target population and the accessible population may not be so easy to identify. The author has the responsibility to mention the broad group of interest (target population) as well as that available group (accessible population) from which the sample was selected.

The section on the sample should identify and describe the specific probability or nonprobability sampling method that was used. This section should also describe the demographic characteristics of the sample and the sample size, and list the percentage of the population represented by the sample. Acknowledgment must be made of any dropout of subjects that occurred during the study and any other potential sampling biases that may have been recognized by the researcher. Finally, the section should discuss the methods taken to protect subjects' rights. Little information is generally provided about ethical issues because of space limitations in published articles. However, anonymity or confidentiality should be mentioned, and the permissions obtained to conduct the study noted.

Collection of Data

Five general questions to ask in evaluating the data-collection section are who?, when?, where?, what?, and how? "Who will collect the data?" "When will the data be collected?" "Where will the data be collected?" "What data will be collected?" and "How will the data be collected?" Use the acronym WWWWH. The specific data-collection method(s) will dictate additional questions that need to be asked. For example, if questionnaires were used, the research report should provide enough information for the reader to determine whether a questionnaire was the most appropriate method to collect data. If interviews were used, the interviewer training process should be explained. Observation research requires that the reader be told how observations were made, who made the observations, and how data were recorded. If physiological instruments were used, the means of assessing the accuracy of these instruments needs to be addressed.

Data-Collection Instruments

All of the data-collection instruments used in a study should be clearly identified and described. Scoring procedures and the range of possible scores on the instrument should also be included, where appropriate.

The characteristics of each instrument should be discussed. If an instrument has been used in previous research, the results of that use should be presented in the discussion of the instrument. The most important characteristics of an instrument concern its reliability and validity. The reader must determine whether the appropriate types of reliability and validity have been reported and if the evidence of the reliability and validity is adequate for use of the instrument in the present study. Pilot study results should be included for any newly developed or revised instrument.

Analysis of Data

Many research consumers cringe when approaching the data analysis section of a research report because they are fearful of the statistics discussed in this section. A beginning knowledge of statistics is sufficient to evaluate the majority of the published research findings. Descriptive statistics on the characteristics of the study sample should be presented first. Next, the subjects' scores on the various instruments need to be reported. Finally, inferential statistics should be presented if the study tested a hypothesis or hypotheses. The author should state whether each of the study hypotheses was supported or not supported. The results of the statistical test, the degrees of freedom, and the probability value should be given. These findings should be clearly presented in both the text and the tables.

Discussion of Findings

In the discussion of findings section of a research report, the author interprets the study results. This material may be more subjective than the information in the findings section. The author should compare the present study findings with those of other studies discussed in the literature review. No new literature sources should be introduced that were not referred to in the review of literature. Study findings should be discussed in light of the theoretical or conceptual framework that was tested. The author must make it clear that the findings either supported or failed to support the study framework.

Both statistical and clinical significance should be discussed. These two types of significance are not always congruent. Findings that are statistically significant may have little or no clinical significance. On the other hand, results that were determined to be statistically nonsignificant could, in fact, have clinical significance. The researcher should also discuss the study limitations and how these limitations are thought to have affected the study results.

Conclusions

Conclusions answer the "So what?" question that might be posed to a researcher at the end of a study. Through the conclusions, the researcher demonstrates the meaning and worth of the research. The study conclusions attempt to make generalizations based on the study findings. Conclusions are often difficult to write, and many authors merely restate the findings or go to the other extreme and overgeneralize.

Conclusions are written tentatively, which means they are not written in stone. Words such as *seems* or *appears* are frequently found at the beginning of a stated conclusion. The findings are bound to the data; the conclusions are based on the data. For example, a finding might be "Postoperative hysterectomy patients who received a backrub at bedtime went to sleep 10.5 minutes faster than postoperative hysterectomy patients who did not receive a backrub." A conclusion related to this finding might be, "It appears that a backrub is an effective means of promoting sleep in postoperative hysterectomy patients." Can you tell, from this conclusion, that the researcher is attempting to generalize beyond the sample that was used in the study?

Implications

The researcher needs to explicitly identify implications for nursing practice, nursing education, or nursing research. The implications section of a research report contains the "shoulds" that result from the research findings. For example, nurse educators should include material in nursing curriculums on the topic of the study or nurse researchers should conduct more research in the area of interest. When the study findings are not statistically or clinically significant, the implications of the study may be that no changes are recommended as the result of the present study.

Recommendations

Although recommendations may be made for nursing practice and nursing education, recommendations found in a research report generally concern future research that is needed. A suggestion can be made that the study be replicated. Another suggestion may concern further development of the instrument or use of a larger sample size. Recommendations should take into consideration the limitations of the present study. The recommendations also should consider the findings of previous studies. Nursing can ill afford to conduct impractical or irrelevant research or to reinvent the wheel, as it were.

Other Considerations

Although the most important areas to evaluate in a research report are the specific components of the research study, other areas also need to be evaluated. Correct grammar, sentence structure, and punctuation are essential. The research consumer may have difficulty concentrating on the merits of the research report if structural errors are found. The author's writing style and use of words, especially limiting the use of complex and technical words, is also important to the reader.

The accuracy and completeness of the reference list is also important. It is very discouraging to the reader to discover a source of interest in the literature review section and then be unable to find this source listed in the reference section. Also, it is not uncommon to find sources in the reference section that were never referred to in the research report. You may also find incomplete references or ones with essential elements missing. The last question to ask is, "After reading this research report, would I refer it to a colleague?"

Finally the reviewer may need guidance in order to determine the scientific merits of the study by evaluating the level and quality of the evidence (Kaplan, 2012). For this type of determination Kaplan recommends that the reader review the Research Toolkit on the American Nurses Association's website.

Critiquing Qualitative Research Reports

The critique of a qualitative study report can be more difficult than the critique of a quantitative study. Your educational preparation likely did not include information about all of the types of qualitative designs and methodologies.

Members of some disciplines, such as sociology and anthropology, often prefer a certain type of design. For example, sociologists may prefer a grounded theory design, whereas anthropologists may choose an ethnographic design. As a whole, nurses do not seem to be attached to any particular design, and many of us have not obtained knowledge about some of the available designs that can be used in qualitative research studies. If you choose to become a qualitative researcher or wish to critique qualitative studies in depth, you may want to seek a mentor. If you are enrolled in a nursing educational program, you will probably have no difficulty in locating a qualitative researcher at your institution. The number of qualitative nurse researchers continues to increase. Qualitative nurse researchers are usually happy to provide support to a nurse who is a novice qualitative researcher or who is interested in qualitative research.

Some of the headings in a qualitative research article are similar to those of a quantitative study, such as the sections named "Background" or "Literature Review," "Methods," and "Findings" or "Results." Some qualitative reports also contain these headings: "Data Collection," "Conclusions," or "Implications." There is less similarity in headings in a qualitative research report than in a quantitative research report.

For guidance in critiquing qualitative research, numerous books and articles are available. Beck published an informative article on critiquing qualitative research in the October 2009 issue of the *AORN (Association of periOperative Registered Nurses) Journal*.

Researcher Qualifications

It may be difficult to critique the expertise of researchers who conduct qualitative studies. Unless you have access to their educational preparation in qualitative research and are familiar with the qualitative research studies they have conducted, you will have no way of determining their qualifications to conduct a particular study. You will probably be able to determine the degrees they have completed and their present place of employment. Some articles contain an email address for the author(s). If so, you may be able to contact them to obtain more information. Also, if the author is affiliated with an educational institution, you may be able to obtain pertinent information about the faculty member on the institution's website.

Title

The title of a qualitative study should indicate the phenomenon to be studied and the types of individuals who will be participants. Sometimes the title of a research study report provides a broad hint as to the type of study being discussed. This is true in both quantitative and qualitative reports. If the title indicates that open-heart surgery patients receiving a particular intervention are being compared to open-heart surgery patients receiving another intervention or the routine treatment, you will have no difficulty determining that you are reading about an experimental study. Another article's title may indicate that the report describes the feelings or emotions of certain people. For example, the title might be "The Lived Experience of Earthquake Survivors." Would you know immediately that you were about to read a qualitative research study report? Read through the table of contents of several issues of research journals, such as *Nursing Research*, and see how many titles clearly indicate quantitative or qualitative research reports.

Abstract

The abstract for a qualitative research report is located in the same place as in a quantitative report—at the top of the article or down the left side of the first page. Abstracts usually contain from 150 to 250 words. The abstract should summarize the main areas of the study, such as the purpose, design, types of participants, sample size, and any major themes uncovered in the data. The abstract is a very important part of a research report because, as mentioned in the section on critiquing quantitative study reports, this section may be the only one that is actually read.

Introduction

This section contains background material about the study and probably contains literature references about the topic. The problem statement, purpose statement, and/or research questions may be found in this introductory section. The main objective in critiquing the introductory section is to determine whether the important components are present and seem appropriate for the study and the material promotes the reader's interest in the report.

Problem of the Study

If the qualitative study report is presented appropriately, you should be able to locate the description of the problem of interest. Try to determine whether the study problem is clear or ambiguous. Does the problem seem significant to nursing? If you are familiar with the research design, does the problem seem to match the research tradition of that particular design? The study problem generally appears in the report's introductory section.

Purpose

The purpose of a research study should always be clear to the reader. The purpose statement is usually presented in a single sentence, and might read something like, "to explore the experience of living in a tent city for 6 months following a 7.0 earthquake that struck the homes of people in Haiti." The purpose may appear in the abstract and also at the end of the introductory section.

Research Question

A qualitative research report may present a broad research question, such as "What were the experiences of survivors of a 7.0 earthquake in Haiti?" The data collection section of the study may also list specific research questions, such as "What were your feelings as you tried to go to sleep in the tent city where you lived for 6 months?" and "What were your concerns about family members when you were separated from them for so long?" Are the research questions appropriate for the problem that was studied? Are they sufficient to gather the information needed for a comprehensive report of the phenomenon under study?

Research Design

This section may be difficult to critique unless you are familiar with all of the various qualitative research designs. The specific design is always mentioned in a research report, usually for the first time in the abstract. Once the design is identified, you may want to go to reference sources (even Wikipedia provides a simple explanation of designs) to gain an understanding of the specific design. This textbook provides some basic information about a number of the more common qualitative research designs. Again, you may want to seek the assistance of a mentor.

Review of the Literature

As you know, quantitative research studies always begin with a review of the literature. However, in order to critique this section of a qualitative research report, you need to be familiar with the study design. As mentioned before, some designs call for an early review of the literature, whereas others call for the review toward the completion of the study. Were classical and current references cited? Were primary sources cited? Does the literature review provide an adequate summary of the existing body of knowledge on the phenomenon of interest? With that in mind, is there evidence to support the need for the study?

Selection of Sample

A purposive sample is usually chosen for a qualitative study. This type of sampling permits the researcher to recruit informants who should be able to provide the best kind of information that relates to the research question (Powers, 2015). Sometimes a convenience sample may be selected. In a qualitative study, the sample is of utmost importance. In a quantitative study, the population from which the sample is chosen is more important than the sample. The sample size in a qualitative study is usually small and the participants have specific inclusion criteria in common. Does the researcher discuss how the decision was made as to the number of participants to include in the study? For example, was the concept of "saturation" or the point when data collection stops providing new information discussed (Powers, 2015)? How were the rights of participants protected? The researcher usually interacts directly with study participants in a qualitative study, and their identities are known. The report should indicate to the reader that the study was subject to external review. The researcher must also demonstrate that risks were minimized. However, as mentioned, because of space limitations, research articles usually contain little information about the protection of subjects' rights.

Collection of Data

The researcher must gain access to the study participants and determine where the data will be collected. Were the data collected in the participants' homes or at some neutral location? Did one researcher collect the data? If more than one researcher collected the data, were they properly trained? Data collection usually involves interviews. Were an adequate number of direct quotes collected to capture the true essence of what the participants were trying to say? These interviews must be recorded in some manner. Were these procedures described in sufficient detail? Were the transcripts of the interviews reviewed for accuracy? What were the qualifications of those individuals who reviewed the transcripts? Was agreement reached on the meaning of the participants' responses from the study participants or from those who collected the data?

Analysis of Data

You may have a difficult time with this section of a qualitative research report. There are many ways to analyze data from a qualitative study. Analysis of data involves an examination of words rather than numbers. Coding is the basic data analysis scheme of qualitative researchers. All qualitative studies involve content analysis procedures. Content analysis varies according to the type of study design. Direct quotes are frequently used. In fact, if you scan a research article and see a number of direct quotes, you will probably conclude that you are examining a qualitative research report. Many qualitative researchers hand-analyze their data, whereas others use computer software in their data analysis. Some of these software programs have been mentioned elsewhere in this textbook. Again, you may need assistance in critiquing this section of a qualitative research report.

Interpretation of Data

The interpretation of the data depends on the research design and research tradition used by the researcher. In the section where the researcher interprets the findings, you may see names like Merleau-Ponty, who focused on people's perceptions of their experiences through their bodily senses (tasting, touching, and hearing). Or you might read about Husserl, a leader of the German phenomenological movement. The researcher may have interpreted the data based on Merlau-Ponty's or Husserl's philosophical beliefs. Qualitative researchers interpret their findings based on the specific type of design used in the study, the ideas of experts in that area of design, and their own qualitative research beliefs. Finally, the research consumer should ask whether the researcher compared the findings to previous study results concerning the phenomenon of interest.

Recommendations

Every researcher makes recommendations based on their study results. Whether they have conducted a quantitative or a qualitative study, researchers generally call for more research on the topic of interest. Most research studies raise further questions that need to be answered. Recommendations are found at the end of each research report.

Other Considerations

The most important areas to evaluate in a qualitative research report are the actual components of the study. However, other areas also need to be evaluated. As in a quantitative report, correct grammar, sentence structure, and punctuation are essential. Was the report organized and easily understood? Was the writing style appealing? Were too many complex words or technical terms used? Would you recommend this research report to a colleague? Would the results of this study help in caring for my patients (Powers, 2015)?

Summary

Most research studies have both strong and weak points. A critical evaluation of all the sections of a research report is essential in determining the usefulness of the research results. Although many additional questions may be raised when examining research reports, this chapter presented some useful guidelines to the beginning researcher as she or he appraises published research reports of quantitative and qualitative studies.

Self-Test

1. Select the most appropriate way to cite another author's findings in a literature review for a quantitative research report.
   A. Use as many direct quotations as space allows in the report.
   B. Paraphrase whenever possible.
   C. Refer the reader to the website of the article with the findings.
   D. Suggest that the reader search for the article in their library.
2. Identify which types of research studies do not use theoretical frameworks. Studies that deal with:
   A. healthcare costs and healthcare delivery.
   B. the reliability and validity of instruments.
   C. patient outcomes, such as management of symptoms.
   D. middle-range theories for nursing research.
3. The researcher plans to survey patients about their alcohol drinking habits. State which assumption appears to be most appropriate for this plan. The patient will:
   A. not understand the question.
   B. truthfully answer the survey question.
   C. not remember how many alcoholic drinks he or she drinks.
   D. lie about his or her drinking habits.
4. Identify when it would be inappropriate to state a directional research hypothesis for a quantitative research study. When:
   A. there is no available research or theory to predict the relationship between the variables.
   B. there is no instrument to empirically test the hypothesis and its variables.
   C. the population is missing from the null hypothesis.
   D. the instrument to collect the data is unreliable.
5. Describe which definitions of terms help researchers who may wish to replicate a study.
   A. Conceptual definitions provide a reflection of the conceptual framework.
   B. Dictionary definitions provide an understanding of the context of the variable.
   C. Operational definitions provide a way to observe and measure the phenomena of interest.
   D. Conceptual definitions provide ambiguous terms that can be used in other studies.
6. What statement in a qualitative research report would indicate that the data collected from interviews represents the participant's views?
   A. The transcripts were reviewed by the data collector.
   B. The transcripts were reviewed for accuracy by the trained researcher.
   C. The data collector replayed the participant's statements.
   D. Both the data collector and the participant agreed on the meaning of the responses.

See answers to Self-Test in the Answer Section at the back of the book.

References

American Psychological Association. (2010). *Publication Manual of the American Psychological Association* (6th ed.). Washington, DC: Author.

Beck, C. T. (2009). Critiquing qualitative research. *Association of periOperative Registered Nurses (AORN), 90*, 543–554. doi: 10.1016/j.aorn.2008.12.023

Fothergill, A., & Lipp, A. (2014). A guide to critiquing a research paper on clinical supervision: Enhancing skills for practice. *Psychiatric and Mental Health Nursing, 21*, 834–840. doi:10.1111/jpm.12161

Ingham-Broomfield, R. (2008). A nurses' guide to the critical reading of research. *Australian Journal of Advanced Nursing, 26*(1), 102–109. http://www.ajan.com.au/

Kaplan, L. (2012). Reading and critiquing a research article. *American Nurse Today, 7*(10). http://www.americannursetoday.com/

Powers, B. A. (2015). Critically appraising qualitative evidence for clinical decision making. In B. M. Melnyk & E. Fineout-Overholt (Eds.), *Evidence-based practice in nursing & healthcare: A guide to best practice* (3rd ed., pp. 139–168). China: Wolters Kluwer Health.

Stevens, K. R. (2011). Critically appraising knowledge for clinical decision making. In B. M. Melnyk & E. Fineout-Overholt (Eds.), *Evidence-based practice in nursing & healthcare: A guide to best practice* (2nd ed., pp. 73–80). China: Wolters Kluwer Health | Lippincott Williams & Wilkins.

Self-Test Answers

Chapter 1

1. C
   Rationale: Scientific research is the most reliable source of nursing knowledge. Without research evidence there is no way to know if an intervention is optimal. Nursing knowledge has come from tradition, authority, and trial and error; however, they are not the most reliable sources of nursing knowledge.
   Chapter: 1
   Learning Objective: 1, Identify the importance of research to nursing.
   Topic/Concept: Importance of Research to Nursing
   Difficulty Level: Easy
   Skill Level: Remembering

2. A
   Rationale: The findings from applied research, which tend to seek solutions to existing problems, often lead to questions that are appropriate for basic research. Applied research does not depend upon the existence of health participants. Applied research does not usually occur in a laboratory. Applied research is based on an immediate practical need.
   Chapter: 1
   Learning Objective: 1, Identify the importance of research to nursing.
   Topic/Concept: Importance of Research to Nursing
   Difficulty Level: Moderate
   Skill Level: Understanding

3. A
   Rationale: The major reason for conducting nursing research is to promote a practice supported by evidence demonstrating that it is the best possible care for the recipient. The major reason for conducting nursing research is not to promote the growth of the nursing profession, document cost-effectiveness of nursing care, or to ensure accountability for nursing practice.
   Chapter: 1
   Learning Objective: 2, Describe four goals for conducting nursing research.
   Topic/Concept: Goals for Conducting Nursing Research
   Difficulty Level: Moderate
   Skill Level: Understanding

4. B
   Rationale: One of the criteria for a profession is the existence of a body of knowledge that is distinct from other disciplines. Through the use of research, nursing is in the process of developing a body of knowledge that is specific to nursing. Borrowing knowledge from the natural sciences does not explain how research establishes the credibility of nursing as a profession. Being identified as having ethical standards does not explain how research establishes the credibility of nursing as a profession. Existing to provide service to society does not explain how research establishes the credibility of nursing as a profession.
   Chapter: 1
   Learning Objective: 2, Describe four goals for conducting nursing research.
   Topic/Concept: Goals for Conducting Nursing Research
   Difficulty Level: Easy
   Skill Level: Understanding

5. A
   Rationale: Quantitative research studies are appropriate for the researcher to collect numerical data that is useful for statistical analysis. Qualitative research is concerned with the subjective meaning of experiences to individuals. Tightly controlled and cost-effective would describe studies but are not types of research.

Chapter: 1
Learning Objective: 3, Compare qualitative and quantitative research.
Topic/Concept: Quantitative and Qualitative Research
Difficulty Level: Easy
Skill Level: Remembering

6. B
   Rationale: In qualitative research studies the participants are invited to freely share their information in a natural setting. *Responses to surveys* or *quiet test settings* does not describe the environment for a qualitative study.
   Chapter: 1
   Learning Objective: 3, Compare qualitative and quantitative research.
   Topic/Concept: Quantitative and Qualitative Research
   Difficulty Level: Easy
   Skill Level: Remembering

7. A, B and C
   Rationale: According to the AACN, graduates of a practice-focused doctoral program should be prepared at the highest level of nursing practice and use their leadership knowledge and skills to evaluate and translate research into practice. Graduates of research-focused doctoral nursing programs are prepared to begin an independent program of research and carry out research.
   Chapter: 1
   Learning Objective: 4, Describe the various roles of nurses in research.
   Topic/Concept: Nurses and Research
   Difficulty Level: Easy
   Skill Level: Remembering

8. A
   Rationale: There are many ways nurses can participate in research studies. They should be able to identify researchable problems because they are at the bedside and know much of what patients need. All nurses are not able to explain the details of a medical research study to potential participants, determine when most study findings are ready for use in nursing practice, or confidently critique the majority of published nursing research studies.
   Chapter: 1
   Learning Objective: 4, Describe the various roles of nurses in research.
   Topic/Concept: Nurses and Research
   Difficulty Level: Easy
   Skill Level: Remembering

9. A
   Rationale: As nurses received advanced degrees, the focus of their research was on education because their degrees were in education. As nurses first began to receive advanced educational preparation and became qualified to conduct research, the studies did not concern the characteristics of nurses, nursing administration, or nursing care.
   Chapter: 1
   Learning Objective: 4, Describe the various roles of nurses in research.
   Topic/Concept: Nurses in Research
   Difficulty Level: Easy
   Skill Level: Remembering

10. A and C
    Rationale: Quality of life and pain were the two highest rated topics in the most recent survey by the Oncology Nurses Society that was used to develop the 2009-2013 Oncology Nursing Society Research Agenda. Falls, domestic violence, and quality assurance were not identified as topics for the Oncology Nurses Society agenda.
    Chapter: 1
    Learning Objective: 5, Summarize the development of nursing research and future priorities.

Topic/Concept: Research Priorities into the Future
Difficulty Level: Easy
Skill Level: Remembering

Chapter 2

1. A
   Rationale: Archie Cochrane is credited with starting the movement toward evidence-based practices after the publication of his book. Sackett wrote an editorial that caused physicians to accept evidence-based medicine. The Cochrane Collaboration is an international nonprofit organization that supports efforts to make well-informed decisions about healthcare. The Agency for Healthcare Research and Quality (AHRQ) is a branch of the U.S. Department of Health and Human Services who promoted the idea of evidence-based practices through the leadership of Evidence-Based Practice Centers (EPCs).
   Chapter: 2
   Learning Objective: 1, Summarize the importance of evidence-based practice in the field of nursing.
   Topic/Concept: Defining Evidence-Based Practice
   Difficulty Level: Easy
   Skill Level: Remembering

2. B
   Rationale: Archie Cochrane, the person who is credited for the concept of an evidence-based practice, was a British medical researcher and epidemiologist. Archie Cochrane was not an American nurse, a male nurse, or an Australian who started the Cochrane Library.
   Chapter: 2
   Learning Objective: 1, Summarize the importance of evidence-based practice in the field of nursing.
   Topic/Concept: Defining Evidence-Based Practice
   Difficulty Level: Easy
   Skill Level: Remembering

3. C
   Rationale: The results from randomized controlled clinical trials (RCCT) are considered the strongest type of evidence for making practice decisions. Thus, RCCTs are the gold standard for supporting evidence-based practice decisions. Patient surveys, patient response during an assessment, or evidence from clinical experiences are not considered the gold standard for practice decisions.
   Chapter: 2
   Module: 1
   Learning Objective: 1, Summarize the importance of evidence-based practice in the field of nursing.
   Topic/Concept: Defining Evidence-Based Practice
   Difficulty Level: Easy
   Skill Level: Remembering

4. A
   Rationale: Sigma Theta Tau International's defined EBP as an integration of the best evidence available, nursing expertise, and the values and preferences of the individuals, families, and communities who are served. A nurse's role as a patient advocate would consider the patient's values while making a clinical decision that is evidence-based. The best evidence and cost-effectiveness would not be the most sensitive to the nurse's role as patient advocate.
   Chapter: 2
   Learning Objective: 1, Summarize the importance of evidence-based practice in the field of nursing.
   Topic/Concept: Defining Evidence-Based Practice
   Difficulty Level: Moderate,
   Skill Level: Understanding

5. D
   Rationale: In addition to using the synthesis of the best evidence from multiple research studies, expert clinicians are also expected to consider the patient's circumstances and values as well as the results that are generated from quality improvement projects. EBP is not necessarily based on changes to practice

over time. EBP is not based upon multiple studies that agree with the clinician's expert opinion. EBP is not based on a combination of research studies and the patient's needs and desires.
Chapter: 2
Learning Objective: 2, Differentiate between research utilization and evidence-based nursing practice.
Topic/Concept: Defining Evidence-Based Practice
Difficulty Level: Easy
Skill Level: Remembering

6. B
Rationale: For nurses, the overall goal of an evidence-based practice is to improve the effectiveness of healthcare processes and patient outcomes with the introduction of current empirically supported knowledge into common care decisions. The overall goal of evidence-based practice is not to improve outcomes with traditional nursing knowledge. The goal of EBP is not to explore how nursing expertise supports the best healthcare for patients. The goal of EBP is not to introduce knowledge gained from patient surveys into clinical decision making.
Chapter: 2
Learning Objective: 2, Differentiate between research utilization and evidence-based nursing practice.
Topic/Concept: Evidence-Based Nursing Practice
Difficulty Level: Easy
Skill Level: Remembering

7. C
Rationale: The Joint Commission, which confers accreditation on healthcare agencies, and the American Nurses Credentialing Center, which provides Magnet Hospital recognition, are two important entities that recognize evidence-based practices in nursing as the best treatment plans for patient care. The Cochrane Library and the National Guideline Clearinghouse store the evidence-based guidelines. David Sackett was instrumental in having evidence-based practice accepted by physicians. Florence Nightingale was not around during the development of evidence-based practice. The AHRQ and the National Quality Strategy do not specifically recognize EBP in nursing as the best treatment plans for patient care.
Chapter: 2
Learning Objective: 2, Differentiate between research utilization and evidence-based nursing practice.
Topic/Concept: Evidence-Based Nursing Practice
Difficulty Level: Moderate
Skill Level: Remembering

8. D
Rationale: The correct answer is *patient satisfaction with pain control*. That is the outcome. The acronym PICOT stands for population (P), intervention of interest (I), comparison or current practice (C), outcome (O), and time (T). "Patients with migraine headaches" is the population (not outcome). Administration of opioids and music therapy are "intervention" vs "comparison intervention" (not outcome).
Chapter: 2
Learning Objective: 2, Differentiate between research utilization and evidence-based nursing practice.
Topic/Concept: Evidence-Based Nursing Practice
Difficulty Level: Moderate
Skill Level: Understanding

9. B
Rationale: According to Hain and Kear (2015), translational research refers to evidence that has been incorporated into guidelines that may be used in clinical settings. The National Guideline Clearinghouse and the Best Practice Information sheets from the Joanna Briggs Institute each provide sources for guidelines that may be practiced in the clinical setting. Translational research can be found in CINAHL but not primary research studies. Translational research can be found in PubMed but not specifically in the Cochrane Library or patient databases.
Chapter: 2
Learning Objective: 3, Discuss the importance of the Cochrane Collaboration and the Cochrane Nursing Care Field to evidence-based practice.

Topic/Concept: Evidence-Based Nursing Practice
Difficulty Level: Moderate
Skill Level: Understanding

10. C
Rationale: The National Quality Forum works to support the Agency for Healthcare Research and Quality. Outcome measures provide a way to assess the results of healthcare that are experienced by patients. Structural measures assess the healthcare infrastructure. Process measures assess the steps that should be followed to provide good care. Composite measures combine multiple measures to produce a single score.
Chapter: 2
Learning Objective: 4, Explain the role of the Agency for Healthcare Research and Quality in evidence-based practice.
Topic/Concept: Agency For Healthcare Research And Quality
Difficulty Level: Easy
Skill Level: Remembering

Chapter 3

1. B
Rationale: The definition of evidence-based practice (EBP) for clinical purposes has evolved to include the concepts of quality and efficiency. Evaluation of the process and structure, patient and family desires, and promotion of outcomes related to hierarchy of evidence are not directly reflected in the definition of EBP for clinical purposes.
Chapter: 3
Learning Objective: 1, Explain how the concept of evidence-based practice (EBP) is evolving in nursing.
Topic/Concept: The Evolving Nature of Evidence-Based Practice
Difficulty Level: Easy
Skill Level: Remembering

2. A
Rationale: Best evidence should include more than the results from randomized controlled clinical trials, but also descriptive and qualitative research as well as knowledge from case studies and scientific principles. Expert opinions, cost-containment data, and traditional preferences are not identified as being research evidence for EBP.
Chapter: 3
Learning Objective: 1, Explain how the concept of evidence-based practice (EBP) is evolving in nursing.
Topic/Concept: The Evolving Nature of Evidence-Based Practice
Difficulty Level: Easy
Skill Level: Remembering

3. C
Rationale: Knowledge-focused triggers relate to new research findings or changes in agency standards (such as federal regulations or standards committee decisions). The incidence of pressure sores, complaints of patients with urinary retention, and fall rates are not considered knowledge-focused triggers for a change to clinical practice.
Chapter: 3
Learning Objective: 2, Describe models that promote the implementation of EBP in nursing practice.
Topic/Concept: Models to Promote Evidence-Based Practice in Nursing
Difficulty Level: Moderate
Skill Level: Analyzing

4. C
Rationale: A problem-focused trigger could include information from a clinical problem or data that relate to risk management, process improvement, benchmarking, and financial issues. HIPAA regulations, Medicare/Medicaid decisions, and CDC regulations would not be problem-focused triggers.

Chapter: 3
Learning Objective: 2, Describe models that promote the implementation of EBP in nursing practice.
Topic/Concept: Models to Promote Evidence-Based Practice in Nursing
Difficulty Level: Moderate
Skill Level: Analyzing

5. A
Rationale: An organizational culture that encourages improved clinical outcomes through the promotion of clinical inquiry and evidence-based changes is essential to building a team to implement EBP. Building a team will take more than individuals who enjoy utilizing research findings. The team will need more than leaders who are experienced at implementing EBP. An effective team will require more than having stakeholders who enjoy the benefits of EBP.
Chapter: 3
Learning Objective: 4, Incorporate ideas into a plan for facilitating the success of an EBP.
Topic/Concept: Facilitators of Evidence-Based Practice
Difficulty Level: Moderate
Skill Level: Applying

6. C
Rationale: EBP is expected to benefit the facility with the standardized care of patients, its anticipated patient outcomes, and value-based healthcare. This may also be tied to reimbursement for their performance. Patient-associated benefits of an EBP promote the belief that patients' treatment decisions are based on knowledge associated with what works and what does not work. The introduction of a newly patented device would not be identified as a benefit to EBP.
Chapter: 3
Learning Objective: 2, Describe models that promote the implementation of EBP in nursing practice.
Topic/Concept: Models to Promote Evidence-Based Practice in Nursing
Difficulty Level: Moderate
Skill Level: Understanding

7. A
Rationale: There is a hierarchy of evidence that ranks the results from a systematic review of randomized controlled trials (RCT) as the highest to the least high level of evidence, which is a consensus opinion. A RCT is the best type of an interventional research design that provides knowledge for a cause-and-effect relationship, while a systematic review of RCTs is a synthesis of a collection of RCT studies with similar interventions. A single study, consensus of opinion, and case-controlled studies are not considered as the highest of the hierarchy of evidence for practice decisions.
Chapter: 3
Learning Objective: 2, Describe models that promote the implementation of EBP in nursing practice.
Topic/Concept: Models to Promote Evidence-Based Practice in Nursing
Difficulty Level: Moderate
Skill Level: Understanding

8. A
Rationale: A care bundle is a series of interventions to reduce the incidence of a disease or condition. They have been used to reduce the incidence of a problem-focused trigger. There is no information to support where care bundles have been used or for what purpose other than to reduce the incidence of a problem-focused trigger.
Chapter: 3
Learning Objective: 2, Describe models that promote the implementation of EBP in nursing practice.
Topic/Concept: Models to Promote Evidence-Based Practice in Nursing
Difficulty Level: Moderate
Skill Level: Understanding

9. B
Rationale: A significant barrier is that there are inadequate numbers of research studies from clinical trials that have compared patient outcomes from new innovative strategies with usual care. Adequate literature reviews, epidemiological databases, or the lack of case studies have not been identified as barriers to EBP.

Chapter: 3
Learning Objective: 3, Identify barriers that could challenge the effective implementation of an EBP.
Topic/Concept: Barriers Associated with EBP
Difficulty Level: Easy
Skill Level: Understanding

10. A
Rationale: Most EBP guidelines have been generated from population-based data. This means that some of the guidelines may not be considered practical for many patients who require individualized healthcare plans because of their unique needs. It is unlikely that CGs are based on old research studies. CGs are considered the gold standard of care. CGs are challenged.
Chapter: 3
Learning Objective: 3, Identify barriers that could challenge the effective implementation of an EBP.
Topic/Concept: Barriers Associated with EBP
Difficulty Level: Moderate
Skill Level: Understanding

11. B
Rationale: Librarians assist with the acquisition of relevant literature from dedicated nursing databases. Librarians will not interpret research data, create outlines for EBP, or provide a rubric to evaluate the evidence for the EBP.
Chapter: 3
Learning Objective: 4, Incorporate ideas into a plan for facilitating the success of an EBP.
Topic/Concept: Facilitators of Evidence-Based Practice
Difficulty Level: Easy
Skill Level: Applying

12. A
Rationale: Schools of nursing have professors who can partner with councils and committees to support the nursing staff and serve as mentors or EBP facilitators. It is unlikely that the professors will establish the budgets, recommend changes in the agency's vision, mission, and goals, or contribute to the agency's journal clubs.
Chapter: 3
Learning Objective: 4, Incorporate ideas into a plan for facilitating the success of an EBP.
Topic/Concept: Facilitators of Evidence-Based Practice
Difficulty Level: Easy
Skill Level: Applying

Chapter 4

1. A
Rationale: Atrocities committed for the sake of research may be found by searching the Nuremberg Trials. The Nuremberg Trials were not triggered by abuses committed on military prisoners in Japan or labor camps in Germany. The need to establish guidelines for researchers would be a positive activity.
Chapter: 4
Learning Objective: 1, Summarize the development of ethical codes and guidelines.
Topic/Concept: Development of Ethical Codes and Guidelines
Difficulty Level: Easy
Skill Level: Remembering

2. B
Rationale: In 1995, six former members of the Japanese biological warfare unit published a book, *The Truth about Unit 731*, to tell about the atrocities they had seen or heard about. Tuskegee Study, the Nuremberg Code, and the Universal Declaration of Human Rights do not focus on the biological warfare experiments conducted in Japan during World War II.
Chapter: 4
Learning Objective: 1, Summarize the development of ethical codes and guidelines.

Topic/Concept: Development of Ethical Codes and Guidelines
Difficulty Level: Easy
Skill Level: Remembering

3. D
Rationale: The three basic principles related to research subjects from the Belmont report are: respect for persons, beneficence, and justice. The Belmont Report did not generate information about informed consent, risk assessments, voluntary consent, conflict of interest, avoid injury, promote benefit, or the Universal Declaration of Human Rights.
Chapter: 4
Learning Objective: 1, Summarize the development of ethical codes and guidelines.
Topic/Concept: Development of Ethical Codes and Guidelines
Difficulty Level: Easy
Skill Level: Remembering

4. B
Rationale: Any institution that receives federal money for research must abide by the DHHS guidelines or risk losing federal money. This federal policy does not address scholarship money, vulnerable human subjects, or the Office of Human Research and Protections.
Chapter: 4
Learning Objective: 1, Summarize the development of ethical codes and guidelines.
Topic/Concept: Development of Ethical Codes and Guidelines
Difficulty Level: Easy
Skill Level: Remembering

5. C
Rationale: IRB approval is a necessity for investigators who wish to do research with human subjects. An intervention on an object does not need IRB approval. A change to a protocol would not need IRB approval. An investigation on outcomes collected by the electronic health record would not need IRB approval.
Chapter: 4
Learning Objective: 2, Describe the role of institutional review boards.
Topic/Concept: Institutional Review Boards
Difficulty Level: Moderate
Skill Level: Analyzing

6. A
Rationale: Attributes associated with QI relate to improvements in healthcare that are not consistently being implemented at a specific site. QI projects would not be more focused on new knowledge that can be translated to other populations of patients. QI projects would not focus on human subjects and their families' concerns. QI projects would not be focused on curing a patient with a complex situation.
Chapter: 4
Learning Objective: 2, Describe the role of institutional review boards.
Topic/Concept: Institutional Review Boards
Difficulty Level: Moderate
Skill Level: Understanding

7. C
Rationale: A full review with a quorum of the IRB voting for approval of the study would be expected for a research study that involves more than minimal risks to the participant. This type of IRB review would be necessary if the study included members from a vulnerable population such as pregnant women, children, fetuses, and infants. A research study could be identified as exempt from requiring IRB review when educational testing or survey procedures do not link the subjects' responses with their identities and the disclosure of their data could not reasonably place the subjects at risk of harm. An expedited review would include a research study protocol that might cause minimal risk to a participant who may identify one's self while responding to survey questions that may relate to somewhat sensitive material. Regular is not a type of review.

Chapter: 4
Learning Objective: 2, Describe the role of institutional review boards.
Topic/Concept: Institutional Review Boards
Difficulty Level: Moderate
Skill Level: Analyzing

8. D
Rationale: A required element of informed consent for a research subject is a statement that describes how the participant's information will be kept confidential. A statement that describes corporate rewards, rationales for the study, or expected results are not required elements of informed consent for a research subject.
Chapter: 4
Learning Objective: 3, Cite examples for the elements of informed consent.
Topic/Concept: Elements of Informed Consent
Difficulty Level: Moderate
Skill Level: Applying

9. A
Rationale: To maintain confidentiality, data are coded and subjects' names and code numbers are kept in a separate location that is accessible only to the researcher or members of the research team. Any list that links subject names with data should be destroyed at the conclusion of the study. Coding of the data is not a part of informed consent. Anonymity occurs when no one, including the researcher, can link subjects with the data they provide. Coding the data is not used to ensure data security.
Chapter: 4
Learning Objective: 3, Cite examples for the elements of informed consent.
Topic/Concept: Elements of Informed Consent
Difficulty Level: Moderate
Skill Level: Applying

10. B
Rationale: Anonymity occurs when no one, including the researcher, can link subjects with the data they provide. In many studies, it is not possible to maintain anonymity. Subjects should be provided with informed consent, confidentiality, and privacy.
Chapter: 4
Learning Objective: 3, Cite examples for the elements of informed consent.
Topic/Concept: Elements of Informed Consent
Difficulty Level: Moderate
Skill Level: Applying

11. A
Rationale: If the subject is a minor or is not able to give informed consent because of mental or physical disability, that subject may provide assent to participate in the study. The child's parents or legal guardians provide informed consent. The terms "consent of a minor" and "minor agreement" are not used.
Chapter: 4
Learning Objective: 3, Cite examples for the elements of informed consent.
Topic/Concept: Elements of Informed Consent
Difficulty Level: Easy
Skill Level: Remembering

12. C
Rationale: Research subjects should always be given the opportunity to obtain the study results. This does not mean that a copy must be sent to all participants. In fact, many participants are not interested in the results. A comment such as "A copy of the study results may be obtained by writing or calling the researcher" should be included. The approximate date when results will be available should also be provided. There is no federal regulation that requires researchers to send a copy of the study results to all participants. There is no firm date when study results should be available to the participants.
Chapter: 4
Learning Objective: 3, Cite examples for the elements of informed consent.

Topic/Concept: Elements of Informed Consent
Difficulty Level: Moderate
Skill Level: Applying

13. A
Rationale: The ANA Code of Ethics for Nurses affirms that the research nurse's role as a patient advocate should include assurances of the fulfillment of human rights through the process of ongoing informed consent, continual assessment of risk versus benefit for research participants, and the prevention of harm. The participant should understand that participation can end at any time. The nurse needs to do more than document adverse events. The nurse researcher would ensure that the IRB has approved the study.
Chapter: 4
Learning Objective: 6, Explain the role of the nurse researcher as a patient advocate.
Topic/Concept: Research Guidelines for Nurses
Difficulty Level: Moderate
Skill Level: Applying

14. B
Rationale: Data fabrication refers to making up data for the purpose of deception. Data falsification refers to the willful distortion of the results of the study or the reported collection of the data. Plagiarism refers to the near or verbatim copying of texts or ideas without identifying the original source of the citation. A ghostwriter is someone who authors a text that is credited to another person.
Chapter: 4
Learning Objective: 5, Analyze issues that threaten integrity in research among nurse researchers.
Topic/Concept: Integrity in Research
Difficulty Level: Moderate
Skill Level: Analyzing

15. D
Rationale: The Office of Research Integrity (ORI) is supported by the U.S. Public Health Services (PHS). This organization promotes integrity in biomedical and behavioral research among institutions that receive research funds from the PHS. The ORI has jurisdiction over allegations of research misconduct that are deemed to be credible and significant. The federal agency for the HIPAA privacy rule, the American Nurses Association and the Nursing and Midwifery Council are not responsible for investigating research misconduct.
Learning Objective: 5, Analyze issues that threaten integrity in research among nurse researchers.
Topic/Concept: Integrity in Research
Difficulty Level: Moderate
Skill Level: Analyzing

16. A
Rationale: Conflict of interest (COI) in research may occur when nurses receive payments from companies that also sponsor their research. When the research is associated with the use of a company's product, there is a risk that this type of relationship could create a bias that relates to the results and dissemination of the findings of the study. Waiting for authorization to use health data, asking a colleague to be a co-author, or disclosing a financial relationship with an industrial manufacturer are not examples of conflict of interest.
Chapter: 4
Learning Objective: 5, Analyze issues that threaten integrity in research among nurse researchers.
Topic/Concept: Integrity in Research
Difficulty Level: Moderate
Skill Level: Analyzing

17. C
Rationale: Advocacy is defined as "the act or process of pleading for, supporting or recommending a cause or a course of action." The research nurse's role as a patient advocate should include assurances of the fulfillment of human rights through the process of ongoing informed consent, continual assessment of risk versus benefit for research participants, and the prevention of harm. Taking extra time to explain more about the details of a study is an example of advocacy. A patient should not be reported for failing to comply with

the expectations of a study. The patient can refuse to participate at any time. The nurse should not discuss any information about other participants. The participants should not be treated as personal friends.
Chapter: 4
Learning Objective: 6, Explain the role of the nurse researcher as a patient advocate.
Topic/Concept: Research Guidelines for Nurses
Difficulty Level: Moderate
Skill Level: Analyzing

18. B
Rationale: Nurses who are not a part of the research team should familiarize themselves with any clinical trials that are being conducted in their work setting in order to be aware if a participant should want to withdraw from participating in the study. Making the care of the patient a priority over the research interventions is not advocacy. This is quality care. Witnessing the informed consent is not advocacy. Data collection is not advocating for the patient.
Chapter: 4
Learning Objective: 6, Explain the role of the nurse researcher as a patient advocate.
Topic/Concept: Research Guidelines for Nurses
Difficulty Level: Moderate
Skill Level: Applying

Chapter 5

1. False
Rationale: The researcher should select a research method because it is best suited to answer the research question. The research should always drive the choice of method, not vice versa.
Chapter: 5
Learning Objective: 1, Differentiate between qualitative and quantitative research.
Topic/Concept: Comparison of Qualitative and Quantitative Research
Difficulty Level: Moderate
Skill Level: Applying

2. False
Rationale: In qualitative research, the researcher often lets the story or participant experience unfold naturally and does not exert control over the study, as would be common in a quantitative or experimental study.
Chapter: 5
Learning Objective: 1, Differentiate between qualitative and quantitative research.
Topic/Concept: Comparison of Qualitative and Quantitative Research
Difficulty Level: Easy
Skill Level: Remembering

3. False
Rationale: With most studies, the researcher should adapt the research in the way that best answers the research question. As long as there is fidelity to concepts of rigor, the steps can be adapted as needed.
Chapter: 5
Learning Objective: 2, Summarize the steps in quantitative research.
Topic/Concept: Steps in Quantitative Research
Difficulty Level: Easy
Skill Level: Remembering

4. True
Rationale: Many research questions are well-suited for study using a mixed methods approach. Using a mixed method or multiple-methods approach allows the researcher to explore a problem from the most comprehensive point of view.
Chapter: 5
Learning Objective: 3, Explain the use of both qualitative and quantitative research methods in a single study.
Topic/Concept: Combining Qualitative and Quantitative Methods

5. False
   Rationale: Generalizability is not a goal of qualitative research.
   Chapter: 5
   Learning Objective: 1, Differentiate between qualitative and quantitative research.
   Topic/Concept: Qualitative Nursing Research
   Difficulty Level: Moderate
   Skill Level: Understanding

6. False
   Rationale: Qualitative studies often have small sample sizes when compared with quantitative or experimental studies.
   Chapter: 5
   Learning Objective: 1, Differentiate between qualitative and quantitative research.
   Topic/Concept: Qualitative Nursing Research
   Difficulty Level: Easy
   Skill Level: Remembering

7. True
   Rationale: Research is not considered complete until the study results are disseminated.
   Chapter: 5
   Learning Objective: 1, Differentiate between qualitative and quantitative research.
   Topic/Concept: Steps in Quantitative Research
   Difficulty Level: Moderate
   Skill Level: Understanding

8. D
   Rationale: Both qualitative and quantitative methods require hard work and attention to detail. The amount of data may vary widely among studies, regardless of the type. The time needed to collect data can vary widely among studies, regardless of the type. In qualitative research, the individual's perspective is very important, whereas in quantitative research, the focus is on the group or population of interest, rather than the individual.
   Chapter: 5
   Learning Objective: 1, Differentiate between qualitative and quantitative research.
   Topic/Concept: Qualitative Nursing Research
   Difficulty Level: Moderate
   Skill Level: Applying

9. B
   Rationale: Any of these responses would be correct for a mixed methods study but for a qualitative study, nonparticipant observations and semi-structured interviews should be used. Closed-ended questions are not useful during a qualitative study. Structured interviews would not be appropriate for a qualitative study. Physiologic measures are more suited to quantitative study. Closed-ended questions and structured interviews are not useful during a qualitative study.
   Chapter: 5
   Learning Objective: 1, Differentiate between qualitative and quantitative research.
   Topic/Concept: Qualitative Nursing Research
   Difficulty Level: Difficult
   Skill Level: Analyzing

10. A
    Rationale: Mixed methods studies involve both qualitative and quantitative methods. Meta-analysis involves examination of data from several studies. Multitrait, multimethod, and methodological plurality are terms that are not commonly accepted in research as descriptive of method.
    Chapter: 5
    Learning Objective: 3, Explain the use of both qualitative and quantitative research methods in a single study.
    Topic/Concept: Combining Qualitative and Quantitative Methods
    Difficulty Level: Easy
    Skill Level: Remembering

Self-Test Answers   **339**

Chapter 6

1. B
   Rationale: The dependent variable is missing. The population and independent variable are present.
   Chapter: 6
   Learning Objective: 3, Compare the criteria to be considered when writing a research question.
   Topic/Concept: Research Question Criteria
   Difficulty Level: Moderate
   Skill Level: Analyzing

2. D
   Rationale: In this statement, the dependent variable is body surface area. The independent variables are weight training and aerobic exercise. The population is men.
   Chapter: 6
   Learning Objective: 3, Compare the criteria to be considered when writing a research question.
   Topic/Concept: Research Question Criteria
   Difficulty Level: Moderate
   Skill Level: Analyzing

3. A
   Rationale: In this statement, the population is missing. Anxiety is the independent variable. Quality of life is the dependent variable.
   Chapter: 6
   Learning Objective: 3, Compare the criteria to be considered when writing a research question.
   Topic/Concept: Research Question Criteria
   Difficulty Level: Moderate
   Skill Level: Analyzing

4. A
   Rationale: The population being studied is missing. The dependent variable is anxiety levels. The independent variable is the gender of the personal trainer.
   Chapter: 6
   Learning Objective: 3, Compare the criteria to be considered when writing a research question.
   Topic/Concept: Research Question Criteria
   Difficulty Level: Moderate
   Skill Level: Analyzing

5. C
   Rationale: Correlational studies do not provide cause and effect findings. Either the independent or dependent variable could be missing. For example, the independent variable could be age and the dependent variable could be experience, or the independent variable could be experience and the dependent variable could be number of patients. The population is personal trainers.
   Chapter: 6
   Learning Objective: 3, Compare the criteria to be considered when writing a research question.
   Topic/Concept: Research Question Criteria
   Difficulty Level: Moderate
   Skill Level: Analyzing

6. B
   Rationale: There are two variables of interest in this study. The dependent variable is quality of life. The independent variable is the type of treatment for renal disease.
   Chapter: 6
   Learning Objective: 3, Compare the criteria to be considered when writing a research question.
   Topic/Concept: Research Question Criteria
   Difficulty Level: Moderate
   Skill Level: Analyzing

7. A
   Rationale: The dependent variable is infection rate. The population is patients receiving hemodialysis.

Chapter: 6
Learning Objective: 3, Compare the criteria to be considered when writing a research question.
Topic/Concept: Research Question Criteria
Difficulty Level: Moderate
Skill Level: Analyzing

8. C
Rationale: The dependent variables are weight, blood pressure, and dialysate. The independent variable is the type of dialysis treatment.
Chapter: 6
Learning Objective: 3, Compare the criteria to be considered when writing a research question.
Topic/Concept: Research Question Criteria
Difficulty Level: Moderate
Skill Level: Analyzing

9. D
Rationale: The dependent variable or how the patients are "different" is not explained or identified. The population is patients. They type of dialysis is the independent variable (either hemodialysis or peritoneal dialysis). This is not a univariate study.
Chapter: 6
Learning Objective: 3, Compare the criteria to be considered when writing a research question.
Topic/Concept: Research Question Criteria
Difficulty Level: Moderate
Skill Level: Analyzing

10. B
Rationale: There is not a cause and effect relationship in correlational studies. However, this study measures two variables. A dependent variable could be considered as level of fatigue. The independent variable could be considered as blood pressure. The population is patients having hemodialysis.
Chapter: 6
Learning Objective: 3, Compare the criteria to be considered when writing a research question.
Topic/Concept: Research Question Criteria
Difficulty Level: Moderate
Skill Level: Analyzing

Chapter 7

1. B
Rationale: There are many purposes for reviewing the literature before you conduct a research study, and the most important one is to find out what is already known about the topic in which you are interested. Research studies can be replicated. This adds more validity to the findings. Classic information can be a starting point for new research. All research studies need a literature review.
Chapter: 7
Learning Objective: 1, Explain the purpose of a literature review.
Topic/Concept: Purposes of the Literature Review
Difficulty Level: Easy
Skill Level: Understanding

2. C
Rationale: An article written by the researcher who conducted a study is a primary source, and an article written by someone summarizing and commenting on that study would be a secondary source. A secondary source may review one or more than one research study. Both are important in a literature review. A primary source is not a type of study that was first identified by the finding tool. All types of sources are included in literature reviews. A primary source is not a summary done on a study topic. A secondary source is a summary or description of a research study done by someone other than the original investigator.

Chapter: 7
Learning Objective: 2, Differentiate among primary and secondary sources and research articles and grey literature.
Topic/Concept: Literature Sources
Difficulty Level: Moderate
Skill Level: Analyzing

3. A
Rationale: Discovering whether the topic has already been researched is a reason to do a literature review. Writing a research question and thesis statement, determining a set of terms and phrases to use for your search, and considering whether your topic should include date parameters are all parts of building a search strategy.
Chapter: 7
Learning Objective: 3, Construct an effectively designed search strategy that includes a concise research question.
Topic/Concept: Search Strategies
Difficulty Level: Moderate
Skill Level: Applying

4. D
Rationale: You can ask for assistance by visiting, emailing, and making an appointment—but occasionally librarians do sleep.
Chapter: 7
Learning Objective: 3, Construct an effectively designed search strategy that includes a concise research question.
Topic/Concept: Search Strategies
Difficulty Level: Easy
Skill Level: Understanding

5. A
Rationale: Most research articles that appear in the journal *Nursing Research* are primary sources. There is no specific journal for secondary sources. Meta-analysis studies and systematic reviews can appear in all research journals.
Chapter: 7
Learning Objective: 2, Differentiate among primary and secondary sources and research articles and grey literature.
Topic/Concept: Literature Sources
Difficulty Level: Easy
Skill Level: Remembering

6. D
Rationale: The Cochrane Database of Systematic Reviews is a leading resource for systematic reviews in healthcare. MEDLINE provides access to journals in the life sciences, with a concentration on biomedicine. CINAHL provides indexing of the top nursing and allied health literature available, including nursing journals and publications from the National League for Nursing and the American Nurses Association Literature. It covers a wide range of topics including nursing, biomedicine, health sciences librarianship, alternative/complementary medicine, consumer health, and allied health disciplines.
Chapter: 7
Learning Objective: 5, Recognize differences in content and accessibility between nursing research databases.
Topic/Concept: Search Strategies
Difficulty Level: Moderate
Skill Level: Analyzing

7. C
Rationale: Databases, catalogs, and search engines are finding tools. Some online databases are available to the general public. Not all databases are online. Databases include other types of literature and search works that may or may not be published.

Chapter: 7
Learning Objective: 5, Recognize differences in content and accessibility between nursing research databases.
Topic/Concept: Search Strategies
Difficulty Level: Moderate
Skill Level: Analyzing

8. D
    Rationale: Grey literature (or gray literature) is included in some databases, but it is not published scholarly articles. Dissertations are examples of grey literature.
    Chapter: 7
    Learning Objective: 2, Differentiate among primary and secondary sources and research articles and grey literature.
    Topic/Concept: Literature Sources
    Difficulty Level: Easy
    Skill Level: Remembering

9. E
    Rationale: All of these questions will help critique a literature review.
    Chapter: 7
    Learning Objective: 6, Evaluate, analyze, and synthesize literature sources for inclusion in a literature review.
    Topic/Concept: Writing the Literature Review
    Difficulty Level: Moderate
    Skill Level: Applying

10. C
    Rationale: Google Scholar includes limiters and options that will allow you to modify and limit your search in order to retrieve authoritative relevant sources. Bing, Scirus, and Web Crawler are not identified as engines to find scholarly articles.
    Chapter: 7
    Learning Objective: 4, Conduct a comprehensive literature search on a given topic.
    Topic/Concept: Search Strategies
    Difficulty Level: Moderate
    Skill Level: Applying

Chapter 8

1. B
    Rationale: Conceptual models contain broad descriptions of abstract concepts and propositions of interest to nursing. A theoretical framework presents a broad, general explanation of the relationships between the concepts of interest in a research study; it is based on one existing theory. A conceptual framework helps explain the relationship between concepts by linking concepts selected from several theories from previous research results or from the researcher's own experiences. Practice models are not used to explain the relationship of concepts and propositions of interest in nursing.
    Chapter: 8
    Learning Objective: 1, Summarize the key terminology for nursing theory.
    Topic/Concept: Theory Terminology
    Difficulty Level: Easy
    Skill Level: Understanding

2. C
    Rationale: A paradigm is a worldview or a set of beliefs about nature and reality. Two examples of paradigms that have impacted nursing research are positivism and postpositivism. A theory is a set of related statements that describes or explains phenomena in a systematic way. A metaparadigm is a core set of concepts and constructs that are interdependent and uniquely defines a discipline. A framework for a research study helps organize the study and provides a context for the interpretation of the study findings.

Chapter: 8
Learning Objective: 1, Summarize the key terminology for nursing theory.
Topic/Concept: Theory Terminology
Difficulty Level: Easy
Skill Level: Understanding

3. D
Rationale: Empirical generalizations. When a similar pattern of events has been found in multiple studies, the pattern of events can be described as an empirical generalization. Critical social theory encourages examination of how individuals or groups of individuals are situated within a social context, and how a particular position in society affects the individual or group of individuals. Relationships among concepts are presented in theoretical statements, called propositional statements. Empirical generalizations summarize the results of several empirical studies.
Chapter: 8
Learning Objective: 1, Summarize the key terminology for nursing theory.
Topic/Concept: Theory Terminology
Difficulty Level: Easy
Skill Level: Understanding

4. C
Rationale: Death is not one of the four concepts of the metaparadigm of nursing. Person, environment, and health, and nursing are the comnmon concepts included in nearly all of the nursing conceptual models.
Chapter: 8
Learning Objective: 2, Compare types and distinguish scopes of nursing theories.
Topic/Concept: Types and Scope of Theories in Nursing Research
Difficulty Level: Easy
Skill Level: Understanding

5. C
Rationale: The health belief model is most appropriate because the nurse would be teaching the patient about healthy eating habits and would want to influence the patient's health beliefs. Anxiety theory would not help with dietary changes. Adult learning theory would focus on teaching and learning. Healthcare system model is not an identified theory.
Chapter: 8
Learning Objective: 2, Compare types and distinguish scopes of nursing theories.
Topic/Concept: Types and Scope of Theories in Nursing Research
Difficulty Level: Moderate
Skill Level: Applying

6. B
Rationale: The uncertainty in illness theory was developed by Mishel (1981, 1990). The social cognitive theory was developed by Bandura. The hierarchy of needs theory was developed by Maslow. The job satisfaction theory was developed by Herzberg.
Chapter: 8
Learning Objective: 3, Describe how theory is integrated into nursing research.
Topic/Concept: Integrating Theory into Nursing Research
Difficulty Level: Easy
Skill Level: Understanding

7. A
Rationale: Grand theories are broad in scope and have abstract constructs and propositions. Middle-range theories are concerned with only a small area of the environment or human experiences. Practice theories have the narrowest focus and produce specific nursing practice guidance for specific patient care situations.
Chapter: 8
Learning Objective: 3, Describe how theory is integrated into nursing research.
Topic/Concept: Integrating Theory into Nursing Research
Difficulty Level: Easy
Skill Level: Understanding

8. C
Rationale: The Health Promotion Model is a middle-range theory that is narrower in scope and contains propositional statements that are concrete and easily testable. Orem's Self-Care Deficit theory and Roy's Adaptation Model are examples of grand theories. Parse was an editor of the *Nursing Science Quarterly* publication.
Chapter: 8
Learning Objective: 3, Describe how theory is integrated into nursing research.
Topic/Concept: Integrating Theory into Nursing Research
Difficulty Level: Easy
Skill Level: Understanding

9. C
Rationale: Both inductive and deductive reasoning are used in the development of theory.
Chapter: 8
Learning Objective: 4, Summarize how nursing theory is developed, tested, and critiqued.
Topic/Concept: Theoretical Development, Testing, and Critique
Difficulty Level: Moderate
Skill Level: Applying

10. A
Rationale: Theory does not prove relationships among variables. It only explains and describes relationships among variables using propositional statements that link concepts.
Chapter: 8
Learning Objective: 4, Summarize how nursing theory is developed, tested, and critiqued.
Topic/Concept: Theoretical Development, Testing, and Critique
Difficulty Level: Moderate
Skill Level: Applying

Chapter 9

1. A
A hypothesis tells the reader what the researcher expects to discover about the relationship between the variables being measured. Answer B is incorrect because the hypothesis might be testing part of a theory; it does not define the theory. Answer C is incorrect because it will be congruent with the problem under study, it will not indicate the source of the problem. Answer D is incorrect because the concepts may be named in the hypothesis, but the hypothesis will not clarify or define the concepts.
Chapter: 9
Learning Objective: 1, Describe the role of hypotheses in research studies.
Topic/Concept: Hypotheses Overview
Difficulty Level: Moderate
Skill Level: Application

2. C
The hypothesis should reflect the main ideas of a theoretical framework. A hypothesis may test one or more propositional statements of a theory. Answer A is incorrect because all studies should have a theoretical framework. Answer B is incorrect because hypothesis and theoretical frameworks are tested. Answer D is incorrect because hypotheses are deductively identified from theoretical frameworks.
Chapter: 9
Learning Objective: 1, Describe the role of hypotheses in research studies.
Topic/Concept: Hypotheses Overview
Difficulty Level: Moderate
Skill Level: Application

3. B
The research question expresses the inquiry of the research problem and the hypothesis is a statement of prediction about what the outcome of the study will be. Answers A and D are incorrect because the research question and hypothesis are different, but related. Answer C is incorrect because the hypothesis is empirically tested.

Chapter: 9
Learning Objective: 1, Describe the role of hypotheses in research studies.
Topic/Concept: Hypotheses Overview
Difficulty Level: Moderate
Skill Level: Application

4. A

Gel pillows cause (causal) reduction (direction). Answer B is incorrect because reduction indicates direction. Answer C is incorrect because gel pillows will reduce is a causal statement. Answer D is incorrect because gel pillows will reduce is a causal statement; if this was an associative hypothesis, it would state that there is a relationship (or association) between use of gel pillows and bilateral head flattening, and reduction indicates direction.
Chapter: 9
Learning Objective: 2, Compare classifications of hypotheses.
Topic/Concept: Classification of Hypotheses
Difficulty Level: Difficult
Skill Level: Application

5. D

There is a relationship (associative) between the use of formula and incidence (no direction indicated) of necrotizing enterocolitis in premature infants. Answer A is incorrect because "There is a relationship" does not indicate causation, and "incidence" does not indicate and increase or decrease in necrotizing enterocolitis. Answer B is incorrect because "There is a relationship" does not indicate causation. Answer C is incorrect because "Incidence" does not indicate and increase or decrease in necrotizing enterocolitis.
Chapter: 9
Learning Objective: 2, Compare classifications of hypotheses.
Topic/Concept: Classification of Hypotheses
Difficulty Level: Difficult
Skill Level: Application

6. B

There are two dependent variables (job turnover rate and job dissatisfaction levels), and one independent variable (length of time in job), which makes the hypothesis complex. The word *higher* indicates direction, and the hypothesis is associative because the researchers are examining the relationship between length of time in job and turnover and satisfaction. Length of time in job does not cause job satisfaction or turnover. Answer A is simple, associative, directional. Answer C is causal (participation in support groups is an intervention that some mothers will get and others will not), directional, and complex. Answer D is associative, directional, and simple.
Chapter: 9
Learning Objective: 2, Compare classifications of hypotheses.
Topic/Concept: Classification of Hypotheses
Difficulty Level: Difficult
Skill Level: Application

7. D

Delayed bath (independent variable) has an effect on breastfeeding attempts (dependent variable), the expected direction of the relationship is not stated, and the hypothesis is testing one independent and one dependent variable. A is incorrect because the hypothesis is causal, complex and directional. B is incorrect because the hypothesis is causal, simple, directional. C is incorrect because the hypothesis is associative, directional, simple.
Chapter: 9
Learning Objective: 2, Compare classifications of hypotheses.
Topic/Concept: Classification of Hypotheses
Difficulty Level: Difficult
Skill Level: Application

8. C

Anxiety is a dependent variable because the measurement of this variable will determine the effect that structured, perioperative support has on the patient's perception of pain. Answer A is incorrect because

the independent variable in this hypothesis is "preoperative pain medication education," which is the manipulated variable. Answers B and D are incorrect because no extraneous or confounding variables are identified in the hypothesis.
Learning Objective: 3, Describe the considerations when developing hypotheses.
Topic/Concept: Developing Hypotheses
Difficulty Level: Difficult
Skill Level: Application

9. A, C, and D
These three are requirements of the structure of a hypothesis. Answer B is incorrect because hypotheses should be written as statements.
Chapter: 9
Learning Objective: 3, Describe the considerations when developing hypotheses.
Topic/Concept: Developing Hypotheses
Difficulty Level: Moderate
Skill Level: Application

10. C
The hypothesis is a declarative statement that includes the independent and dependent variable, the population of interest, and indicates the direction of the anticipated relationship. Answer A is incorrect because it does not indicate the direction of the anticipated relationship. Answer B is incorrect because it is phrased as a question and does not indicate the direction of the anticipated relationship. Answer D is incorrect because it is phrased as a question.
Chapter 9
Learning Objective: 3, Describe the considerations when developing hypotheses.
Topic/Concept: Developing Hypotheses
Difficulty Level: Moderate
Skill Level: Application

Chapter 10

1. C
Rationale: The selection bias threat occurs when study results are attributed to the experimental treatment or the researcher's manipulation of the independent variable when, in fact, the results are related to subject differences before the independent variable was manipulated. The threat of history occurs when some event besides the experimental treatment occurs during the course of a study, and this event influences the dependent variable. Testing refers to the influence of the pretest or knowledge of baseline data on the post-test scores. The Hawthorne effect occurs when study participants respond in a certain manner because they are aware that they are being observed.
Chapter: 10
Learning Outcome: 2, Distinguish between the types of internal and external valdity and threats to each seen in experimental designs.
Topic/Concept: Experimental Research
Difficulty Level: Moderate
Skill Level: Analyzing

2. B
Rationale: Testing refers to the influence of the pretest or knowledge of baseline data on the posttest scores. The threat of history occurs when some event besides the experimental treatment occurs during the course of a study, and this event influences the dependent variable. The selection bias threat occurs when study results are attributed to the experimental treatment or the researcher's manipulation of the independent variable when, in fact, the results are related to subject differences before the independent variable was manipulated. The Hawthorne effect occurs when study participants respond in a certain manner because they are aware that they are being observed.
Chapter: 10
Learning Outcome: 2, Distinguish between the types of internal and external valdity and threats to each seen in experimental designs.

Topic/Concept: Experimental Research
Difficulty Level: Moderate
Skill Level: Analyzing

3. D
   Rationale: The Hawthorne effect occurs when study participants respond in a certain manner because they are aware that they are being observed. The threat of history occurs when some event besides the experimental treatment occurs during the course of a study, and this event influences the dependent variable. Testing refers to the influence of the pretest or knowledge of baseline data on the posttest scores. The selection bias threat occurs when study results are attributed to the experimental treatment or the researcher's manipulation of the independent variable when, in fact, the results are related to subject differences before the independent variable was manipulated.
   Chapter: 10
   Learning Outcome: 2, Distinguish between the types of internal and external valdity and threats to each seen in experimental designs.
   Topic/Concept: Experimental Research
   Difficulty Level: Moderate
   Skill Level: Analyzing

4. D
   Rationale: The Rosenthal effect is used to indicate the influence of an interviewer on respondents' answers. It has been shown that researcher characteristics such as gender, dress, and type of jewelry may influence study participants' answers to questions in nonexperimental studies. The threat of history occurs when some event besides the experimental treatment occurs during the course of a study, and this event influences the dependent variable. Testing refers to the influence of the pretest or knowledge of baseline data on the posttest scores. The selection bias threat occurs when study results are attributed to the experimental treatment or the researcher's manipulation of the independent variable when, in fact, the results are related to subject differences before the independent variable was manipulated.
   Chapter: 10
   Learning Outcome: 2, Distinguish between the types of internal and external valdity and threats to each seen in experimental designs.
   Topic/Concept: Experimental Research
   Difficulty Level: Moderate
   Skill Level: Analyzing

5. A
   Rationale: The threat of history occurs when some event besides the experimental treatment occurs during the course of a study, and this event influences the dependent variable. Testing refers to the influence of the pretest or knowledge of baseline data on the posttest scores. The selection bias threat occurs when study results are attributed to the experimental treatment or the researcher's manipulation of the independent variable when, in fact, the results are related to subject differences before the independent variable was manipulated. The Rosenthal effect is used to indicate the influence of an interviewer on respondents' answers. It has been shown that researcher characteristics such as gender, dress, and type of jewelry may influence study participants' answers to questions in nonexperimental studies.
   Chapter: 10
   Learning Outcome: 2, Distinguish between the types of internal and external valdity and threats to each seen in experimental designs.
   Topic/Concept: Experimental Research
   Difficulty Level: Moderate
   Skill Level: Analyzing

6. C
   Rationale: One criterion for true experiemental research is the random assignment of subjects to groups. Quasi-experimental designs are those in which there is either no comparison group or subjects are not randomly assigned to groups. Sample size, nonprobability sample, or an experimental treatment does not distinguish true experimental research from quasi-experimental research.

Chapter: 10
Learning Outcome: 3, Distinguish among true, quasi- and pre-experimental designs.
Topic/Concept: Types of Experimental Designs
Difficulty Level: Moderate
Skill Level: Analyzing

7. A
Rationale: In this study there is no control group however there is a pretest and posttest. A pretest would be needed to determine if the exercises made an impact. This is not a case study.
Chapter: 10
Learning Outcome: 3, Distinguish among true, quasi- and pre-experimental designs.
Topic/Concept: Types of Experimental Designs
Difficulty Level: Difficult
Skill Level: Analyzing

8. B
Rationale: The Solomon four-group design controls for the reactive effects of the pretest. Sensitization to the pretest canoccur in the pretest-posttest control group design. In a one-shot case study, a single group is exposed to an experimental treatment and observed after the treatment. In a time-series design, the researcher periodically observes or measures the subjects. The experimental treatment is administered between two of the observations.
Chapter: 10
Learning Outcome: 3, Distinguish among true, quasi- and pre-experimental designs.
Topic/Concept: Types of Experimental Designs
Difficulty Level: Difficult
Skill Level: Applying

9. D
Rationale: The threat of history occurs when some event besides the experimental treatment occurs during the course of a study, and this event influences the dependent variable. The researcher may not be able to determine if the teaching about a heart attack or the CDC report influenced the participants. It is unclear if the television celebrity did any teaching about how the heart functions. People dropping out of the study will not be the greatest affect to this study's validity. A change in the price of a heart model will not affect the validity of the study.
Chapter: 10
Learning Outcome: 2, Distinguish between the types of internal and external valdity and threats to each seen in experimental designs.
Topic/Concept: Experimental Research
Difficulty Level: Difficult
Skill Level: Analyzing

10. C
Rationale: Quasi-experimental designs are those in which there is either no comparison group or subjects are not randomly assigned to groups. Administering a pretest, using random sampling, and using a longitudinal design will not influence the use of a true experimental design.
Chapter: 10
Learning Outcome: 3, Distinguish among true, quasi- and pre-experimental designs.
Topic/Concept: Types of Experimental Designs
Difficulty Level: Difficult
Skill Level: Applying

Chapter 11

1. False
Rationale: This is a description of grounded theory. Phenomenological studies examine human experiences through the descriptions provided by the people involved.
Chapter: 11
Module: 1

Learning Objective: 1, Summarize the important features of six common types of qualitative designs.
Topic/Concept: Qualitative Research Designs
Difficulty Level: Easy
Skill Level: Remembering

2. False
Rationale: This is a description of bracketing. Reflexivity is required for effective bracketing.
Chapter: 11
Learning Objective: 1, Summarize the important features of six common types of qualitative designs.
Topic/Concept: Qualitative Research Designs
Difficulty Level: Easy
Skill Level: Remembering

3. True
Rationale: Ethnography is a form of qualitative research that focuses on social relationships and the context in which they occur
Chapter: 11
Learning Objective: 1, Summarize the important features of six common types of qualitative designs.
Topic/Concept: Qualitative Research Designs
Difficulty Level: Easy
Skill Level: Remembering

4. True
Rationale: When a researcher is interested in an area in which little research has been done or in which existing theories are not sufficient, grounded theory studies are a good choice. The outcome of a grounded theory study is a theory that is grounded in data from the study.
Chapter: 11
Learning Objective: 1, Summarize the important features of six common types of qualitative designs.
Topic/Concept: Qualitative Research Designs
Difficulty Level: Moderate
Skill Level: Applying

5. True
Rationale: In grounded theory, data analysis is done using the constant comparison method where data are constantly compared to data that have already been gathered.
Chapter: 11
Learning Objective: 1, Summarize the important features of six common types of qualitative designs.
Topic/Concept: Qualitative Research Designs
Difficulty Level: Moderate
Skill Level: Applying

6. False
Rationale: Generally speaking, qualitative studies have a smaller sample size.
Chapter: 11
Learning Objective: 1, Summarize the important features of six common types of qualitative designs.
Topic/Concept: Qualitative Research Designs
Difficulty Level: Easy
Skill Level: Remembering

7. True
Rationale: Because healthcare is complex, mixed methods research is increasingly popular as a way to explore complex problems that influence health and health outcomes.
Chapter: 11
Learning Objective: 2, Discuss the main principles and purposes that guide researchers to use more than one method.
Topic/Concept: Mixed Methods Research
Difficulty Level: Easy
Skill Level: Remembering

8. B
   Rationale: The sequential exploratory strategy involves an initial period of qualitative data collection and analysis followed by a quantative data collection and analysis. Purposive sampling involves choosing participants who can fill in gaps in the data. Concurrent triangulation involves collecting qualitative and qualitative data simultaneously. Sequential exploratory strategy involves an initial period of qualitative data collection and analysis followed by a quantative data collection and analysis
   Chapter: 11
   Learning Objective: 3, Describe the strategies a researcher might use in a mixed method study.
   Topic/Concept: Strategies for Mixed Methods Research
   Difficulty Level: Moderate
   Skill Level: Applying

9. B
   Rationale: In qualitative studies, participant observations and semistructured interviews are the data collection methods most likely to be considered. Closed-ended questions, structured interviews, and physiologic measures are most appropriate for quantitative studies.
   Chapter: 11
   Learning Objective: 1, Summarize the important features of six common types of qualitative designs.
   Topic/Concept: Qualitative Research Designs
   Difficulty Level: Difficult
   Skill Level: Applying

10. C
    Rationale: Phenomenology is interested in the lived experiences of participants. When a researcher is interested in an area in which little research has been done or in which existing theories are not sufficient, grounded theory studies are a good choice. Action research is a type of qualitative research that actively engages the community of interest in solving a problem. Case studies are in-depth examinations of people or groups of people.
    Chapter: 11
    Learning Objective: 1, Summarize the important features of six common types of qualitative designs.
    Topic/Concept: Qualitative Research Designs
    Difficulty Level: Moderate
    Skill Level: Applying

Chapter 12

1. False
   Rationale: Simple random sample is the most unbiased of the probability methods.
   Chapter: 12
   Learning Objective: 1, Summarize the concepts related to populations and samples in research design.
   Topic/Concept: Populations
   Difficulty Level: Moderate
   Skill Level: Applying

2. False
   Rationale: In nonprobability sampling, the sample elements are chosen from the population by nonrandom methods. Nonrandom methods of sampling are more likely to produce a biased sample than are random methods.
   Chapter: 12
   Learning Objective: 1, Summarize the concepts related to populations and samples in research design.
   Topic/Concept: Populations
   Difficulty Level: Moderate
   Skill Level: Analyzing

3. True
   Rationale: Although researchers are always interested in populations, an entire population is generally not used in a research study. The researcher probably cannot gain access to a population of potential research participants. Also, the accuracy gained when all members are included is often not worth the time and money involved.

Chapter: 12
Learning Objective: 2, Differentiate among various types of probability and nonprobability sampling methods.
Topic/Concept: Samples and Sampling
Difficulty Level: Moderate
Skill Level: Applying

4. True
   Rationale: A sampling frame is a listing of all elements of a population.
   Chapter: 12
   Learning Objective: 2, Differentiate among various types of probability and nonprobability sampling methods.
   Topic/Concept: Samples and Sampling
   Difficulty Level: Moderate
   Skill Level: Applying

5. A
   Rationale: Convenience sampling is also referred to as accidental or incidental, and involves choosing readily available people or objects for a study.
   Chapter: 12
   Learning Objective: 2, Differentiate among various types of probability and nonprobability sampling methods.
   Topic/Concept: Samples and Sampling
   Difficulty Level: Moderate
   Skill Level: Applying

6. B
   Rationale: In cluster random sampling, large groups, or clusters, become the sampling units.
   Chapter: 12
   Learning Objective: 2, Differentiate among various types of probability and nonprobability sampling methods.
   Topic/Concept: Samples and Sampling
   Difficulty Level: Moderate
   Skill Level: Applying

7. F
   Rationale: Snowball sampling describes a method of sampling that involves the assistance of study subjects to help obtain other potential subjects.
   Chapter: 12
   Learning Objective: 2, Differentiate among various types of probability and nonprobability sampling methods.
   Topic/Concept: Samples and Sampling
   Difficulty Level: Moderate
   Skill Level: Applying

8. C
   Rationale: Systematic random sampling involves selecting every kth element of the population, such as every fifth, eighth, or twenty-first element.
   Chapter: 12
   Learning Objective: 2, Differentiate among various types of probability and nonprobability sampling methods.
   Topic/Concept: Samples and Sampling
   Difficulty Level: Moderate
   Skill Level: Applying

9. E
   Rationale: Simple random sampling is a type of probability sampling method that ensures each element of the population has an equal and independent chance of being chosen.

352 Self-Test Answers

Chapter: 12
Learning Objective: 2, Differentiate among various types of probability and nonprobability sampling methods.
Topic/Concept: Samples and Sampling
Difficulty Level: Moderate
Skill Level: Applying

10. D
Rationale: Quota sampling is similar to stratified random sampling, in that the first step involves dividing the population into homogeneous strata and selecting sample elements from each of these strata.
Chapter: 12
Learning Objective: 2, Differentiate among various types of probability and nonprobability sampling methods.
Topic/Concept: Samples and Sampling
Difficulty Level: Moderate
Skill Level: Applying

Chapter 13

1. A
Rationale: Mutually exclusive means the categories are distinct from each other. The other choices do not provide categories that are distinct from each other.
Chapter: 13
Learning Objective: 1, Differentiate among the four levels of measurement.
Topic/Concept: Measurement
Difficulty Level: Moderate
Skill Level: Applying

2. C
Rationale: Data collected at the ratio level of measurement is considered the highest or most precise level of data. Rating pain on a scale provides the most precise data. The other choices are subjective and cannot be quantified.
Chapter: 13
Learning Objective: 1, Differentiate among the four levels of measurement.
Topic/Concept: Measurement
Difficulty Level: Moderate
Skill Level: Analyzing

3. B
Rationale: The amount of money is a bank account would be considered ratio data because it is possible to be zero. Temperature would be interval data. Age and weight would be nominal data.
Chapter: 13
Learning Objective: 1, Differentiate among the four levels of measurement.
Topic/Concept: Measurement
Difficulty Level: Moderate
Skill Level: Analyzing

4. A
Rationale: Anytime more than one person is involved in data collection, assurances must be made that the data are being gathered in the same manner. Training will be needed for the data collectors, and checks should be made on the reliability of the collected data. The data collectors are not being trained to promote the validity of the instruments, promote the correct level of measurement use, or to promote the statistical analysis of the data.
Chapter: 13
Learning Objective: 2, Compare data-collection methods and instruments.
Topic/Concept: Data-Collection Process
Difficulty Level: Moderate
Skill Level: Applying

5. C
    Rationale: An outcome measurement that is relevant and sensitive to nursing interventions is symptom management. Physical therapy is a different discipline. Infection is a disease process. Addiction is a health problem. Physical therapy, infection, and addiction would not be as relevant and sensitive to nursing interventions.
    Chapter: 13
    Learning Objective: 2, Compare data-collection methods and instruments.
    Topic/Concept: Data-Collection Process
    Difficulty Level: Moderate
    Skill Level: Analyzing

6. B
    Rationale: The stability reliability of an instrument refers to its consistency over time. Construct reliability is not a type of instrument reliability. Interrater is determined by the degree to which two or more independent raters or observers are in agreement. Internal consistency reliability, or scale homogeneity, addresses the extent to which all items on an instrument measure the same variable.
    Chapter: 13
    Learning Objective: 3, Compare and contrast the concepts of reliability and validity.
    Topic/Concept: Criteria for Selection of a Data-Collection Instrument
    Difficulty Level: Moderate
    Skill Level: Applying

7. D
    Rationale: Construct validity involves the measurement of a variable that is not directly observable. A construct cannot be directly observed, is not concrete, or composed of items directly related to each other.
    Chapter: 13
    Learning Objective: 3, Compare and contrast the concepts of reliability and validity.
    Topic/Concept: Criteria for Selection of a Data-Collection Instrument
    Difficulty Level: Moderate
    Skill Level: Analyzing

8. A
    Rationale: Factor analysis is a method used to identify clusters of related items on an instrument or scale. Predictive validity examines the ability of an instrument to predict behavior of subjects in the future. Concurrent validity compares an instrument's ability to obtain a measurement of participants' behavior that is comparable to some other criterion of that behavior. Known groups is a type of construct validity.
    Chapter: 13
    Learning Objective: 3, Compare and contrast the concepts of reliability and validity.
    Topic/Concept: Criteria for Selection of a Data-Collection Instrument
    Difficulty Level: Moderate
    Skill Level: Analyzing

9. B
    Rationale: The research report should include a description of the data collection instruments. The biographical information about the authors of the study is not a part of the research report. Information about the statistician or marital status of the participants are not included in the research report.
    Chapter: 13
    Learning Objective: 4, Explain the factors and issues that impact data collection.
    Topic/Concept: Utilizing the Data
    Difficulty Level: Moderate
    Skill Level: Applying

10. B
    Rationale: The research article should include if the instrument was tested for reliability when used with the sample. The research article does not need to include if permission to report on the validity of the instrument was obtained. The age of the instrument and the uses of the instrument are not a part of the research article.

Chapter: 13
Learning Objective: 4, Explain the factors and issues that impact data collection.
Topic/Concept: Utilizing the Data
Difficulty Level: Moderate
Skill Level: Applying

Chapter 14

1. B
   Rationale: During an interview, the subject is more likely to respond appropriately to the question. Interviews can be more expensive because they are labor-intensive. Data collectors need to be trained to conduct the interviews. Data is not easily collected through interviews.
   Chapter 14
   Learning Outcome: 2, Explain the important concepts in using interviews as a data-collection method.
   Topic/Concept: Interviews
   Difficulty Level: Medium
   Skill Level: Analyzing

2. C
   Rationale: The Delphi technique is a data-collection technique that employs several rounds of questions to seek a consensus on a particular topic from a group of experts. Projective technique is used when conducting a personality inventory. The observation method would not be appropriate for this research study. The semantic differential asks subjects to indicate their position or attitude about some concept along a continuum between two adjectives or phrases that are presented in relation to the concept being measured.
   Chapter 14
   Learning Outcome: 6, Compare and contrast other types of data-collection methodologies.
   Topic/Concept: Other Data Collection Methods
   Difficulty Level: Medium
   Skill Level: Applying

3. B
   Rationale: In a projective technique, individuals are presented with stimuli designed to be ambiguous. Responses reflect internal feelings of the subjects that are projected on the external stimuli. An attitude scale, self-report questionnaire, or an interview are not the most likely approaches to prevent participants from providing socially acceptable responses to questions.
   Chapter 14
   Learning Outcome: 5, Explain roles of physiological and psychological data-collection methods.
   Topic/Concept: Physiological and Psychological Measures
   Difficulty Level: Easy
   Skill Level: Understanding

4. D
   Rationale: The Likert scale asks the participant to respond to an item ranging from strongly agree to strongly disagree. In a projective technique, a respondent is presented with stimuli designed to be ambiguous or to have no definite meaning. The semantic differential asks subjects to indicate their position or attitude about some concept along a continuum between two adjectives or phrases that are presented in relation to the concept being measured. The Q sort is a means of obtaining data in which subjects sort statements into categories according to their attitudes toward, or rating of, the statements. The Delphi technique describes a data-collection technique that employs several rounds of questions to seek a consensus on a particular topic from a group of experts.
   Chapter 14
   Learning Outcome: 4, Compare the characteristics and implications of the Likert and the Semantic Differential attitude scales.
   Topic/Concept: Attitude Scales
   Difficulty Level: Medium
   Skill Level: Analyzing

5. A
Rationale: The semantic differential asks subjects to indicate their position or attitude about some concept along a continuum between two adjectives or phrases that are presented in relation to the concept being measured. In a projective technique, a respondent is presented with stimuli designed to be ambiguous or to have no definite meaning. The Q sort is a means of obtaining data in which subjects sort statements into categories according to their attitudes toward, or rating of, the statements. The Likert scale asks the participant to respond to an item ranging from strongly agree to strongly disagree. The Delphi technique describes a data-collection technique that employs several rounds of questions to seek a consensus on a particular topic from a group of experts.
Chapter 14
Learning Outcome: 4, Compare the characteristics and implications of the Likert and the Semantic Differential attitude scales.
Topic/Concept: Attitude Scales
Difficulty Level: Medium
Skill Level: Analyzing

6. C
Rationale: The Q sort is a means of obtaining data in which subjects sort statements into categories according to their attitudes toward, or rating of, the statements. The semantic differential asks subjects to indicate their position or attitude about some concept along a continuum between two adjectives or phrases that are presented in relation to the concept being measured. In a projective technique, a respondent is presented with stimuli designed to be ambiguous or to have no definite meaning. The Likert scale asks the participant to respond to an item ranging from strongly agree to strongly disagree. The Delphi technique describes a data-collection technique that employs several rounds of questions to seek a consensus on a particular topic from a group of experts.
Chapter 14
Learning Outcome: 6, Compare and contrast other types of data-collection methodologies.
Topic/Concept: Other Data Collection Methods
Difficulty Level: Medium
Skill Level: Analyzing

7. B
Rationale: In a projective technique, a respondent is presented with stimuli designed to be ambiguous or to have no definite meaning. The semantic differential asks subjects to indicate their position or attitude about some concept along a continuum between two adjectives or phrases that are presented in relation to the concept being measured. The Q sort is a means of obtaining data in which subjects sort statements into categories according to their attitudes toward, or rating of, the statements. The Likert scale asks the participant to respond to an item ranging from strongly agree to strongly disagree. The Delphi technique describes a data-collection technique that employs several rounds of questions to seek a consensus on a particular topic from a group of experts.
Chapter 14
Learning Outcome: 5, Explain roles of physiological and psychological data-collection methods.
Topic/Concept: Physiological and Psychological Measures
Difficulty Level: Medium
Skill Level: Analyzing

8. E
Rationale: The Delphi technique describes a data-collection technique that employs several rounds of questions to seek a consensus on a particular topic from a group of experts. The semantic differential asks subjects to indicate their position or attitude about some concept along a continuum between two adjectives or phrases that are presented in relation to the concept being measured. In a projective technique, a respondent is presented with stimuli designed to be ambiguous or to have no definite meaning. The Q sort is a means of obtaining data in which subjects sort statements into categories according to their attitudes toward, or rating of, the statements. The Likert scale asks the participant to respond to an item ranging from strongly agree to strongly disagree.
Chapter 14
Learning Outcome: 6, Compare and contrast other types of data-collection methodologies.

Topic/Concept: Other Data Collection Methods
Difficulty Level: Medium
Skill Level: Analyzing

Chapter 15

1. A
   Rationale: SD is the symbol for the standard deviation of a sample. Sigma is the symbol of the summation sign. μ is the symbol for the mean of a population measurement. X is the symbol for the mean of a sample measurement.
   Chapter: 15
   Learning Objective: 1, Summarize the key concepts related to statistical symbols and classification.
   Topic/Concept: Key Concepts in Statistics
   Difficulty Level: Easy
   Skill Level: Applying

2. B
   Rationale: The mode is the category or value that occurs most often in a set of data under consideration. 20/30 occurs most often in this set of data. 20/20 appears only one time. 20/40 appears twice. 20/100 appears only one time.
   Chapter: 15
   Learning Objective: 2, Compare the four classifications of descriptive statistics.
   Topic/Concept: Descriptive Statistics
   Difficulty Level: Easy
   Skill Level: Understanding

3. C
   Rationale: The mean represents the average sum of a set of values. The mode represents the most frequently occurring value of the data. The median represents the middle score or value in a group of data. Correlations describe how two variables vary.
   Chapter: 15
   Learning Objective: 2, Compare the four classifications of descriptive statistics.
   Topic/Concept: Descriptive Statistics
   Difficulty Level: Moderate
   Skill Level: Applying

4. D
   Rationale: Standard deviation is the average deviation or variation of all the values in a set of values from the mean value of those data. Skewness represents a nonsymmetrical distribution in which the distribution has an off-center peak. Correlations are measures of relationships between variables. Measures of central tendency are measures are statistics that describe the average, typical, or most common value for a group of data.
   Chapter: 15
   Learning Objective: 2, Compare the four classifications of descriptive statistics.
   Topic/Concept: Descriptive Statistics
   Difficulty Level: Easy
   Skill Level: Applying

5. B
   Rationale: Based on the information given the score is 2.5 SDs higher than the average or mean of the test grades. There is not enough information given to support that all of the scores on the test are high. A 2.5 standard deviation above the mean does not suggest the existence of an error. There is no z-score given.
   Chapter: 15
   Learning Objective: 2, Compare the four classifications of descriptive statistics.
   Topic/Concept: Descriptive Statistics
   Difficulty Level: Moderate
   Skill Level: Analyzing

6. **B**

    Rationale: The standard deviation is a measure of variability that indicates the average deviation or variability of all the values from the mean of a set of values. The mode is only a crude estimate of the average value of the data. The graph that shows the relationship between two variables is a scattergram. The range of a group of scores figured by adding the highest and lowest numbers is a measure of variability.
    Chapter: 15
    Learning Objective: 2, Compare the four classifications of descriptive statistics.
    Topic/Concept: Descriptive Statistics
    Difficulty Level: Moderate
    Skill Level: Understanding

7. **D**

    Rationale: A correlation concerns the extent to which values of one variable (X) with the value on another variable (Y). Correlations are computed through pairing the value of each subject on one variable (X) with the value on another variable (Y). Correlation does not equate with causation. X and Y are different variables to be compared.
    Chapter: 15
    Learning Objective: 3, Discuss how measures of relationships are different from the other three classifications of descriptive statistics.
    Topic/Concept: Measures of Relationships
    Difficulty Level: Easy
    Skill Level: Understanding

8. **C**

    Rationale: $r = -.50$ indicates a strong negative (inverse) relationship between the two variables. $r = .30$ indicates both variables are increasing/decreasing together, but this correlation is not as strong as another choice. $r = -.30$ indicates a negative (inverse) relationship but is not as strong as another choice. Correlation coefficients can only vary between -1.00 and $+1.00$.
    Chapter: 15
    Learning Objective: 3, Discuss how measures of relationships differ from the other three classifications of statistics.
    Topic/Concept: Measures of Relationships
    Difficulty Level: Moderate
    Skill Level: Analyzing

9. **D**

    Rationale: The children weigh more than 0% of the population and weigh less than 10% of the population. There is not enough information to determine if the children are eating enough. The subject group is at the 90th percentile, not above. The subject group is at the 90th percentile, not below.
    Chapter: 15
    Learning Objective: 2, Compare the four classifications of descriptive statistics.
    Topic/Concept: Descriptive Statistics
    Difficulty Level: Moderate
    Skill Level: Analyzing

10. **B**

    Rationale: The median would represent the middle income of the participants. This statistic does not describe an average of the incomes, but the most frequently occurring income of a sample. The mean of the participants' incomes might not represent an accurate distribution of incomes since it could be influenced by very high incomes. This statistic measures how two variables would vary with each other.
    Chapter: 15
    Learning Objective: 1, Summarize the key concepts related to statistical symbols and classifications.
    Topic/Concept: Key Concepts in Statistics
    Difficulty Level: Moderate
    Skill Level: Applying

Chapter 16

1. C
   Rationale: The level of significance was reached. Finding statistical significance may not be clinically significant. Sample sizes may be small. The hypothesis is never tested statistically.
   Chapter: 16
   Learning Objective: 1, Summarize the two broad purposes of statistics.
   Topic/Concept: Purposes of Inferential Statistics
   Difficulty Level: Easy
   Skill Level: Understanding

2. A
   Rationale: Rejection of the null hypothesis provides support for the research hypothesis. The research hypothesis is never tested statistically. The null hypothesis should be rejected which would provide support for the research hypothesis.
   Chapter: 16
   Learning Objective: 1, Summarize the two broad purposes of inferential statistics.
   Topic/Concept: Purposes of Inferential Statistics
   Difficulty Level: Easy
   Skill Level: Understanding

3. A
   Rationale: Pulse rates are an example of ratio data. Religious affiliation, blood type, and identification numbers are examples of nominal data.
   Chapter: 16
   Learning Objective: 2, Discuss the three factors affecting choice of statistical measures.
   Topic/Concept: Factors Affecting Choice of Statistical Measures
   Difficulty Level: Easy
   Skill Level: Understanding

4. A
   Rationale: Nonparametric statistical tests may be used with nominal and ordinal data. Nonparametric tests make no assumptions about the distribution of the population. Nonparametric tests maybe used when sample sizes are small.
   Chapter: 16
   Learning Objective: 2, Discuss the three factors affecting choice of statistical measures.
   Topic/Concept: Factors Affecting Choice of Statistical Measures
   Difficulty Level: Easy
   Skill Level: Understanding

5. B
   Rationale: The null hypothesis has been proven statistically significant. The hypothesis is never tested statistically. .04 is statistically significant. The data can be tested.
   Chapter: 16
   Learning Objective: 1, Summarize the two broad purposes of inferential statistics.
   Topic/Concept: Purposes of Inferential Statistics
   Difficulty Level: Moderate
   Skill Level: Analysis

6. C
   Rationale: ANOVA is a parametric statistical test and is based on the assumption that data are interval or ratio level. The level of measurement is not nominal, ordinal, or a percentage.
   Chapter: 16
   Learning Objective: 3, Describe statistical tests commonly reported in nursing studies.
   Topic/Concept: Statistical Tests Used in Nursing Research
   Difficulty Level: Moderate
   Skill Level: Applying

7. C
   Rationale: There are three groups: A) 30 diploma school graduates, B) 30 associate degree graduates, and C) 30 baccalaureate graduates. The pairings for testing would be A+B, A+C, and B+C.
   Chapter: 16
   Learning Objective: 3, Describe statistical tests commonly reported in nursing studies.
   Topic/Concept: Statistical Tests Used in Nursing Research
   Difficulty Level: Moderate
   Skill Level: Applying

8. B
   Rationale: The analysis of variance (ANOVA) test is used to compare more than two groups. A dependent t test is used to examine the mean values of some variable in two groups. An independent t test is used when there is no association or connection between the scores of the groups that are being observed. Chi-square test is used compare sets of data that are in the form of frequencies or percentages (nominal data).
   Chapter: 16
   Learning Objective: 3, Describe statistical tests commonly reported in nursing studies.
   Topic/Concept: Statistical Tests Used in Nursing Research
   Difficulty Level: Moderate
   Skill Level: Applying

9. C
   Rationale: The probability level of .03 indicates there is a significant difference between the means of at least two of the groups, but does not tell exactly where the difference occurs. Other statistical tests are needed.
   Learning Objective: 3, Describe statistical tests commonly reported in nursing studies.
   Topic/Concept: Statistical Tests Used in Nursing Research
   Difficulty Level: Hard
   Skill Level: Analyzing

10. B
    Rationale: Given an α of .05, any $p \leq .05$ would support the research hypothesis, thus using the language of "fail to reject" the null hypothesis. The $p = .03$ given is less than .05, indicating that these results would only occur by chance 3 times in 100. Stating that the researcher would "reject the null hypothesis" indicates that there was no statistical difference determined by this test. As the p value is .03, and .03 is less than .05, a difference was observed. There is no information given that an error in calculation occurred. This printout is typical of the results reported following a t test.
    Chapter: 16
    Learning Objective: 3, Describe statistical tests commonly reported in nursing studies.
    Topic/Concept: Statistical Tests Used in Nursing Research
    Difficulty Level: Moderate
    Skill Level: Applying

Chapter 17

1. A
   Rationale: A is the best answer because the narrative should appear before the table if the researcher refers to the table in the narrative. B is incorrect because a blank space does not necessarily indicate to the reader that data are missing and may lead the reader to believe that the data were inadvertently left out—instead, a dash should be used. C is incorrect because the statistical test used in the study should be listed in the narrative description of the findings. D is not the best answer because information can be presented in both the narrative and the table, but if both are used, the text in the narrative should not be presented in its entirety in the table.
   Chapter: 17
   Learning Objective: 1, Summarize the parts of a presentation.
   Topic/Concept: Presentation of Findings of The Study
   Difficulty Level: Easy
   Skill Level: Understanding

2. D
Rationale: Qualitative studies generally involve analyzing verbatim responses from the participants. A is incorrect because *statistical studies* is not a classification of nursing research studies. B is incorrect because descriptive studies generally do not involve analyzing subjective data with direct quotes from participants. C is incorrect because quantitative studies do involve analyzing subjective data with direct quotes from participants.
Chapter: 17
Learning Objective: 1, Summarize the parts of a presentation.
Topic/Concept: Presentation of Findings of the Study
Difficulty Level: Moderate
Skill Level: Understanding

3. B
Rationale: B is the best answer because according to APA style, a table is not needed when the narrative already has presented the information in its entirety. A is incorrect because highlights or important items are included in a table only when they are not presented entirely in the narrative. C is incorrect because a table and a narrative are appropriate when the narrative does not repeat the information entirely in the table.
D is incorrect because the table should not include everything that was presented in the table in its entirety.
Chapter: 17
Learning Objective: 1, Summarize the parts of a presentation.
Topic/Concept: Presentation of Findings of the Study
Difficulty Level: Easy
Skill Level: Remembering

4. B
Rationale: B is correct because clinical significance is not associated with statistical significance; they are independent of each other. A is incorrect because probability levels is not a factor in determining clinical significance. It is determined by the usefulness of the findings in the clinical settings. C is incorrect because clinical significance is not related to statistical significance. D is incorrect because clinical and statistical significance are not mutually exclusive.
Chapter: 17
Learning Objective: 2, Explain the discussion of findings, study hypotheses, and statistical and clinical significance.
Topic/Concept: Discussion of Findings and Significance
Difficulty Level: Difficult
Skill Level: Analyzing

5. A
Rationale: A is correct. If the null hypothesis is rejected through statistical analysis, support is provided for the research hypothesis. B is incorrect. If the null hypothesis is not rejected, it would be inappropriate to say that the research hypothesis was supported. C is incorrect. To say that the research hypothesis was rejected is the opposite of saying that the findings of the study support the intervention. D is incorrect. This statement is similar to saying the research hypothesis failed to support the findings of the study.
Chapter: 17
Learning Objective: 2, Explain the discussion of findings, study hypotheses, and statistical and clinical significance.
Topic/Concept: Discussion of Findings and Significance
Difficulty Level: Difficult
Skill Level: Applying

6. C
Rationale: The null hypothesis was accepted with no statistical difference between the groups, but there was clinically important difference between the two groups. A is incorrect. To say that the null hypothesis was rejected is to say that there was a statistical difference between the groups. However, in this case there

was a statistically *nonsignificant difference* between the groups. B is incorrect. The research hypothesis was not supported. D is incorrect. The research hypothesis was not supported, but the findings were clinically important.
Chapter: 17
Learning Objective: 2, Explain the discussion of findings, study hypotheses, and statistical and clinical significance.
Topic/Concept: Discussion of Study Hypothesis
Difficulty Level: Difficult
Skill Level: Evaluating

7. A
Rationale: The conclusion should be based on the findings. B is incorrect. The review of the literature provides information on the background of the study. C is incorrect. The conclusions of the study support the implications; they are not based on the implications. D is incorrect. The conclusions of the study support recommendations for future research; they are not based on the recommendations.
Chapter: 17
Learning Objective: 3, Describe the purpose of conclusions, implications, and recommendations for research studies.
Topic/Concept: Conclusions, Implications and Recommendations
Difficulty Level: Moderate
Skill Level: Understanding

8. A
Rationale: Concluding there is a positive relationship between children's anxiety and failure to cooperate with physical exams suggests nurses should try to assess anxiety. B is incorrect. Concluding there is a positive relationship between children's anxiety and failure to cooperate with physical exams does not necessarily mean nurses should investigate a causal relationship between anxiety levels and children's failure to cooperate with physical examinations. C is incorrect. Despite the existence of anxiety, children must have physical examinations. D is incorrect. Nothing about the conclusions of the research suggests parents should remain with the child.
Chapter: 17
Learning Objective: 3, Describe the purpose of conclusions, implications, and recommendations for research studies.
Topic/Concept: Conclusions, Implications and Recommendations
Difficulty Level: Moderate
Skill Level: Understanding

9. B
Rationale: B is correct. Recommendations from a study should include a discussion of how to extend the study in future research. A is incorrect. A discussion of the findings of the study relate more to the details of the statistical findings associated with the study. C is incorrect. Comparisons of the results of the study with other research findings is more appropriate in the discussion or conclusion section. D is incorrect. The means of implementing the study findings relate to how you might apply the findings into practice.
Chapter: 17
Learning Objective: 3, Describe the purpose of conclusions, implications, and recommendations for research studies.
Topic/Concept: Conclusions, Implications and Recommendations
Difficulty Level: Easy
Skill Level: Understanding

Chapter 18

1. B
Rationale: Journal articles generally are widely disseminated to nurses through publication. Dissertations mostly are housed in the libraries of the schools or universities in which they were published. Conference oral presentations generally are limited to conference participants. Poster presentations generally are limited to the participants who attend the poster sessions.

362 Self-Test Answers

   Chapter: 18
   Learning Objective: 1, Describe the means of communicating nursing research findings.
   Topic/Concept: Communication of Nursing Research Findings
   Difficulty Level: Moderate
   Skill Level: Understanding

2. D
   Rationale: Poster presentations are less intimidating to beginning researchers. Manuscripts that are submitted by beginning researchers are less likely to be accepted for publication. Oral presentations at a conference can be intimidating to beginning researchers. Presenting a research paper at a conference can be intimidating to beginning researchers.
   Chapter: 18
   Learning Objective: 1, Describe the means of communicating nursing research findings.
   Topic/Concept: Communication of Nursing Research Findings
   Difficulty Level: Easy
   Skill Level: Remembering

3. B
   Rationale: Submitting a manuscript is time wasted if the editors are not interested in the subject matter. Most manuscripts require revisions before they are accepted for publication. Formats of research articles vary among journals. Most journals do not restrict submission of manuscripts to beginning researchers.
   Chapter: 18
   Learning Objective: 1, Describe the means of communicating nursing research findings.
   Topic/Concept: Communication of Nursing Research Findings
   Difficulty Level: Moderate
   Skill Level: Understanding

4. A
   Rationale: Public sources, such as National Institutes of Nursing Research, have provided most of the funding for nursing research. Though private foundations, such as Robert Wood Johnson, fund some nursing research, they are not the major supporters of nursing research. Though some businesses, such as Apple fund nursing research, they are not the major supporters of nursing research. Though some philanthropists may be approached for funding of nursing research, they are not the major supporters of nursing research.
   Chapter: 18
   Learning Objective: 1, Describe the means of communicating nursing research findings.
   Topic/Concept: Communication of Nursing Research Findings
   Difficulty Level: Moderate
   Skill Level: Understanding

5. B
   Rationale: Researchers have found that a significant barrier to research utilization is that most research findings are not published. Nurses' lack of knowledge of research findings is the most frequently cited barrier to research utilization. Nurses' lack of knowledge of research findings is the most frequently cited reason for the lack of nursing research utilization. Most research findings are not ready for use in practice which is a significant barrier to research utilization.
   Chapter: 18
   Learning Objective: 2, Summarize issues related to research utilization.
   Topic/Concept: Utilization of Nursing Research Findings
   Difficulty Level: Moderate
   Skill Level: Understanding

6. B
   Rationale: The nurse uses the intervention in practice or applies it indirectly in the implementation stage of the Rogers's Innovation-Diffusion Model. The nurse becomes aware of a research-based nursing intervention in the knowledge stage of the Rogers's Innovation-Diffusion Model. The nurse forms a positive or negative attitude toward the intervention in the persuasion stage of Rogers's Innovation-Diffusion

Model. The nurse evaluates effectiveness of the intervention in the confirmation stage of Rogers's Innovation-Diffusion Model.
Chapter: 18
Learning Objective: 2, Summarize issues related to research utilization.
Topic/Concept: Utilization of Nursing Research Findings
Difficulty Level: Moderate
Skill Level: Applying

Chapter 19

1. A
   Rationale: Nursing is the most highly rated profession in the United States. This is a result of the survey.
   Chapter: 19
   Learning Objective: 1, Explain economic terms that have an impact on nursing.
   Topic/Concept: Healthcare Economics and Nursing
   Difficulty Level: Easy
   Skill Level: Remembering

2. A
   Rationale: The demand curve for nursing labor is a derived demand that depends on, i.e. is derived from, the demand for the product (or service).
   Chapter: 19
   Learning Objective: 1, Explain economic terms that have an impact on nursing.
   Topic/Concept: Healthcare Economics and Nursing
   Difficulty Level: Moderate
   Skill Level: Understanding

3. A
   Rationale: This is the general finding of most studies.
   Chapter: 19
   Learning Objective: 2, Determine the cost-effectiveness of nursing care based on the results of selected nursing research studies.
   Topic/Concept: Nursing Research Cost-Effectiveness Studies
   Difficulty Level: Easy
   Skill Level: Remembering

4. F
   Rationale: Healthcare is generally jointly produced with other health professionals, and thus the individual contribution by nurses is difficult to isolate.
   Chapter: 19
   Learning Objective: 1, Explain economic terms that have an impact on nursing.
   Topic/Concept: Healthcare Economics and Nursing
   Difficulty Level: Moderate
   Skill Level: Understanding

5. F
   Rationale: The level of reimbursement for nurses depends on the perceived value of their contribution to the services provided which in turn requires continual assessment of that contribution.
   Chapter: 19
   Learning Objective: 1, Explain economic terms that have an impact on nursing.
   Topic/Concept: Healthcare Economics and Nursing
   Difficulty Level: Easy
   Skill Level: Understanding

6. T
   Rationale: Because the production of more service (e.g. treating more patients) brings in more revenues, but also entails greater expenses, profit from one more unit of service can only increase if marginal benefit exceeds marginal expense. The marginal profit will decrease if marginal expense exceeds marginal benefit.

Chapter: 19
Learning Objective: 1, Explain economic terms that have an impact on nursing.
Topic/Concept: Healthcare Economics and Nursing
Difficulty Level: Difficult
Skill Level: Understanding

7. T
Rationale: Hospital-acquired pneumonia, the prevention of which would decrease length of stay in the hospital, was one of eleven medical conditions Dall studied as a cost-effective measure that nursing care could be expected to favorably impact.
Chapter: 19
Learning Objective: 2, Determine the cost-effectiveness of nursing care based on the results of selected nursing research studies.
Topic/Concept: Nursing Research Cost-Effectiveness Studies
Difficulty Level: Moderate
Skill Level: Remembering

8. F
Rationale: Where appropriate, the PPACA explicitly requires the practice of evidence-based medicine especially with respect to preventive care.
Chapter: 19
Learning Objective: 3, Summarize the impact of governmental agencies and related organizations on nurses and the cost of healthcare.
Topic/Concept: Impacts of Governmental Agencies and Related Organizations
Difficulty Level: Moderate
Skill Level: Remembering

Chapter 20

1. B
Rationale: Paraphrasing is preferred rather than the use of many direct quotations. The reader does not need to be referred to the website or the library to learn more about a study being cited in a literature review.
Chapter: 20
Learning Objective: 1, Summarize the guidelines for critiquing a quantitative research report.
Topic/Concept: Critiquing Quantitative Research Reports
Difficulty level: Moderate
Skill Level: Applying

2. A
Rationale: Theoretical frameworks are not used for health services research, a branch of research which studies issues related to access to care, healthcare costs, and healthcare delivery. Theoretical frameworks are used for the reliability and validity of instruments, studies that evaluation outcomes and symptoms, and for middle-range theories.
Chapter: 20
Learning Objective: 1, Summarize the guidelines for critiquing a quantitative research report.
Topic/Concept: Critiquing Quantitative Research Reports
Difficulty level: Moderate
Skill Level: Applying

3. B
Rationale: The researcher may make a commonsense assumption that is necessary to proceed with the research. Such an assumption might be, "The respondents will answer the questions honestly." Not understanding the question, not remembers alcohol intake, or being deceptive about drinking habits are not assumptions.
Chapter: 20
Learning Objective: 1, Summarize the guidelines for critiquing a quantitative research report.

Topic/Concept: Critiquing Quantitative Research Reports
Difficulty level: Moderate
Skill Level: Analyzing

4. A

Rationale: Directional research hypotheses are preferred however are not to be used when there is no available research or theory that predicts the relationship between the variables being examined. Directional research hypotheses are not contingent upon the use of an instrument, a missing population from the null hypothesis, or based upon the reliability of the instrument.
Chapter: 20
Learning Objective: 1, Summarize the guidelines for critiquing a quantitative research report.
Topic/Concept: Critiquing Quantitative Research Reports
Difficulty level: Moderate
Skill Level: Understanding

5. C

Rationale: Operational definitions indicate the observable, measurable phenomena associated with the study variables. A conceptual framework is needed. Definitions about variables should be included and not expected to be found in a dictionary. Conceptual definitions are concrete information for the particular study. Definitions of key terms in a research report are necessary to make explicit what is being studied. Replication of a study is aided by clear definitions of terms.
Chapter: 20
Learning Objective: 1, Summarize the guidelines for critiquing a quantitative research report.
Topic/Concept: Critiquing Quantitative Research Reports
Difficulty level: Moderate
Skill Level: Understanding

6. D

Rationale: In a qualitative study, agreement needs to be reached on the meaning of the participants' responses between both the data collector and the participant. The participant's view won't necessarily be represented by the data collector or researcher reviewing the transcripts. Replaying the participant's statements may be done without the participant in attendance.
Chapter: 20
Learning Objective: 2, Summarize the guidelines for critiquing a qualitative research report.
Topic/Concept: Critiquing Qualitative Research Reports
Difficulty level: Moderate
Skill Level: Analyzing

Appendix A
Consent Form

Consent to Act as a Subject for Research and Investigation

I. I hereby authorize _____ to perform the following investigation:
The study will involve my 4-year-old child participating in an experiment. The investigation will consist of a physical examination of the eyes, ears, throat, elbow, and knee reflexes. Blood pressure and temperature will also be checked. The physical examination will require about 15 minutes. The child will receive a play session before the physical examination, or not, depending on the group to which he (she) is randomly assigned. If the child does not receive the play session before the physical examination, he (she) may receive the same play session after the physical examination. The physical examination and the play sessions will be conducted by registered nurses. The examining nurse will be experienced in the examination of children. The play sessions will be conducted by the researcher, who is experienced in working with children and with play techniques. Another registered nurse will observe the child during the physical examination.

II. The procedure or investigation listed in Paragraph I has been explained to me by _____.

III. I understand that the procedures or investigations described in Paragraph I involve the following possible risks or discomforts:
  1. Confidential information from the study results might be accidentally released.
  2. The child may feel anxious about the physical examination procedure.

IV. I understand that my child's rights and welfare will be protected as follows:
  1. Safeguards against the accidental release of data will include the use of a code number, and only the investigator will know the name and the code number of each child. No names or code numbers will be used in the final research report. Only group statistics will be reported. There will be no way a reader of the final report can identify any of the participants. Any information pertaining to the identity of the participants will be destroyed when the study is completed.
  2. The child will not be pressured into participating in the physical examination procedure. If the child does not want to participate in the activity, the child will not be examined.
  3. The participation or nonparticipation of the child in the study will not influence care received at the day-care center. The child's participation in the study is strictly voluntary. The child may be withdrawn from the study at any time, without any penalty.
  4. The participants who do not receive the play session before the physical examination will be given the opportunity for the play session in small groups after their physical examinations are done. The registered nurse conducting the play periods with the physical examination equipment is experienced in working with children and various play techniques.

V. I understand that the procedures and investigations described in Paragraph I have the following potential benefits to myself and others:
  1. By participation in this study, the child will become more familiar with possible frightening equipment that is routinely used during physical examinations.

2. Because the child is more familiar with the equipment used, the child may be less anxious and more cooperative during the examination described in paragraph 1.
3. The results of physical examinations are more accurate if the child is not resistive during the procedures.
4. The child may have increased self-esteem because the child is better able to control behavior during the examination described in paragraph 1.
5. Participation in this study will help produce new knowledge that will assist child-care workers in dealing with young children.

VI. I understand that no medical service or compensation will be provided to the subjects by the university as a result of injury from participation in the research described in paragraph 1.

VII. An offer has been made to answer all of my questions regarding the study. If alternative procedures are more advantageous to me, they have been explained. I understand that I may terminate my child's participation in the study at any time. The subject is a minor (age ____).

Signatures (One Required)

_____   _____
Father   Date

_____   _____
Mother   Date

_____   _____
Guardian   Date

Appendix B
Critiquing Exercise

Retrieve the following article:

Horner, J. K., Piercy, B. S., Eure, L., & Woodward, E. K. (2014). A pilot study to evaluate mindfulness as a strategy to improve inpatient nurse and patient experiences. *Applied Nursing Research, 27*, 198–201. doi:10.1016/j.apnr.2014.01.003

Based on the information learned while reading this book, critique the article and answer the following questions:

1. **Title**
   - Is the title clear?
   - Does it contain the population and the variables?
   - Is the length appropriate?
   - Are there any extraneous or unnecessary words?

2. **Researcher Qualifications**
   - Are you able to determine the researchers' educational and research qualifications to conduct the study?
   - One of the four researchers has "RN" after her name. What disciplines do you think the other three individuals represent, and what roles did they have in the study?
   - Do you think one of these four individuals might have expertise in statistics?
   - Was any funding obtained for this study?
   - Conduct a computer search and see what information you can obtain about the researchers.

3. **Abstract**
   - Is the length appropriate?
   - What elements of the study are contained in the abstract (Purpose? Hypotheses or Research Questions? Methods? Identification of participants? Major findings?)?
   - Does the abstract gain your attention and make you want to read the article?

4. **Introduction**
   - Does the Introduction section present pertinent information about the study problem?
   - Is the significance of the research clearly identified?
   - What components of the study are contained in this section of the report?
   - Is appropriate background information presented?

5. **Purpose**
   - Is the purpose of the study made clear?
   - Is the population identified?
   - Are the major study variables included?

6. **Review of the Literature**
    - The review of the literature was included in the Background. Is this the only location of literature sources?
    - Are the literature sources pertinent to the study?
    - Are direct quotes or paraphrases used?
    - Are you able to determine if primary sources have been cited?
    - What are the most recent and oldest references cited?
    - The article was published in 2014; would you expect some references from 2013 and 2014 (notice the date of acceptance for publication)?

7. **Theoretical/Conceptual Framework**
    - This article does not identify a theoretical framework section.
    - Has the title concept of "mindfulness" been linked to a conceptual framework?
    - Does this concept seem appropriate for the study?

8. **Assumptions**
    - Can you identify at least three assumptions made by the researchers (beliefs or assertions that were not documented from literature sources)?

9. **Limitations**
    - What are some of the study limitations identified by the researchers?
    - Did you identify additional limitations of the study?
    - Is it appropriate to discuss threats to internal and external validity in this type of study?
    - What do you think is the greatest weakness of this study?

10. **Hypothesis(es)**
    - Did the researchers have any basis (from the framework or the literature) for predicting study outcomes in the form of hypotheses?
    - How many hypotheses were actually tested, based on data found in Table 1?

11. **Definition of Terms**
    - Determine what variables needed to be defined, then search for the definitions provided by the researchers.
    - Are both conceptual and operational definitions provided for the main study variables?
    - Do the definitions provide observable, measurable criteria?
    - Would you be able to replicate the study based on the definitions provided?

12. **Research Design**
    - The design section clearly lists the study as a "quasi-experimental study design." What makes this design "quasi-experimental"?
    - Do you believe the design could be classified as any other type?
    - How were students assigned to the two simulation groups?
    - Was random assignment used?

13. **Setting**
    - Is there reference to the setting?
    - Do you think the study might have been conducted at the place where the researchers were employed?

14. **Population and Sample**
    - Are the target populations and accessible populations identified?
    - Is the sample clearly identified?
    - What type of sampling method was used to select the sample?
    - Does the sample size seem adequate?
    - Was power analysis used to determine sample size?
    - Was permission to conduct the study obtained from the appropriate authorities? Were nurses' rights protected?

15. **Data Collection**
    - Who collected the data (researchers or research assistants)?
    - When were the data collected (time period—how long)?
    - Where were the data collected (location of data collection)?
    - What data were collected (data to determine errors committed)?
    - How were the data collected (data-collection method)?

16. **Data-Collection Instruments**
    - What type of instrument was used to collect data?
    - Was the instrument appropriate to gather the data for the study?
    - How were reliability and validity of the instrument assessed?

17. **Analysis of Data**
    - Are the statistical findings presented clearly?
    - What types of statistics were used to present the data?
    - Were demographic statistics presented on the sample?
    - What statistic was used to present the number of errors made by students?
    - Why was a 2-tailed t-test and one-way ANOVA statistic used as an inferential statistical test? (*Hint*: What was the level of measurement of the data?)
    - Based on Table 1, how many findings were significant?

18. **Discussion of Findings**
    - Were additional literature sources cited in this section?
    - Were the findings discussed in regard to other studies in the literature?
    - Were the findings related back to the theoretical framework?

19. **Discussions**
    - Were you able to pick out a conclusion or conclusions in this section that was/were based on the study findings?

20. **Implications**
    - What implications are pointed out by the researchers?
    - Identify other possible implications of this study.
    - Do you think this study has broad implications for many areas of nursing, such as nursing education, nursing practice, or nursing administration?

21. **Recommendations**
    - What recommendations were made by the researchers?
    - Were recommendations found in one location in the article?
    - Were study limitations considered in the recommendations made by the researchers?
    - Are there other recommendations that you think could have been made by the researchers?

22. **Other Considerations**
    - What was the "lag time" for publication of this article?
    - Was the article easy to read and understand?
    - Was the use of technical terms limited?
    - Were the tables and figures appropriate?
    - Were the references cited in the article also listed on the reference page?
    - Were references cited complete and in APA format?
    - Are there additional comments that you would like to make concerning this article?
    - Would you recommend this article to a colleague?

Glossary

abstracts (research abstracts). Brief summaries of research studies; generally contain the purpose, methods, and major findings of the study.

accessible population. The group of people or objects that is available to the researcher for a particular study.

action research. A type of qualitative research that actively engages the community of interest in solving a problem.

alpha (α). See level of significance, also type I error.

alternate forms reliability (parallel forms reliability). Results are compared using two forms or versions of the same instrument.

alternative hypothesis. See research hypothesis.

ambiguous questions. Questions containing words that may be interpreted in more than one way.

analysis of covariance (ANCOVA). A statistical test that allows the researcher to control statistically for some variable(s) that may have an influence on the dependent variable.

analysis of variance (ANOVA). A statistical test used to compare the difference between the means of two or more groups or sets of values.

analyze. Determine what evidence or information is given in each source to support the points, inferences, or arguments about your topic.

anonymity. The identity of research subjects is unknown, even to the study investigator.

applied research. Research that is conducted to find a solution to an immediate practice problem.

assent. Agreement to participate in research by someone, especially a child older than 7 years, who is not capable cognitively of giving informed consent.

assumptions. Beliefs that are held to be true but have not necessarily been proven; assumptions may be explicit or implicit.

attitude scales. Self-report data-collection instruments that ask respondents to report their attitudes or feelings on a continuum.

attribute variables. See demographic variables.

attrition (dropout, subject dropout). Study participant withdraws from a study.

bar graph. A figure used to represent a frequency distribution of nominal or ordinal data.

basic research. Research that is conducted to generate knowledge rather than to solve immediate problems.

beneficence. Research participants should be protected from harm.

beta (β). See type II error.

bimodal distribution. A frequency distribution that contains two identical high-frequency values.

bivariate study. A research study in which the relationship between two variables is examined.

blind review. Manuscript reviewers are not made aware of the author's identity before the manuscript is evaluated.

bracketing. A process in which qualitative researchers put aside their own feelings or beliefs about a phenomenon that is being studied to keep from biasing their observations.

call for abstract. A request for a summary of a study that the researcher wishes to present at a research conference.

canonical correlation. Examines the correlation between two or more independent variables and two or more dependent variables.

case studies. Research studies that involve an in-depth examination of a single person or a group of people. A case study might also examine an institution.

catalogs. Indexes of the materials held by a library or organization.

cause-and-effect relationship. One thing or event makes some other thing or event happen.

cells. Boxes in a table that are formed by the intersection of rows and columns.

central limit theorem. The phenomenon in which sample values tend to be normally distributed around the population value.

chi-square test (χ^2). A nonparametric statistical test used to compare sets of data that are in the form of frequencies or percentages (nominal level data).

class interval. A group of scores in a frequency distribution.

clinical nursing research. Nursing research studies involving clients or that have the potential for affecting clients.

clinical trials. Research studies conducted to evaluate new treatments, new drugs, and new or improved medical equipment.

closed-ended questions. Questions that require respondents to choose from given alternatives.

cluster random sampling. A random sampling process that involves two or more stages. The population is first listed by clusters or categories (e.g., hospitals) and then the sample elements (e.g., hospital administrators) are randomly selected from these clusters.

coefficient alpha. See Cronbach's alpha.

coefficient of determination (r^2, R^2). A statistic obtained by squaring a correlation coefficient and is interpreted as the percentage of variance shared by two variables.

cohort study. A special type of longitudinal study in which subjects are studied who have been born during one particular period or who have similar backgrounds.

collectively exhaustive categories. Categories are provided for every possible answer.

comparative studies. Studies in which intact groups are compared on some dependent variable. The researcher is not able to manipulate the independent variable, which is frequently some inherent characteristic of the subjects, such as age or educational level.

comparison group. A group of subjects in an experimental study that does not receive any experimental treatment or receives an alternate treatment such as the "normal" or routine treatment.

complex hypothesis. A hypothesis that concerns a relationship where two or more independent variables, two or more dependent variables, or both are being examined.

computer-assisted literature searches. The use of a computer to obtain bibliographic references that have been stored in a database.

computerized database. A compilation of information that can be retrieved by computer.

concept. A word picture or mental idea of a phenomenon.

conceptual definition. A dictionary or theoretical definition of an abstract idea that is being studied by the researcher.

conceptual framework. A background or foundation for a study; a less well-developed structure than a theoretical framework; concepts are related in a logical manner by the researcher.

conceptual model. Symbolic presentation of concepts and the relationships between these concepts.

concurrent validity. A type of criterion validity in which a determination is made of the instrument's ability to obtain a measurement of subjects' behavior that is comparable to some other criterion used to indicate that behavior.

confidence interval. A range of values that, with a specified degree of probability, is thought to contain the population value.

confidentiality. The identity of the research subjects is known only to the study investigator(s).

confounding variable. See extraneous variable.

constant comparison. Data gathered in a qualitative study are constantly or continually compared to data that have already been gathered.

construct. A highly abstract phenomenon that cannot be directly observed but must be inferred by certain concrete or less abstract indicators of the phenomenon.

construct validity. The ability of an instrument to measure the construct that it is intended to measure.

content analysis. A data collection method that examines communication messages that are usually in written form.

content validity. The degree to which an instrument covers the scope and range of information that is sought.

contingency questions. Questions that are relevant for some respondents and not for others.

contingency table. A table that visually displays the relationship between sets of nominal data.

control group. A group of subjects in an experimental study that does not receive the experimental treatment (see comparison group).

convenience sampling (accidental sampling). A nonprobability sampling procedure that involves the selection of the most readily available people or objects for a study.

correlation. The extent to which values of one variable (X) are related to the values of a second variable (Y). Correlations may be either positive or negative.

correlational studies. Research studies that examine the strength of relationships between variables.

correlation coefficient. A statistic that presents the magnitude and direction of a relationship between two variables. Correlation coefficients range from –1.00 (perfect negative relationship) to +1.00 (perfect positive relationship).

criterion validity. The extent to which an instrument corresponds or correlates with some criterion measure of the information that is being sought; the ability of an instrument to determine subjects' responses at present or predict subjects' responses in the future.

critical region (region of rejection). An area in a theoretical sampling distribution that contains the critical values, which are values considered to be statistically significant.

critical value. A scientific cutoff point that denotes the value in a theoretical distribution at which all obtained values from a sample that are equal to or beyond that point are said to be statistically significant.

critique (research critique). Assesses the strengths and weaknesses of a study.

Cronbach's alpha (coefficient alpha). Provides an estimate of the reliability of a written instrument when considering all possible ways to divide the items on the instrument into two halves.

cross-sectional study. A research study that collects data on subjects at one point in time.

data. The pieces of information or facts collected during a research study.

database. See computerized database.

debriefing. A meeting with research participants at the conclusion of a study that ensures their understanding of the reasons and the justification for the procedures used in the study.

deductive reasoning. A reasoning process that proceeds from the general to the specific, from theory to empirical data.

degrees of freedom (df). A concept in inferential statistics that concerns the number of values that are free to vary.

Delphi technique. A data-collection method that uses several rounds of questions to seek a consensus on a particular topic from a group of experts on the topic.

demographic questions. Questions that gather data on characteristics of the subjects (see demographic variables).

demographic variables. Subject characteristics such as age, educational levels, and marital status.

dependent t test. A form of the t test that is used when one set of scores or values is associated or dependent on another set of scores or values.

dependent variable. The "effect"; a response or behavior that is influenced by the independent variable; sometimes called the criterion variable.

derived demand. The demand for labor is *derived* from the demand for the product (or service) that the firm produces and sells.

descriptive statistics. The group of statistics that organizes and summarizes numerical data obtained from populations and samples.

descriptive studies. Research studies in which phenomena are described or the relationship between variables is examined; no attempt is made to determine cause-and-effect relationships.

design. See research design.

diminishing marginal returns. As more of a variable input (like labor) is hired, and the amount of capital is fixed, the marginal product of a worker declines.

directional research hypothesis. A type of hypothesis in which a prediction is made of the type of relationship that exists between variables.

discovery systems. Expanded library catalogs that not only index the materials held by a library or organization but also include links to materials from databases.

disproportional stratified sampling. Random selection of members from population strata where the number of members chosen for each stratum is not in proportion to the size of the stratum in the total population.

double-barreled questions. Questions that ask two questions in one.

double-blind experiment. An experiment in which neither the researcher nor the research participants know which participants are in the experimental and control groups.

dropout. Study participant withdraws from a study.

effect size. How useful a treatment or intervention was in several studies as indicated by the difference between data from control groups and experimental groups.

e-journal. A journal that can be accessed online.

element. A single member of a population.

empirical data. Objective data gathered through the sense organs.

empirical generalization. A summary statement about the occurrence of phenomena that is based on empirical data from a number of different research studies.

equivalence reliability. The degree to which two forms of an instrument obtain the same results or two or more observers obtain the same results when using a single instrument to measure a variable.

ethnographic studies (ethnography). Research studies that involve the collection and analysis of data about cultural groups.

event sampling. Observations made throughout the entire course of an event or behavior.

evidence-based practice (EBP) (sometimes called *evidence-based nursing practice*). Nursing practice that is based on the best available evidence, particularly research findings.

experimental design. See quasi-experimental, pre-experimental, and true experimental designs.

experimenter effect. A threat to the external validity of a research study that occurs when the researcher's behavior influences the subjects' behavior in a way that is not intended by the researcher.

explanatory studies. Research studies that search for causal explanations; usually experimental.

exploratory studies. Research studies that are conducted when little is known about the phenomenon being studied.

ex post facto studies. Studies in which the variation in the independent variable has already occurred in the past, and the researcher is trying to determine after the fact if the variation that has occurred in the independent variable has any influence on the dependent variable being measured in the present.

external criticism (external appraisal, external examination). A type of examination of historical data that is concerned with the authenticity or genuineness of the data. External criticism might be used to determine if a letter was actually written by the person whose signature appeared on the letter.

external validity threats. The degree to which study results can be generalized to other people and other research settings.

extraneous variable. A type of variable that is not the variable of interest to a researcher but that may influence the results of a study. Other terms for extraneous variable are intervening variable and confounding variable.

e-zine. A magazine that can be accessed online.

face validity. A subjective determination that an instrument is adequate for obtaining the desired information; on the surface or the face of the instrument it appears to be an adequate means of obtaining the desired data.

factor analysis. A type of validity used to identify clusters of related items on an instrument or scale.

field studies. Research studies that are conducted in the field or in a real-life setting.

filler questions. Questions used to distract respondents from the purpose of other questions that are being asked.

focus group. A small group of individuals who meet together and are asked questions by a moderator about a certain topic or topics.

framework. See conceptual framework and theoretical framework.

frequency distribution. A listing of all scores or numerical values from a set of data and the number of times each score or value appears; scores may be listed from highest to lowest or lowest to highest.

frequency polygon. A graph that uses dots connected with straight lines to represent the frequency distribution of interval or ratio data. A dot is placed above the midpoint of each class interval.

galley proofs. Sheets of paper that show how an article or book will appear in typeset form.

generalization. See empirical generalization.

grand theories. Theories that are concerned with a broad range of phenomena in the environment or in the experiences of humans.

grey literature. Literature produced by the government, academics, businesses, and industry not traditionally controlled by a commercial publisher. Examples include reports, conference proceedings, technical documentation and policy briefs. In recent years researchers have realized the value of this information and it has become much easier to access.

grounded theory studies. Research studies in which data are collected and analyzed, and then a theory is developed that is grounded in the data.

Hawthorne effect. A threat to the external validity of a research study that occurs when study participants respond in a certain manner because they are aware that they are involved in a research study.

histogram. A graph used to represent the frequency distribution of variables measured at the interval or ratio level.

historical studies. Research studies that are concerned with the identification, location, evaluation, and synthesis of data from the past.

history threat. A threat to the internal validity of an experimental research study; some event in addition to the experimental treatment occurs between the pretreatment and posttreatment measurement of the dependent variable, and this event influences the dependent variable.

hypothesis. A statement of the predicted relationship between two or more variables.

impact factor. A number used to evaluate the influence of a particular journal article.

independent *t* test. A form of the *t* test that is used when there is no association between the two sets of scores or values being compared.

independent variable. The "cause" or the variable thought to influence the dependent variable; in experimental research it is the variable manipulated by the researcher.

indexes. Compilations of reference materials that provide information on books and periodicals.

inductive reasoning. A reasoning process that proceeds from the specific to the general, from empirical data to theory.

inferential statistics. That group of statistics concerned with the characteristics of populations and uses sample data to make an inference about a population.

informed consent. A subject voluntarily agrees to participate in a research study in which he or she has full understanding of the study before the study begins.

institutional review board (IRB). Every agency or institution that receives federal money for research must have an IRB to review research proposals.

instrument. A data-collection tool.

instrumentation change. A threat to the internal validity of an experimental research study that involves changes from the pretest measurements to the posttest measurements as a result of inaccuracy of the instrument or the judges' ratings rather than as a result of the experimental treatment.

integrative review. See systematic review.

interaction effect. The result of two variables acting in conjunction with each other.

internal consistency reliability (scale homogeneity). The extent to which all items of an instrument measure the same variable.

internal criticism. A type of examination of historical data that is concerned with the accuracy of the data. Internal criticism might be used to determine if a document contained an accurate recording of events as they actually happened.

internal validity threats. The degree to which changes in the dependent variable (effect) can be attributed to the independent or experimental variable (cause) rather than to the effects of extraneous variables.

interobserver reliability. See interrater reliability.

interquartile range. Contains the middle half of the values in a frequency distribution.

interrater reliability (interobserver reliability). The degree to which two or more independent judges are in agreement about ratings or observations of events or behaviors.

interval level of measurement (interval data). Data can be categorized, ranked, and the distance between the ranks can be specified; pulse rates and temperature readings are examples of interval data.

intervening variable. See extraneous variable.

interview. A method of data collection in which the interviewer obtains responses from a subject in a face-to-face encounter or through a telephone call.

interview schedule. An instrument containing a set of questions, directions for asking these questions, and space to record the respondents' answers.

judgmental sampling. See purposive sampling.

key informant. A person who is knowledgeable about the culture that is being studied in ethnographic research.

known-groups procedure. A research technique in which a research instrument is administered to two groups of people whose responses are expected to differ on the variable of interest.

laboratory studies. Research studies in which subjects are studied in a special environment that has been created by the researcher.

level of measurement. Indicates the precision with which data can be gathered and the mathematical operations that can be used with the data; the four levels of measurement are nominal, ordinal, interval, and ratio.

level of significance (probability level). The probability of rejecting a null hypothesis when it is true; symbolized by lowercase Greek letter alpha (α); also symbolized by p.

Likert scale. An attitude scale named after its developer, Rensis Likert. These scales usually contain five or seven responses for each item, ranging from "strongly agree" to "strongly disagree."

limitations. Weaknesses in a study; uncontrolled variables.

literature sources. Sources of written information, such as books, journals, reference materials, reports, and dissertations.

longitudinal study. Subjects are followed during a period in the future; data are collected at two or more different time periods.

manipulation. The independent or experimental variable is controlled by the researcher to determine its effect on the dependent variable.

marginal benefit. Also known as the marginal revenue product of a worker; has two components: (a) the marginal product of labor—the additional output produced by an additional worker, and (b) the marginal revenue—the additional revenue generated by selling an additional unit of output.

marginal expense. The additional cost of hiring one more worker.

marginal product. The additional output produced by an additional worker.

marginal revenue. The additional revenue generated by selling an additional unit of output.

maturation. A threat to the internal validity of an experimental research study that occurs when changes that take place within study subjects as a result of the passage of time (growing older, taller) affect the study results.

mean (M). A measure of central tendency; the average of a set of values that is found by adding all values and dividing by the total number of values. The population symbol is μ, and the sample symbol is $\bar{x}$.

measurement. A process in scientific research that uses rules to assign numbers to objects.

measures of central tendency. Statistics that describe the average, typical, or most common value for a group of data.

measures of relationship. Statistics that present the correlation between variables.

measures of variability. Statistics that describe how spread out values are in a distribution of values (e.g., range, standard deviation).

measures to condense data. Statistics that are used to condense and summarize data.

median (Md, Mdn). A measure of central tendency; the middle score or value in a group of data.

meta-analysis. A technique that combines the results of several similar studies on a topic and statistically analyzes the results as if only one study had been conducted.

metasynthesis. A technique used in summarizing reports of two or more qualitative studies that cover the same topic.

methodological studies. Research studies that are concerned with the development, testing, and evaluation of research instruments and methods.

middle-range theories. Theories that have a narrow focus; concerned with only a small area of the environment or of human experiences.

mixed methods research. The combination of quantitative and qualitative methods in one study.

modal class. The category with the greatest frequency of observations; used with nominal and ordinal data.

mode (Mo). A measure of central tendency; the category or value that occurs most often in a set of data.

model. A symbolic representation of some phenomenon or phenomena.

monopsony. A large buyer of an input, such as the only hospital in town, that can therefore set wages.

mortality threat. A threat to the internal validity of an experimental research study that occurs when either the subject dropout rate is different, or characteristics are different, between those who drop out of the experimental group and those who drop out of the comparison group.

multimodal. A frequency distribution in which more than two values have the same high frequency.

multiple regression. A statistical procedure used to determine the influence of more than one independent variable on the dependent variable.

multivariate analysis of variance (MANOVA). A statistical test that examines the difference between the mean scores of two or more groups on two or more dependent variables that are measured at the same time.

multivariate study. A research study in which more than two variables are examined.

mutually exclusive categories. Categories are uniquely distinct; no overlap occurs between categories.

narrative inquiry. Research in which one understands, through the stories people tell, the way people create meaning in their lives.

negatively skewed. A frequency distribution in which the tail of the distribution points to the left.

negative relationship (inverse relationship). A relationship between two variables in which there is a tendency for the values of one variable to increase as the values of the other variable decrease.

network sampling. See snowball sampling.

nominal level of measurement (nominal level of data). The lowest level of measurement; data are "named" or categorized, such as race and marital status.

nondirectional research hypothesis. A type of research hypothesis in which a prediction is made that a relationship exists between variables, but the type of relationship is not specified.

nonequivalent control group design. A type of quasi-experimental design; similar to the pretest-posttest control group experimental design, except that there is no random assignment of subjects to groups.

nonexperimental research. Research in which the researcher does not manipulate or control the independent variable.

nonparametric tests (distribution-free statistics). Types of inferential statistics that are not concerned with population parameters; requirements for their use are less stringent; can be used with nominal and ordinal data and small sample sizes.

nonparticipant observer (covert). Research observer does not identify herself or himself to the subjects who are being observed.

nonparticipant observer (overt). Research observer openly identifies that she or he is conducting research and provides subjects with information about the type of data that will be collected.

nonprobability sampling. A sampling process in which a sample is selected from elements or members of a population through nonrandom methods; includes convenience, quota, and purposive.

nonrefereed journal. A journal that uses editorial staff members or consultants to review manuscripts.

nonsignificant results. Study results do not allow rejection of the null hypothesis.

nonsymmetrical distribution (skewed distribution). Frequency distribution in which the distribution has an off-center peak. If the tail of the distribution points to the right, the distribution is said to be positively skewed; if the tail of the distribution points to the left, the distribution is said to be negatively skewed.

normal curve. A bell-shaped curve that graphically depicts a normally distributed frequency distribution (see normal distribution).

normal distribution. A symmetrical bell-shaped theoretical distribution; has one central peak or set of values in the middle of the distribution.

null hypothesis (H_0). A statistical hypothesis that predicts there is no relationship between variables; the hypothesis that is subjected to statistical analysis.

nursing research. A systematic, objective process of analyzing phenomena of importance to nursing.

observation research. A data-collection method in which data are collected through visual observations.

one-group pretest-posttest design. A type of pre-experimental design; compares one group of subjects before and after an experimental treatment.

one-shot case study. A type of pre-experimental design; a single group of subjects is observed after a treatment to determine the effects of the treatment. No pretest measurement is made.

one-tailed test of significance. A test of statistical significance in which the critical values (statistically significant values) are sought in only one tail of the theoretical sampling distribution (either the right or the left tail).

open-ended questions. Questions that allow respondents to answer in their own words.

operational definition. The definition of a variable that identifies how the variable will be observed or measured.

ordinal level of measurement (ordinal data). Data can be categorized and placed in order; small, medium, and large is an example of a set of ordinal data.

outcomes research. Research that examines the outcomes or results of patient care interventions.

parallel forms reliability. See alternate forms reliability.

parameter. A numerical characteristic of a population (e.g., the average educational level of people living in the United States).

parametric statistical tests. Types of inferential statistics that are concerned with population parameters. When parametric tests are used, assumptions are made that (a) the level of measurement of the data is interval or ratio, (b) data are taken from populations that are normally distributed on the variable being measured, and (c) data are taken from populations that have equal variances on the variable being measured.

participant observation. Involves the direct observation and recording of information in a study and requires that the researcher become a part of the setting in which the person, group, or culture is being observed.

participant observer (covert). Research observer interacts with the subjects and observes their behavior without their knowledge.

participant observer (overt). Research observer interacts with subjects openly and with the full awareness of those people who are observed.

participatory action research. A special kind of community-based action research in which there is collaboration between the study participants and the researcher in all steps of the study: determining the problem, the research methods to use, the analysis of data, and how the study results will be used.

pecuniary terms. Expressed in monetary values.

peer review. The review of a research manuscript by professional colleagues who have content or methodological expertise concerning the material presented in the manuscript.

percentage (%). A statistic that represents the proportion of a subgroup to a total group, expressed as a percentage ranging from 0% to 100%.

percentile. A data point below which lies a certain percentage of the values in a frequency distribution.

personality inventories. Self-report measures used to assess the differences in personality traits, needs, or values of people.

phenomenological studies (phenomenology). Research studies that examine human experiences through the descriptions of the meanings of these experiences provided by the people involved.

pilot study. A small-scale trial run of an actual research study.

population. A complete set of persons or objects that possess some common characteristic of interest to the researcher.

positively skewed. A frequency distribution in which the tail of the distribution points to the right.

positive relationship (direct relationship). A relationship between two variables in which the variables tend to vary together; as the values of one variable increase or decrease, the values of the other variable increase or decrease.

posttest. Data are collected after the researcher has administered the experimental treatment.

posttest-only control group design. True experimental design in which subjects in the experimental and comparison groups are given a posttest after the experimental group receives the study treatment.

power analysis. A procedure that is used to determine the sample size needed to prevent a type II error.

power of a statistical test. The ability of a statistical test to reject a null hypothesis when it is false (and should be rejected).

predictive validity. A type of criterion validity of an instrument in which a determination is made of the instrument's ability to predict behavior of subjects in the future.

pre-existing data. Existing information that has not been collected for research purposes.

pre-experimental design. A type of experimental design in which the researcher has little control over the research situation; includes the one-shot case study and the one-group pretest-posttest design.

pretest. Data are collected before the researcher has administered the experimental treatment; data obtained in the pretest may also be called baseline data.

pretest-posttest control group design. True experimental design in which subjects in the experimental and comparison groups are given a pretest before and a posttest after the administration of the study treatment to the experimental group.

primary source. In the research literature, an account of a research study that has been written by the original researcher(s); in historical studies, firsthand information or direct evidence of an event.

principal investigator. The lead researcher; the person who has the primary responsibility for the study.

probability level (p). See level of significance.

probability sampling. The use of a random sampling procedure to select a sample from elements or members of a population; includes simple, stratified, cluster, and systematic random sampling techniques.

probes. Prompting questions that encourage the respondent to elaborate on the topic being discussed.

production function. Output that can be produced with a given set of input.

projective technique. Self-report measure in which a subject is asked to respond to stimuli that are designed to be ambiguous or to have no definite meaning. The responses reflect the internal feelings of the subject that are projected on the external stimuli.

proportional stratified sampling. Random selection of members from population strata where the number of members chosen from each stratum is in proportion to the size of the stratum in the total population.

propositional statement (theoretical statement). A statement or assertion of the relationship between concepts.

prospective studies. Studies in which the independent variable or presumed cause is identified at the present time and then subjects are followed for some time in the future to observe the dependent variable or effect.

purposive sampling (judgmental sampling). A nonprobability sampling procedure in which the researcher uses personal judgment to select subjects considered to be representative of the population.

p value. See level of significance.

Q sort (Q methodology). A data-collection method in which subjects are asked to sort statements into categories according to their attitudes toward, or rating of, the statements.

qualitative research. Research that is concerned with the subjective meaning of an experience to an individual.

quantitative research. Research that is concerned with objectivity, tight controls over the research situation, and the ability to generalize findings.

quasi-experimental design. A type of experimental design in which there is either no comparison group or no random assignment of subjects to groups; includes the nonequivalent control group design and time-series design.

query letter. A letter of inquiry sent to a journal to determine the editor's interest in publishing a manuscript. The letter usually contains an outline of the manuscript and important information about the content of the manuscript.

questionnaire. A self-report instrument, often paper-and-pencil, used to gather data from subjects.

quota sampling. A nonprobability sampling procedure in which the researcher selects the sample to reflect certain characteristics of the population.

r. The symbol for a correlation coefficient.

random assignment. A procedure used in an experimental study to ensure that each study subject has an equal chance of being placed into any one of the study groups.

random sampling. See probability sampling.

range. A measure of variability; the distance between the highest and lowest value in a group of values or scores.

ratio level of measurement (ratio data). Data can be categorized, ranked, the distance between ranks specified, and a "true" or natural zero point identified; the amount of money in a checking account or number of requests for pain medication are examples of ratio data.

reactive effects of the pretest. A threat to the external validity of a research study that occurs when subjects are sensitized to the experimental treatment by the pretest.

refereed journal. A journal that uses experts in a given field to review manuscripts.

reflexivity. The process of identifying and setting aside personal beliefs about the subject of the study.

region of rejection. See critical region.

reliability. The consistency and dependability of a research instrument to measure a variable; types of reliability are stability, equivalence, and internal consistency.

replication study. A research study that repeats or duplicates an earlier research study, with all of the essential elements of the original study held intact. A different sample or setting may be used.

research design. The overall plan for gathering data in a research study.

research hypothesis (H_1). An alternative hypothesis to the statistical null hypothesis; predicts the researcher's actual expectations about the outcome of a study; also called scientific, substantive, and theoretical.

research instruments (research tools). Devices used to collect data in research studies.

research problem. An area where knowledge is needed to advance the practice of nursing.

research question. The specific question that the researcher expects to be answered in a study.

research report. A written or oral summary of a research study.

research utilization. The implementation of research findings into practice.

respondent. A person in a study who provides answers or responses to the researcher.

retrospective studies. Studies in which the dependent variable is identified in the present (e.g., a disease condition) and an attempt is made to determine the independent variable (e.g., cause of the disease) that occurred in the past.

Rosenthal effect. The influence of interviewers on respondents' answers.

sample. A subset of the population that is selected to represent the population.

sampling bias. The difference between sample data and population data that can be attributed to a faulty selection process; a threat to the external validity of a research study that occurs when subjects are not randomly selected from the population.

sampling distribution. A theoretical frequency distribution that is based on an infinite number of samples. Sampling distributions are based on mathematical formulas and logic.

sampling error. Random fluctuations in data that occur when a sample is selected to represent a population.

sampling frame. A listing of all the elements of the population from which a sample is to be chosen.

saturation. The researcher hears a repetition of themes or ideas as additional participants are interviewed in a qualitative study.

scatter plot (scatter diagram, scattergram). A graphic presentation of the relationship between two variables. The graph contains variables plotted on an X axis and a Y axis. Pairs of scores are plotted by the placement of dots to indicate where each pair of Xs and Ys intersect.

search engine. Finding tool used to look for information on the internet.

secondary source. In the research literature, an account of a research study that has been written by someone other than the study investigators; in historical studies, secondhand information or data provided by someone who did not observe the event.

selection bias. A threat to the internal validity of an experimental research study that occurs when study results are attributed to the experimental treatment when, in fact, the results may be related to pretreatment differences between the subjects in the experimental and comparison groups.

semantic differential. Attitude scale that asks subjects to indicate their position or attitude about some concept along a continuum between two adjectives or phrases that are presented in relation to the concept being measured.

semiquartile range. Determined by dividing the interquartile range in half (see interquartile range).

semistructured interviews. Interviewers ask a certain number of specific questions, but additional questions or probes are used at the discretion of the interviewer.

simple hypothesis. A hypothesis that predicts the relationship between one independent and one dependent variable.

simple random sampling. A method of random sampling in which each element of the population has an equal and independent chance of being chosen for the sample.

simulation studies. Laboratory studies in which subjects are presented with a description of a case study or situation intended to represent a real-life situation.

skewed. A frequency distribution that is nonsymmetrical.

snowball sampling (network sampling). A sampling method that involves the assistance of study subjects to help obtain other potential subjects.

Solomon four-group design. True experimental design that minimizes threats to internal and external validity.

stability reliability. The consistency of a research instrument over time; test-retest procedures and repeated observations are methods to test the stability of an instrument.

standard deviation (SD; s). A measure of variability; the statistic that indicates the average deviation or variation of all the values in a set of data from the mean value of that data.

standard error of the mean ($s_{\bar{x}}$). The standard deviation of the sampling distribution of the mean.

statistic. A numerical characteristic of a sample (e.g., the average educational level of a random sample of people living in the United States).

stratified random sampling. A random sampling process in which a sample is selected after the population has been divided into subgroups or strata according to some variable of importance to the research study.

structured interviews. Interviewers ask the same questions in the same manner of all respondents.

structured observations. The researcher determines the behaviors to be observed before data collection. Usually some kind of checklist is used to record behaviors.

study limitations. Weaknesses in a study that are not controlled by the researcher (e.g., educational level and age of participants).

subject dropout. See attrition; dropout.

survey studies. Research studies in which self-report data are collected from a sample to determine the characteristics of a population.

symmetrical distributions. Frequency distributions in which both halves of the distribution are the same.

synthesize. Combine the points, inferences, or arguments from different sources to provide readers with information about the existing research on your topic.

systematic random sampling. A random sampling process in which every kth (e.g., every fifth) element or member of the population is selected for the sample.

systematic review. A rigorous scientific approach that combines results from a group of research studies and looks at the studies as a whole; also called an integrative review, can summarize many studies at once while focusing on a single area of interest.

table of random numbers. A list of numbers that have been generated in such a manner that there is no order or sequencing of the numbers. Each number is equally likely to follow any other number.

target population. The entire group of people or objects to which the researcher wishes to generalize the findings of a study.

telephone interviews. Data are collected from subjects through the use of phone calls rather than in face-to-face encounters.

testing (threat to internal validity). A threat to the internal validity of a research study that occurs when a pretest is administered to subjects; the effects of taking a pretest on responses on the posttest.

test-retest reliability. See stability reliability.

theoretical framework. A study framework based on propositional statements from a theory.

theoretical statement. See propositional statement.

theory. A set of related statements that describes or explains phenomena systematically.

time sampling. Observations of events or behaviors that are made during certain specified time periods.

time-series design. Quasi-experimental design in which the researcher periodically observes subjects and administers an experimental treatment between two of the observations.

triangulation. The use of two or more different sampling strategies, data collectors, data collection procedures, or theories in one study.

true experimental design. An experimental design in which the researcher (a) manipulates the experimental variable, (b) includes at least one experimental and one comparison group in the study, and (c) randomly assigns subjects to either the experimental or the comparison group; includes the pretest-posttest control group design, posttest-only control group design, and Solomon four-group design.

t test (t). A parametric statistical test that examines the difference between the means of two groups of values. Types of t tests are the independent t test (independent samples t test) and the dependent t test (paired t test).

two-tailed test of significance. A test of statistical significance in which critical values (statistically significant values) are sought in both tails of the sampling distribution; used when the researcher has not predicted the direction of the relationship between variables.

type I error (α). A decision is made to reject the null hypothesis when it is actually true; a decision is made that a relationship exists between variables when it does not.

type II error (β). A decision is made not to reject the null hypothesis when it is false and should be rejected; a decision is made that no relationship exists between variables when, in fact, a relationship does exist.

unimodal. A frequency distribution that contains one value that occurs more frequently than any other.

univariate study. A research study in which only one variable is examined.

unstructured interviews. The interviewer is given a great deal of freedom to direct the course of the interview; the interviewer's main goal is to encourage the respondent to talk freely about the topic being explored.

unstructured observations. The researcher describes behaviors as they are viewed, with no preconceived ideas of what will be seen.

validity (of instruments). The ability of an instrument to measure the variable that it is intended to measure. See also internal validity threats and external validity threats of experimental studies.

variable. A characteristic or attribute of a person or object that differs among the persons or objects being studied (e.g., age, blood type).

variance (SD^2; s^2). A measure of variability; the standard deviation squared.

visual analogue scale. Subjects are presented with a straight line anchored on each end with words or phrases that represent the extremes of some phenomenon, such as pain. Subjects are asked to make a mark on the line at the point that corresponds to their experience of the phenomenon. Either a horizontal or vertical line may be used.

volunteers. Subjects who have asked to participate in a study.

z score. A standard score that indicates how many standard deviations that a particular value is from the mean of the set of values.

Credits

Chapter 1: Page 2: From Polit, D. F., & Beck, C. T. (2012). *Nursing research: Generating and assessing evidence for nursing practice* (9th ed.). Philadelphia: Wolters Kluwer. © 2012; Page 2: From Grove, S. K., Burns, N., & Gray, J. (2013). Discovering the World of Nursing Research. In *The practice of nursing research: Appraisal, synthesis, and generation of evidence* (7th ed.). Published by Elsevier Health Sciences. © 2013; Page 13: From Research Priorities for Public Health Nursing in *Public Health Nursing, 27*(1), 94–100. Published by John Wiley and Sons. © 2010.

Chapter 2: Page 19: From Sackett, D. L., Rosenberg, W. M., Gray, J. A., Haynes, R. B., & Richardson, W. S. (1996). Evidence based medicine: What it is and what it isn't. *British Medical Journal, 312*, 71–72. Published by BMJ Publishing Group Ltd. © 1996; Page 19: From *Evidence-based Nursing Position Statement*. Published by Sigma Theta Tau International. © 2005.

Chapter 3: Pages 32: From Grove, S., Burns, N., & Gray, J. (2013). Evolution of Research in Building Evidence-Based Nursing Practice. In *The practice of nursing research: Appraisal, synthesis generation of evidence* (7th ed.) St. Louis, MO: Saunders Elsevier. © 2013; Pages 32: From Titler, M. (2014). Overview of evidence-based practice and translation science. *Nursing Clinics of North America, 49*(3), 269–274. Published by Elsevier, Inc. © 2014.

Chapter 4: Page 45: Code of Federal Regulations: Title 45 Public Welfare. Published by U.S. Department of Health & Human Service; Page 52: Code of Ethics for Nurses with Interpretive Statements by Margaret Hegge. Published by American Nurses Association. © 2015; Page 43: From Shearer, L. (1982, October 17). Now it can be told. *Dallas Morning News*. 10–11. © 1982.

Chapter 5: Page 61: From Downs, F. (1994). Hitching the research wagon to theory. *Nursing Research, 43*(4), 195. Published by Wolters Kluwer Health Inc. © 1994.

Chapter 6: Page 78: From Bridges, E., McNeill, M., & Munro, N. (2016). Research in review: Driving critical care practice change. *American Journal of Critical Care, 25*(1), 76–84. Published by American Association of Critical-Care Nurses. © 2016; Pages 82: From *To a Mouse* by Robert Burns; Pages 86–87: From Read, C. Y., & Ward, L. D. (2016). Faculty performance on the Genomic Nursing Concept Inventory. *Nursing Scholarship, 48*(1), 5–13. Published by John Wiley and Sons. © 2016; Page 87: From Hernon, P., & Schwartz, C. (2007). What is a problem statement? *Library & Information Science Research, 29*, 307–309. Published by Elsevier Inc. © 2009.

Chapter 7: Pages 95: From Federer, L. (2013). The librarian as research informationist: A case study. *Medical Library Association, 101*(4), 298–302. Published by Medical Library Association. © 2013; Page 93: From Health Services Research and Health Policy Grey Literature Project: Summary Report. Published by National Institute of Health; Page 95: From Federer, L. (2013). The librarian as research informationist: A case study. *Medical Library Association, 101*(4), 298–302. Published by Medical Library Association. © 2003.

Chapter 8: Page 104: From Kerlinger, F. (1973). *Foundations of behavioral research* (2nd ed.). New York: Holt, Rinehart & Winston. © 1973; Page 104: From Grove, S., Burns, N., & Gray, J. (2013). *The practice of nursing research: Appraisal, synthesis generation of evidence* (7th ed.). St. Louis, MO: Saunders Elsevier. © 2013; Page 105: Grove, S., Burns, N., & Gray, J. (2013). *The practice of nursing research: Appraisal, synthesis generation of evidence* (7th ed.). St. Louis, MO: Saunders Elsevier. © 2013; Page 105: From Bush, H. (1979). Models for nursing. *Advances in Nursing Science, 1*(2), 13–21. Published by Wolters Kluwer Health Inc. © 1979; Page 107: From Fawcett, J., & Desanto-Madeya, S. (2013). *Contemporary nursing knowledge: Analysis and evaluation of nursing models and theories* (3rd ed.). Philadelphia: F. A. Davis. © 2013; Page 108: From Rogers, M. (1980).

Nursing: A science of unitary man. In J. P. Riehl and C. Roy (Eds.), *Conceptual models for nursing practice* (2nd ed.). New York: Appleton-Century-Crofts. © 1980; Page 108: From Farren, A. T. (2010). Power, uncertainty, self-transcendence, and quality of life in breast cancer survivors. *Nursing Science Quarterly, 23*, 63–71. Published by Sage Publications. © 2010; Page 110: From Pipe, T. B., Bortz, J. J., & Dueck, A. (2009). Nurse leader mindfulness meditation program for stress management: A randomized controlled trial. *Nursing Administration, 39*, 130–137. Published by Wolters Kluwer Health Inc. © 2009; Page 116: From Maslow, A. (1970). *Motivation and personality* (2nd ed.). New York: Harper & Row. © 1970.

Chapter 9: Page 124: From Kerlinger, F. (1986). *Foundations of behavioral research* (3rd ed.). New York: Holt, Rinehart & Winston; Page 129: From Fisher, R. (1951). *The design of experiments* (6th ed.). New York: Hafner. © 1951; Page 124: From Polit, D. F., & Beck. C. T. (2012). *Nursing research: Principles and methods* (9th ed.). © 2012. Philadelphia: Lippincott Williams & Wilkins; Page 129: From Polit, D. F., & Beck. C. T. (2012). *Nursing research: Principles and methods* (9th ed.). Philadelphia: Lippincott Williams & Wilkins. © 2012.

Chapter 11: Page 164: From Creswell, J., Klassen, A. C., Plano Clark, V. L., Clegg Smith, K. (n.d.). *Best practices for mixed methods research in the health sciences*. Office of Behavioral and Social Sciences Research, National Institutes of Health; Page 160: From Leininger, M. M. (Ed.). (1985). *Qualitative research methods in nursing*. Orlando, FL: Grune & Stratton. © 1985; Page 162: From Rowniak, S. (2015). PrEP: A case study. *American Association of Nurse Practitioners, 27*(6), 296–299. Published by John Wiley and Sons. © 2015; Page 164: Creswell, J. (2003). *Research design: Qualitative, quantitative and mixed method approaches*. Thousand Oaks, CA: Sage. © 2003.

Chapter 12: Page 178: Massive nurses' health study in seventh year, reports first findings on disease links in women. (1983). *American Journal of Nursing, 83*(17), 998–999. Published by Lippincott Williams & Wilkins. © 1983.

Chapter 14: Page 205: From Oppenheim, A. (1966). *Questionnaire design and attitude measurement*. New York: Basic Books. © 1966.

Chapter 15: Pages 241–242: From Roscoe, J. (1975). *Fundamental research statistics for the behavioral sciences* (2nd ed.). New York: Holt, Rinehart & Winston. © 1975.

Chapter 16: Page 251: From Spatz, C., & Johnston, J. (1984). *Basic statistics: Tales of distribution* (3rd ed.). Monterey, CA: Brooks/Cole. © 1984; Page 256: From Elzey, F. (1974). *A first reader in statistics* (2nd ed.). Monterey, CA: Brooks/Cole. © 1974.

Chapter 17: Page 280: From Polit, D. F. & Beck, C. F. (2010). Generalization in quantitative and qualitative research: Myths and strategies. *International Journal of Nursing Studies 47*(11), 1451–1458. Published by Elsevier. © 2010.

Chapter 18: Page 288: From Northam, S., Yarbrough, S., Haas, B., & Duke, G. (2010). Journal editor survey information to help authors publish. *Nurse Educator, 35*(1), 29–36. Published by Lippincott Williams & Wilkins Inc, © 2010; Page 294: From Burns, N., & Grove, S. K. (2009). *The practice of nursing research: Appraisal, synthesis, and generation of evidence* (6th ed.). St. Louis, MO: Saunders Elsevier. © 2009.

Chapter 19: Page 304: From Chen, C., McNeese-Smith, D., Cowan, M., Upenieks, V., & Afifi, A. (2009). Evaluation of a nurse practitioner-led care management model in reducing inpatient drug utilization and cost. *Nursing Economics, 27*(3), 160–169. Published by Jannetti Publications Inc. © 2009; Page 305: From Laurant, M., Reeves, D., Hermens, R., Braspenning, J., Grol, R. & Sibbald, B. (2005). Substitution of doctors by nurses in primary care. *Cochrane Database Systematic Review*, April 18. Published by John Wiley and Sons, © 2005; Pages 305–306: From Cryer, L., Shannon, S. B., Van Amsterdam, M., & Leff, B. (2012). Costs for "hospital at home" patients were 19 percent lower, with equal or better outcomes compared to similar inpatients. *Health Affairs, 31*(6), 1237–1243. Published by Project HOPE. © 2012; Page 306: From Buerhaus, P., Welton, J., & Rosenthal, M. (2010). Health care payment reform: Implications for nurses. *Nursing Economics, 28*(1), 49–54. Published by Anthony J. Jannetti Inc. © 2010.

Index

Note: Page numbers followed by *e*, *f*, *t*, or *b* represent study examples, figures, tables, or boxes respectively. Page numbers in **bold** indicates Glossary terms.

A

Abscissa, 235
Abstract, 287, 315, 321, **372**
   call for, 287, 296, **372**
   critiquing guidelines for, 315
   dissertation, 94
Accessible population, 64, 170, 170*e*, 183, 318, **372**
Accidental sampling, **374**. *See also* Convenience sampling
Accountability for nursing practice, 5, 14
ACE Center for Advancing Clinical Excellence, 27
Action research, 68*t*, 163, 163*e*, **372**
   participatory, 163, **380**
   type of qualitative research, 68*t*
Administrative support, 82
Advocacy, defined, 52
Affordable Care Act, 307–308
Agency for Healthcare Research and Quality (AHRQ), 23–26
   evidence-based practice centers (EPC), 24–25
   National Guideline Clearinghouse (NGC), 25–26
   U.S. Preventive Services Task Force (USPSTF), 25
Alpha (α), 195, 257, **372**
Alternate forms reliability, 194, **372**
Alternative hypothesis, 129, **372**
Ambiguous questions, 207, 224, **372**
American Association of College of Nursing (AACN), 7
American Nurses Association (ANA) Research and Studies Commission, 52
American Nurses Credentialing Center (ANCC), 20
American Nurses Foundation (ANF), 4, 10, 11, 292
American Psychological Association (APA), 96, 98, 230, 274
American Society for Parenteral and Enteral Nutrition (A.S.P.E.N.) guidelines, 37

Analysis of covariance (ANCOVA), 266–267, 266*e*, **372**
Analysis of variance (ANOVA), 262–263, 263*e*, **372**
Analyze, 99, **372**
Anonymity, **372**
   as element of informed consent, 49
   in qualitative research, 70
Applied research, 3, 14, **372**
Article preparation, 289
Assent, 50, **372**
Association of Community Health Nursing Educators (ACHNE), 13
Association of Critical Care Nurses, 38
Associative research hypothesis, 128–129, 129*e*
Assumptions, 62, 316, **372**
Attitude scales, 216, **372**
   Likert scale, 216–217, 217*e*, 217*f*
   semantic differential scales, 218, 218*e*, 218*f*
Attribute variables, 207, **372**
Attrition, 141, 154, **372**

B

Bar graph, 234, 235*f*, **372**
Basic research, 3, 4, 4*e*, 11, 14, 48, **372**
Basic social processes, 161
Belmont Report, 44
Beneficence, 45, **372**
Best Practice Recommendation, 27
Beta (β), 261, **372**
Bimodal class, 237, 247
Bimodal distribution, 237, 247, **372**
Bivariate study, 84, **372**
Blind review, 291, **372**
Bracketing, 159, **372**
Brown Report, The, 10, 15

C

Calculated value/critical value, comparison, 258–259
Call for abstract, 287, **372**
Canonical correlation, 267, **372**
Case studies, 162–163, 163*e*, **372**

Catalogs, 96–97, **372**
Causal research hypothesis, 128, 128*e*
Cause-and-effect relationship, 139, **373**
Cells, 275, **373**
Center for Disease Control and Prevention (CDC), 34
Centers for Medicare & Medicaid Services (CMS), 307
Central limit theorem, 179, 251, 269, **373**
Central tendency. *See* Measures of central tendency
Chi-square test, 263–265, 264*t*, 265*e*, **373**
CINAHL. *See* Cumulative Index to Nursing and Allied Health Literature
Class interval, 231, **373**
Clinical nursing research, 2, **373**
Clinical significance, 277, 277*e*
Clinical trials, 19, 52, 267, **373**
Closed-ended questions, 207–208, **373**
Cluster random sampling, 173–174, 174*e*, **373**
Cochrane Centers, 23
Cochrane Central Register of Controlled Trials (CENTRAL), 22, 98
Cochrane Collaboration (CC), 12. *See also* Evidence-based nursing practice (EBNP)
  Cochrane Centers, 23
  Cochrane Database, 22
  Cochrane Library, 22
  Cochrane Nursing Care Field (CNCF), 23
Cochrane Database, 22
Cochrane Database of Systematic Reviews (CDSR), 22, 98
Cochrane Library, 22, 98
Cochrane Methodology Register (CMAR), 22, 98
Cochrane Nursing Care (CNC), 12, 23
Cochrane Nursing Care Field (CNCF), 12, 15, 23
Cochrane Nursing Care Network (CNCN), 12, 15
Cochrane Reviews, 12, 22, 23, 28
Code of Ethics for Nurses with Interpretative Statements, 52
Coding, 72, 199, 323
Coefficient alpha, 195, **373**
Coefficient of determination, 242, 242*t*, 248, **373**
Cohort study, 177, **373**

Collectively exhaustive categories, 207, 224, **373**
Communication of nursing research findings
  journal article, publishing, 288–290
  paper presentation, 287–288
  poster presentation, 288
  refereed and nonrefereed journals, 290–292
  research report preparation, 286
  research reports for funding agencies, 292
  research result presentation at professional conferences, 286–287
Comparative statements, research questions, 85
Comparative studies, 150–151, 150*e*, **373**
Comparison group, 144, **373**
Complex hypothesis, 126–127, 127*t*, **373**
Composite measures, 26
Computer-assisted literature searches, 61, **373**
Computerized database, 97, **373**
Concept, 34, 104, **373**
Conceptual definition, 63, **373**
Conceptual framework, 61–62, 115, **373**
Conceptual model, 106, **373**
Conclusions, 278–279, 319
Concurrent validity, 197, 197*e*, **373**
Conduct and Utilization of Research in Nursing (CURN) project, 20, 294–295
Confidence interval, 252–255, **373**
Confidentiality, 49, **373**
Confirmability, 71
Conflicts of interest (COI), 52
Confounding variable, 153, **373**
Consent. *See* Informed consent
Constant comparison method, 161, **373**
Construct, 105, **374**
Construct validity, 197, 198, 198*e*, **374**
Content analysis, 72, **374**
Content validity, 196, 196*e*, **374**
Contingency questions, 208–209, **374**
Contingency table, 243, 244*f*, **374**
Control group, 144, **374**
Convenience sampling, 175–176, 176*e*, **374**
Correlated samples *t* test. *See* Dependent *t* test
Correlation, 149, **374**
Correlational statements, research questions, 85
Correlational studies, 149, 150*e*, **374**

Correlation coefficient, 241–245, 242*t*, 243*f*, **374**
  contingency table, 243
  correlational procedures, types of, 243–244
  Pearson *r* test, 244–245, 245*e*
  scatter plot, 242–243, 243*f*
  significance of, 265–266
  Spearman rho, 245, 245*e*
Cost-effectiveness of nursing care, 5–6
Cost-effectiveness studies, 303–306
  need for research studies on nursing care, 306–307
  telenursing (TN), 305–306
Cost of research projects, 82
Cover letter, 209, 224
Credibility
  of nursing profession, 5
  qualitative study, 71
Criterion validity, 196, 197*e*, **374**
Critical region, 258, **374**
Critical value, 258–259, **374**
Critique (research critique), 313, 314, **374**
Cronbach's alpha (coefficient alpha), 195, **374**
Cross-sectional study, 177, 178*e*, **374**
Cumulative Index to Nursing and Allied Health Literature (CINAHL), 21, 38, 97

D
Dall study, 302–303
Data, **374**
  coding, 199
  defined, 65
  empirical, 3, 14, 85, 87, 88, 116*f*, **375**
  fabrication, 51
  interpretation, 323
    as step in qualitative research, 72
  organization for analysis, 65–66
Data analysis, 161, 319, 323
  as step in qualitative research, 72
  as step in quantitative research, 66
Database of Abstracts of Reviews of Effects (DARE), 22
Databases, 97, **374**
Databases, Cochrane, 22
Databases for nursing students. *See also* Literature review
  CINAHL databases, 97
  Cochrane databse of Systematic Review, 98
  MEDLINE databases, 97
  Ovid Nursing Database, 98
  ProQuest Dissertations & Theses Database (PQDT), 98
  PsychINFO, 98
  Science Direct, 98–99
  Scopus, 99
  Search engines, 99
Data collection, 161, 178, 318, 323
  as step in qualitative research, 70–71
  as step in quantitative research, 65
Data-collection instruments, 318
Data-collection methods
  attitude scales
    Likert scale, 216–217, 217*e*, 217*f*
    semantic differential scales, 218, 218*e*, 218*f*
  completion instructions, 209
  cover letter, 209
  critiquing guidelines, 222–223, 223*b*
  Delphi technique, 221, 221*e*
  factors influencing response rates, 210
  interview
    advantages, 214
    disadvantages, 214
    instruments, 212
    interviewer guidelines, 213
    interviewers on respondents, 213–214
    interviewer training, 212–213
    questions, 212
    semistructured, 211–212
    structured, 211
    timing and setting for, 213
    unstructured, 211
  language and reading level of questions, 205–206
  length of questionnaire and questions, 206
  observation methods
    behaviors to be observed, 214
    event sampling, 215
    nurse *vs.* researcher, 216
    observer and subjects, relationship, 215–216
    research observers, 214–215
    structured/unstructured observations, 215
    time sampling, 215
  physiological measures, 219
  preexisting data, 222
  psychological tests

personality inventories, 219
projective technique, 219–220, 220*e*
Q Sort, 220, 220*e*
questionnaires, 204–205
  advantages of, 210
  disadvantages of, 210–211
  distribution of, 210
  overall appearance of, 205
questions, placement of, 209
questions, types of
  closed-ended questions, 207–208
  contingency questions, 208–209
  demographic questions, 207
  filler questions, 209
  open-ended questions, 208
visual analogue scale (VAS), 221, 221*e*
wording of questions, 207
Data-collection process
  critiquing, 199–200, 200*t*
  instruments
    development of, 192
    existing instruments, 191–192
    pilot study, 192
  methods, 190–191
Data utilization
  error sources in data collection, 199
  preparing data for analysis, 199
Debriefing, 48, 51, 54, **374**
Declaration of Helsinki, 44
Declarative form, research question, 83
Declarative statement, 130
Deductive processes in theory generation/
    development, 116*t*
Deductive reasoning, 116, 119, **374**
Degrees of freedom, 259, **374**
Delphi technique, 221, 221*e*, **374**
Demographic questions, 207, **374**
Demographic variables, 207, **374**
Dependability, 71
Dependent *t* test, 262, 262*e*, **374**
Dependent variable, 63, **375**
Derived demand, 301, **375**
Descriptive statistics, **375**
  critiquing descriptive statistics,
    246, 246*b*
  measures of central tendency,
    236–238
    mean, 238
    median, 237
    mode, 237
  measures of relationships, 240–246

  correlation coefficients, 241–245,
    242*t*, 243*f*
  intraocular method of data analysis,
    245–246
measures of variability, 238–240
  percentile, 239
  range, 239
  standard deviation, 239–240
  variance, 240
  z-scores, 240
measures to condense data
  frequency distributions, 231–234, 231*t*,
    232*f*, 232*t*, 233*f*
  graphic presentations, 126*f*, 234–236, 235*f*
Descriptive studies, 138, **375**
Diaries, 222, 222*e*
Digital object identifier (DOI), 96
Diminishing marginal returns, 301, **375**
Directional research hypothesis, 63, 128,
  128*e*, **375**
Discovery catalogs. *See* Discovery systems
Discovery systems, 97, **375**
Discussion of study findings
  statistical and clinical significance,
    277–278, 277*e*
  study hypotheses, 276–277
  study limitations, 276
Disproportional stratified sampling,
  172, **375**
Double-barreled questions, 207, **375**
Double-blind experiment, 142, **375**
Dropout, 141, 154, **375**

E

Edwards Personal Preference Schedule
    (EPPS), 219
Effect size, 267, **375**
e-journal, 96, **375**
Element, 170, **375**
Empirical data, 3, 14, 85, 87, 88, 116*f*, **375**
Empirical generalization, 105, 116, 119,
  126, **375**
Empirically testable hypothesis, 85, 131,
  133, 317
Entry to research site, gaining, 70
Equivalence reliability, 194, 201, **375**
Ethical codes and guidelines
  ethical research guidelines, 44–45
  historical overview, 42–43
  unethical research in United States,
    43–44

Ethical issues, 80
　critiquing guidelines, 53, 53b
　ethical codes and guidelines, 42–45
　informed consent, elements of, 47–51
　institutional review board (IRB), 45–47
　integrity in research, 51–52
　in presentation of study findings, 274
　research guidelines for nurses, 52–53
Ethical research, founding principles of, 44–45
Ethnographic studies, 160–161, 161e, **375**
Event sampling, 215, 224, **375**
Evidence-based nursing practice (EBNP), 4–5
　Agency for Healthcare Research and Quality (AHRQ), 23–26, 26e
　　Evidence-Based Practice Centers, 24–25
　　National Guideline Clearinghouse (NGC), 25–26
　　U.S. Preventive Services Task Force (USPSTF), 25
　benefits of, 20–21
　clinical questions, 21
　Cochrane Collaboration (CC)
　　Cochrane Centers, 23
　　Cochrane Database, 22
　　Cochrane Library, 22
　　Cochrane Nursing Care Field (CNCF), 23
　defined, 18
　research utilization (RU) vs., 20
　sources for, 21
　use of evidence in nursing, 19
Evidence-based nursing practice centers, 26–28
　ACE Center for Advancing Clinical Excellence, 27
　Joanna Briggs Institute (JBI), 27
　Sarah Cole Hirsh Institute (SCHI), 27–28
Evidence-based practice (EBP), 14, 19, 294, **375**
　barriers associated with, 36
　evolving nature of, 32–33
　facilitators of, 36–37
　Iowa model, application of, 37–38
　models
　　Iowa model, 33
　　Iowa model concepts, 34–36
　　Stetler model, 33
Evidence-based practice centers (EPC), 24–25
Evidence summaries, 21
Existing theories, as source of nursing research problems, 79
Experiences measures, 26

Experimental design, 64, **375**
Experimental research
　pre-experimental designs, 147–148
　symbolic presentation of research designs, 143
　threats to external validity, 142–143
　threats to internal validity, 140–142
　validity of, 139–140
Experimenter effect, 142, **375**
Explanatory studies, 138, **375**
Exploratory studies, 138, **375**
Ex post facto studies, 150, **375**
External validity, 139
External validity, threats to, **376**
　experimenter effect, 142
　Hawthorne effect, 142, 142e
　reactive effects of pretest, 142–143
Extraneous variables, 62, 139, **376**

F

Face validity, 195–196, 196e, **376**
Factor analysis, 198, 198e, **376**
Fawcett's metaparadigm of nursing, 107
Feasibility of study
　administrative support, 82
　availability of subjects, 82
　cost, 82
　equipment and supplies, 82
　peer support, 82
　time, 81
Field notes, 161
Field studies, 152, **376**
Figures, in presentation of study findings, 275
Filler questions, 209, **376**
Finding tools
　catalogs, 96–97
　databases, 97
Focus group, 71, 71e, **376**
Framework, 61, 115, 118b, **376**
Frequency distribution, 231–234, 231t, 232f, 232t, 233f, 252t, **376**
Frequency polygon, 235, **376**

G

Galley proofs, 289, **376**
Generalization. *See* Empirical generalization
Governmental agencies/related organizations
　Affordable Care Act, 307–308
　public health, 308
　regulatory agencies, 308

Grand theories, 119, **376**
Graphic presentations, 126*f*, 234–236, 235*f*
Gray literature. *See* Grey literature
Grey literature, 93–94, **376**
Grounded theory, 161, 161*e*, **376**

H

Hawthorne effect, 49, 142, 142*e*, **376**
Health and Human Services (HHS), U. S., 23
Health care economics and nursing
  Dall study, 302–303
  market forces affecting nurses, 301–302
  value of nursing, determining, 302
Healthcare quality improvement, 14
Healthcare unit (HCU), 303
Health Insurance Portability and Accountability Act (HIPAA) Privacy Rule, 52
Health Technology Assessment Database (HTA), 22
Heart failure self-care, theory of, 111, 111*e*
Histogram, 235, **376**
Historical studies, 42–43, **376**
History threat, 140, **376**
Human Rights Guidelines for Nurses in Clinical and Other Research, 52
Human subjects, 45
Hypothesis(es), 62, 105, 317, **376**
  classifications of
    associative research hypothesis, 128–129, 129*e*
    causal research hypothesis, 128, 128*e*
    complex hypothesis, 126–127, 127*t*
    directional research hypothesis, 128, 128*e*
    nondirectional research hypothesis, 127, 127*e*
    null hypothesis, 129, 130, 130*e*
    research hypothesis, 129
    simple hypothesis, 126
  development of
    critiquing hypotheses, 132–133, 133*b*
    empirically testable, 131
    hypotheses and theory testing, 132
    hypothesis format, 131–132
    population, 131
    problem statement, 131
    purpose statement, 131
    research question, 131
    variables, 131
    written in declarative statement, 130
    written in present tense, 130
  for, support for, 259
  formulation, 62–63
  overview, 124–126
    purposes of, 125
    sources or rationale for, 125–126
  for study, 255–256
  study, discussion, 276–277
  testing of, 255

I

Impact factor (IF), 290, **376**
Implications, 279, 319
Incidental sampling. *See* Convenience sampling
Independent *t* test, 261, 261*e*, **376**
Independent variable, 62, **377**
Indexes, 97, 98, 290, **377**, 116*t*
Inductive reasoning, 116, 116*t*, **377**
Inferential statistics, 230, **377**
  critiquing guidelines, 268, 268*b*
  purposes of
    calculated value/critical value, comparison, 258–259
    confidence intervals, 253–255
    hypothesis for study, 255–256
    level of significance, 257
    one-tailed test of significance, 257
    population parameters estimation, 251–252, 252*t*
    sampling distribution of mean, 252–253
    statistical test, choice of, 256
    study hypothesis, support for, 259
    testing of hypotheses, 255
    test statistic calculation, 258
    two-tailed test of significance, 257–258
  statistical measures, factors on
    nonparametric tests, 259–260
    parametric statistical tests, 259–260
    power of statistical test, 260
    type I/type II errors, 260–261, 260*f*
  statistical tests in nursing research
    analysis of covariance (ANCOVA), 266, 266*e*, 267
    analysis of variance (ANOVA), 262–263, 263*e*
    chi-square test, 263–265, 264*t*, 265*e*
    meta-analysis, 267, 267*e*

394 Index

Inferential statistics (*continued*)
    metasynthesis, 267, 267*e*
    multiple regression, 266, 266*e*
    multivariate analysis of variance (MANOVA), 267
    significance of correlation coefficients, 265–266
    t test, 261–262
Informants' rights, 45
Information extraction from literature sources, 99
Information sources, 92
Informed consent, **377**
  anonymity, 49
  benefits, description of, 48
  confidentiality, 49
  contact information for questions, 49–50
  disclosure of appropriate alternative procedures, 48–49
  documentation of, 50–51
  purpose of study/study procedures, 47–48
  unforeseeable injuries, 49
  unforeseeable risks, description of, 48
  voluntary participation in nursing research, 50
Institute of Emergency Nursing Research, 13
Institutional review board (IRB), 45–46, **377**
  IRB approval, 46–47
  members of, 46
Instrument, 191, **377**
Instrumentation change, 141, **377**
Instruments, data collection
  criteria for selection
    practicality of instrument, 192
    reliability and validity, relationship, 198
    reliability of instrument, 191–193
    validity of instrument, 195–198
  development of, 192
  existing instruments, 191–192
  pilot study, 192
Instruments, interview, 212
Instruments for Clinical Health-Care Research, 191
Integrative review, 22
Integrity in research, 51–52
Interaction effect, 127, **377**
Internal consistency reliability, 194–195, 195*e*, **377**
Internal validity, 139
Internal validity, threats to, **377**
  history threat, 140
  instrumentation change, 141
  maturation, 140
  mortality, 141–142
  selection bias, 140
  testing threats, 141, 141*e*
Interobserver reliability, 194, **377**
Interpretivism, 107
Interquartile range (IQR), 239, **377**
Interrater reliability, 194, 194*e*, **377**
Interrogative sentence form, 83
Interval level of measurement, 188, **377**
Interview
  advantages, 214
  data-collection method, 70
  disadvantages, 214
  instruments, 212
  interviewer guidelines, 213
  interviewers on respondents, 213–214
  interviewer training, 212–213
  questions, 212
  schedule, 212, **377**
  semistructured, 211–212
  structured, 211
  timing and setting for, 213
  unstructured, 211
Interviewer
  guidelines, 213
  on respondents, 213–214
  training, 212–213
Intraocular method of data analysis, 245–246
Iowa model, 33
  application of, 37–38
  concepts, 34–36

J

Joanna Briggs Institute (JBI), 27, 98
Journal article, publishing, 288–290
Journal selection, 290
Judgmental sampling. *See* Purposive sampling
Justice, 44

K

Key informant, 70, **377**
Knowledge, nursing, 2–3
Known-groups procedure, 197, **377**

L

Laboratory studies, 152, **377**
Leadership responsibilities, 35

Learning process, 115
Level of measurement, **377**
   appropriate level, determining, 189
   data conversion to lower level, 189
   defined, 188
   interval, 188
   nominal, 188
   ordinal, 188
   ratio, 189
Level of significance, 257, **377**
Librarian, 95–96
Likert scale, 216–217, 217*e*, 217*f*, **378**
Limitations, study, 62, 276, 276*e*, 280, 317, **378**
Literature review, 322
   components of, 100, 100*b*
   critiquing, in research article, 100
   databases for nursing students
      CINAHL databases, 97
      Cochrane Databse of Systematic Review, 98
      MEDLINE databases, 97
      Ovid Nursing Database, 98
      ProQuest Dissertations & Theses Database (PQDT), 98
      PsychINFO, 98
      Science Direct, 98–99
      Scopus, 99
      Search engines, 99
   extracting information from literature sources, 99
   finding tools
      catalogs, 96–97
      databases, 97
   and librarian, 95–96
   literature sources
      grey literature, 93–94
      information sources, 92
      primary source, 92
      and search tools, 93
      secondary source, 92
   purposes, 91–92
   search strategy development, 94–95, 95*f*
   as step in qualitative research, 69
   as step in quantitative research, 61
Literature sources, 78, **378**
   grey literature, 93–94
   information sources, 92
   of nursing research problems, 78
   primary source, 92
   and search tools, 93
   secondary source, 92

Lived experiences, 159
Longitudinal study, 177, **378**

M

Magnet recognition (MR), 20
Managed care organization (MCO), 304
Manipulation, 143, **378**
Manuscript rejection, 291–292
Marginal benefit, 301, 302, 306, 309, **378**
Marginal expense, 301, **378**
Marginal product , 301, 309, **378**
Marginal revenue, 301, **378**
Maturation, 140, **378**
Mean, 238, 252–253, **378**
Measurement, 187–189, **378**
   appropriate level of measurement, determining, 189
   converting data to lower level of measurement, 189
   defined, 188
   level of, 188–189
Measurement scale, 188. *See also* Level of measurement
Measures of central tendency, 236–238, **378**
   mean, 238
   median, 237
   mode, 237
Measures of relationships, 240–246, **378**
   correlation coefficients, 241–245, 242*t*, 243*f*
   intraocular method of data analysis, 245–246
Measures of variability, 238–240, **378**
   percentile, 239
   range, 239
   standard deviation, 239–240
   variance, 240
   z-scores, 240
Measures to condense data, **378**
   frequency distributions, 231–234, 231*t*, 232*f*, 232*t*, 233*f*
   graphic presentations, 126*f*, 234–236, 235*f*
Median, 237, **378**
MEDLINE databases, 97
Mental health nursing, 13
Mental Measurement Yearbooks (MMYs), 191
Meta-analysis, 267, 267*e*, **378**
Metaparadigm, 106–107
Metasynthesis, 267, 267*e*, **378**
Methodological studies, 151, **378**

Middle-range theories, 110, **378**
Mindfulness meditation course (MMC), 110
Minnesota Multiphasic Personality Inventory (MMPI), 219
Misconduct, research, 51
Mishel's uncertainty in illness theory, 110, 110*e*
Mixed methods study, 73, 73*e*, 164–165
Modal class, 237, **378**
Mode, 237, 247, **378**
Model, defined, 105, **378**
Monetary compensation, 48
Monopsony, 301, 309, **378**
Mortality, 141–142
Mortality threat, 141, **378**
Multimodal class, 237, **378**
Multiple regression, 266, 266*e*, **379**
Multiple-variable studies, 84–85
Multistage sampling, 174
Multivariate analysis of variance (MANOVA), 267, **379**
Multivariate study, 84, **379**
Mutually exclusive categories, 208, **379**

N

Narrative inquiry, 162, 162*e*, **379**
Narrative presentation, in presentation of study findings, 274–275
National Association of Orthopaedic Nurses, 12
National Center for Nursing Research (NCNR), 11, 12
National Database of Nursing Quality Indicators (NDNQI), 191
National Guideline Clearinghouse (NGC), 25–26
National Institute for Nursing Research (NINR), 4, 11
National Institutes of Health (NIH), 11
National Library of Medicine (NLM), 97
National Quality Forum (NQF), 29
National Quality Strategy (NQS), 24
Negatively skewed distribution, 232, 233*f*, **379**
Negative relationship, 149
Negative words, 207
Neuman's Systems Model, 109
NHS Economic Evaluation Database (EED), 22
Nominal level of measurement, 188, **379**

Nondirectional research hypothesis, 127, 127*e*, 257, **379**
Nonequivalent control group design, 146–147, **379**
Nonexperimental research designs, 64, **379**
  comparative studies, 150–151, 150*e*
  correlational studies, 149, 150*e*
  methodological studies, 151
  secondary analysis studies, 151–152, 151*e*
  settings for research, 152
  survey studies, 148–149
  types of, 139*t*, 148
Nonparametric inferential technique, 263
Nonparametric statistical tests, 259–260, **379**
Nonparticipant observer (covert), 215, **379**
Nonparticipant observer (overt), 215, **379**
Nonprobability sampling, 175, **379**
  convenience sampling, 175–176, 176*e*
  purposive sampling, 177, 177*e*
  quota sampling, 176–177, 177*e*
Nonrefereed journal, 290–292, **379**
Nonsignificant result, 277, **379**
Nonsymmetrical distributions, 232, 247, **379**
Normal curve, 233, **379**
Normal distribution, 233, **379**
Null hypothesis, 129, 130, 130*e*, 255–256, **379**
Nuremberg Code, 48, 50
Nurse researcher as patient advocate, 52–53
Nurse *vs.* researcher, 216
Nursing conceptual models, 107
Nursing knowledge, sources of, 2–3
Nursing research, **379**
  Cochrane Collaboration (CC) and Cochrane Nursing Care Field, 12
  defined, 2
  funding for, 4
  goals for conducting
    accountability for nursing practice, 5
    cost-effectiveness of nursing care, 5–6
    credibility of nursing profession, 5
    evidence-based nursing practice (EBNP), 4–5
  history of, 8–11
  National Institute of Nursing Research (NINR), 11
  nursing knowledge, sources of, 2–3
  priorities for future
    Association of Community Health Nursing Educators (ACHNE), 13
    healthcare quality improvement, 14

Institute of Emergency Nursing
  Research, 13
 mental health nursing, 13
 National Association of Orthopaedic
  Nurses, 12
 nursing education, research in, 13–14
 Oncology Nursing Society (ONS), 13
 purposes of, 3–4
 qualitative research, 6
 quantitative research, 6
 roles of nurses and, 7–8
 scientific research, 3
Nursing research problems
 considerations for
  ethical issues, 80
  feasibility of study, 81–82
  personal motivation, 81
  researcher qualifications, 81
  significance for nursing, 80–81
 critiquing
  problem statement, 86–87, 88*b*
  purpose statement, 87, 88*b*
  research questions, 87, 88*b*
 factors to consider
  empirically testable, 85
  population, 83
  variable(s), inclusion of, 83–85
  written in interrogative sentence form, 83
 research question format, 85–86
 sources of
  existing theories, 79
  literature sources, 78
  personal experiences, 78
  previous research, 79–80

O

Observation methods
 behaviors to be observed, 214
 event sampling, 215
 nurse *vs.* researcher, 216
 observer and subjects, relationship, 215–216
 research observers, 214–215
 structured/unstructured observations, 215
Observation research, 214–215, 222, 318, **380**
Office of Human Research and Protections (OHRP), 45
Office of Research Integrity (ORI), 51
Oncology Nursing Society (ONS), 13
One-group pretest-posttest design, 147–148, 148*e*, **380**
One-shot case study, 147, **380**

One-tailed test of significance, 257, **380**
One-variable studies, 83–84
Open-ended questions, 208, 209, **380**
Operational definitions, 63, **380**
Ordinal level of measurement, 188, **380**
Ordinate, 235
Orem's self-care model, 107–108, 108*e*
Outcome measures, 26
Ovid Nursing Database, 98

P

Paired *t* test. *See* Dependent *t* test
Paradigm, 106–107
Parallel forms reliability, 194, **380**
Parameter, 230, **380**
Parametric statistical tests, 259–260, **380**
Participant compensation, 48
Participant observation, 71, **380**
Participant observer (covert), 216, **380**
Participant observer (overt), 216, **380**
Participants, 45, 48
Participants' rights protection, 70
Participatory action research (PAR), 163, **380**
Patient-Centered Outcome Research (PCOR), 24
Patient engagement, 26
Patient Protection and Affordable Care Act (PPACA), 24, 307
Pearson *r* test, 244, 245, 245*e*
Pecuniary terms, 301, **380**
Peer review, 291, 296, **380**
Peer support, 82
Pender's Health Promotion Model (HPM), 110, 110*e*
Percentage, 236, **380**
Percentile, 239, **380**
Personal experiences, 78
Personality inventories, 219, **380**
Personal motivation, 81
Phenomenology, 159–160, 160*e*, **380**
PICOT, format for asking clinical questions, 21
Pilot study, 65, 192, **380**
Population, 131
 accessible, 170, 170*e*
 defined, 64
 identification, 64
 member, 170
 parameters estimation, 251–252, 252*t*
 in research question, 83
 target, 170, 170*e*

Positively skewed distribution, 232, 232f, **380**
Positive relationship, 149, **381**
Positivism, 106
Poster, presentation of, 288
Postpositivism, 106
Posttest, 141, **381**
Posttest-only control group design, 145, 145e, **381**
Power analysis, 180, 180e, **381**
Power of statistical test, 260, **381**
Practice theories, 111
Predictive validity, 197, **381**
Pre-experimental design, **381**
    one-group pretest-posttest design, 147–148
    one-shot case study, 147
Prescriptive theory of acute pain management, 111, 111e
Presentation of study findings
    critiquing guidelines, 281, 281b
    ethical issues in, 274
    figures, 275
    findings of quantitative study, 274
    narrative presentation, 274–275
    tables, 275
Pretest, 141, 381
Pretest, reactive effects of, 142–143
Pretest-posttest control group design, 144–145, 145e, **381**
Previous research, 79–80
Primary evidence, 21
Primary source, 92, **381**
Principal investigator, 7, 8, 14, 211, 287, **381**
Probability samples, 65
Probability sampling, 171, **381**
    cluster random sampling, 173–174, 174e
    simple random sampling, 171–172, 172e
    stratified random sampling, 172–173, 173e, 173t
    systematic random sampling, 174–175, 175e
Probes, 211, 224, **381**
Problem identification, 68
Problem statement, 86–87, 88b, 131
Production function, 301, **381**
Projective technique, 219–220, 220e, **381**
Proportional stratified sampling, 172, **381**
Propositional statement, 104, 105, **381**
ProQuest Dissertations & Theses Database (PQDT), 98
Prospective studies, 150, **381**

PsychINFO, 98
Psychological tests
    personality inventories, 219
    projective technique, 219–220, 220e
Public health, 308
PubMed, 97
Purpose of study
    qualitative research, 69
    quantitative research, 60–61
    stating, 69
Purpose statement, 87, 88b, 131
Purposive sampling, 177, 177e, **381**

Q

Q sort, 220, 220e, **381**
Qualitative data analysis software (QDAS), 72
Qualitative research, 6, 67–73, 68b, **382**
    combining with quantitative methods, 73
    in nursing research development, 6
    and quantitative research, comparison, 58–59, 59t
    steps in
        data analysis, 72
        data collection, 70–71
        data interpretation, 72
        entry to research site, gaining, 70
        problem identification, 68
        purpose, stating, 69
        review of literature, 69
        rights of participants, protecting, 70
        sample selection, 69
        study results, communicating, 72
        study results, utilizing, 73
    types of, 68, 68t
Qualitative research designs. *See also* Mixed methods research
    action research studies, 163, 163e
    case studies, 162–163, 1663e
    ethnographic studies, 160–161, 161e
    grounded theory, 161, 161e
    narrative inquiry, 162, 162e
    phenomenology, 159–160, 160e
Quality improvement (QI), 33, 46
Quantitative research, 6, **382**
    combining with qualitative research method, 73
    and qualitative research, comparison, 58–59, 59t
    steps in, 59–67, 60b

data analysis, 66
data collection, 65
data organization for analysis, 65–66
findings, communicating, 66–67
findings, interpretation of, 66
findings, utilizing, 67
hypothesis formulation, 62–63
limitations of study, 62
literature review, 61
pilot study, 65
population identification, 64
purpose of study, determination, 60–61
research design selection, 63–64
research problem identification, 60
research question formulation, 61
sample selection, 64–65
study assumptions identification, 62
study variables/terms, defining, 63
theoretical/conceptual framework development, 61–62

Quantitative research designs
critiquing, 152, 153b
descriptive studies, 138
experimental research
external validity, threats to, 142–143
internal validity, threats to, 140–142
pre-experimental designs, 147–148
quasi-experimental designs, 146–147
symbolic presentation of, 143
true experimental designs, 143–146
validity of, 139–140
explanatory studies, 138
exploratory studies, 138
nonexperimental research designs
comparative studies, 150–151, 150e
correlational studies, 149, 150e
methodological studies, 151
secondary analysis studies, 151–152, 151e
settings for research, 152
survey studies, 148–149
types of, 139t, 148
research design, 138, 139t

Quantitative research reports, 314–315
abstract, 315
assumptions, 316–317
conclusions, 319
critiquing, 313–324
abstract, 321
researcher qualifications, 321
title, 321
data analysis, 319, 323
data collection, 318, 323
data-collection instruments, 318
data interpretation, 323
discussion of findings, 319
hypothesis(es), 317
implications, 319
limitations of study, 317
literature review, 316, 322
population and sample, 318
problem identification, 315–316
problem of study, 321
purpose, 316, 322
recommendations, 320, 323
research design, 317–318, 322
researcher qualifications, 315
research question, 322
sample selection, 322
setting for research project, 318
terms, definition of, 317
theoretical/conceptual framework, 316
title, 315

Quasi-experimental design, 146, **382**
nonequivalent control group design, 146–147
time-series design, 147

Query letter, 291, **382**

Questionnaire, 190, **382**
advantages of, 210
defined, 204
disadvantages of, 210–211
distribution of, 210
interview, 212
language and reading level of, 205–206
length of, 206
overall appearance of, 205
placement of, 209
types of
ambiguous, 207, 224
closed-ended questions, 207–208
contingency questions, 208–209
demographic questions, 207
double-barreled, 207
double negative, 207
filler questions, 209
open-ended questions, 209
wording of, 207

Quota sampling, 176–177, 177e, **382**

R

Random assignment, 143, 145, 182, **382**
Randomization procedures in research, 182, 182*f*
Randomized controlled trials (RCT), 34
Random sampling, 182, **382**
Range, 239, **382**
Ratio level of measurement, 189, **382**
Reactive effects of pretest, 142–143, 154, **382**
Recommendations, 279, 320, 323
Record references accurately (RRA), 96
Refereed journals, 290–292, **382**
Reflexivity, 159, **382**
Region of rejection, 259, **382**
Regulatory agencies, 308
Reliability, **382**
  of instrument
    equivalence reliability, 194
    internal consistency reliability, 194–195, 195*e*
    stability reliability, 193–194
  and validity, relationship, 198
Replication study, 79, 80, 80*e*, 279–280, **382**
Research
  conflicts of interest (COI) in, 52
  design, 63–64, 138, 139*t*, 322, **382**
  design selection, 63–64
  hypothesis, 129
  misconduct, 51
  observers, 214–215
  scientific, 3
  tools (*See* Research instruments)
Researcher qualifications, 81, 315, 321
Research hypothesis, 63, 66, **382**
  associative, 128–129, 129*e*
  causal, 128, 128*e*
  directional, 128, 128*e*
  nondirectional, 127, 127*e*
  null and, 129–130
Research instruments, 191, **382**. *See also* Instruments, data collection
Research problem, **382**
  defined, 60
  identification, 60
Research question, 61, 87, 88*b*, 131, 322, **382**
  format, 85–86
  formulation, 61
Research report, **382**
  defined, 286
  preparation, 286
  presentation at professional conferences, 286–287
  presentation of research findings
    figures, 275
    narrative, 274–275
    poster, 288
    tables, 275
Research utilization (RU), 8, 20, 294, 296*e*, **382**
Research variables, 84, 187
Respect for persons, 45
Respondent, 45, **382**
Retain, 256
Retrospective studies, 150, **382**
Review of literature, 61, 69
Rights of participants, protecting, 70
Rogers's innovation-diffusion model, 295
Rogers's science of unitary human beings, 108, 108*e*
Rosenthal effect, 142, **382**
Roy's Adaptation Model (RAM), 108–109, 109*e*

S

Sample, **383**
  defined, 64
  selection, 64–65, 69, 322
  size, 179–180
Samples and sampling, 170–178
  critiquer, 182, 183*b*
  nonprobability sampling methods
    convenience sampling, 175–176, 176*e*
    purposive sampling, 177
    quota sampling, 176–177, 177*e*
  probability sampling methods
    cluster random sampling, 173–174, 174*e*
    simple random sampling, 171–172, 172*e*
    stratified random sampling, 172–173, 173*e*, 173*t*
    systematic random sampling, 174–175, 175*e*
  time frame for studying sample, 177–178
Sampling bias, 181, 184, **383**
Sampling concepts and factors
  randomization procedures in research, 182, 182*f*
  sample size, 179–180
  sampling bias, 181
  sampling error, 181, 181*t*
Sampling distribution of mean, 252–253, **383**
Sampling error, 181, 181*t*, **383**
Sampling frame, 170, 171, **383**

Sarah Cole Hirsh Institute (SCHI), 27–28
Saturation, 69, 70, 70*e*, **383**
Scatter diagram. *See* Scatter plot
Scattergram. *See* Scatter plot
Scatter plot, 242–243, 243*f*, 244*f*, **383**
Science Direct, 98–99
Scientific research, 3, 64
Scopus, 99
Search engine, 93*t*, 99, **383**
Search tools, 93
Secondary analysis studies, 151–152, 151*e*
Secondary source, 92, **383**
Selection bias, 140, 147, **383**
Self-efficacy theory, 114
Self-reflection process, 159
Semantic differential scales, 218, 218*e*, 218*f*, **383**
Semiquartile range (SQR), 239, **383**
Semistructured interview, 211–212, **383**
Sigma Theta Tau International (STTI), 19
Significance
    clinical, 277, 277*e*
    of correlation coefficients, 265–266
    level of, 257
    one-tailed test of, 257
    statistical, 277–278, 277*e*
    two-tailed test of, 257–258
Simple hypothesis, 126, **383**
Simple random sampling, 171–172, 172*e*, **383**
Simulation studies, 152, 152*e*, **383**
Skewed distribution, 232, **383**
Snowball sampling, 176, 176*e*, **383**
Solomon four-group design, 146, 146*e*, **383**
Spearman rho, 245, 245*e*
Stability reliability, 193–194, **383**
Standard deviation, 239–240, **383**
Standard error of mean, 252–253, 269, **383**
Statistical measures, factors on
    nonparametric statistical tests, 259–260
    parametric statistical tests, 259–260
    power of statistical test, 260
    type I/type II errors, 260–261, 260*f*
Statistical significance, 277–278, 277*e*
Statistical symbols, 230
Statistical test
    choice of, 256
    in nursing research
        analysis of covariance (ANCOVA), 266–267, 266*e*
        analysis of variance (ANOVA), 262–263, 263*e*
        chi-square test, 263–265, 264*t*, 265*e*
        meta-analysis, 267, 267*e*
        metasynthesis, 267, 267*e*
        multiple regression, 266, 266*e*
        multivariate analysis of variance (MANOVA), 267
        significance of correlation coefficients, 265–266
        t test, 261–262
    power of, 260
Statistics, classifications of, 230
Statistics for the Terrified, 229
Stetler model, 33
Stratified random sampling, 172–173, 173*e*, 173*t*, **384**
Structural measures, 26
Structured interview, 211, **384**
Structured observations, 215, **384**
Student *t* test. *See t* test
Study assumptions identification, 62
Study findings
    conclusions, 278–279
    discussion of
        statistical and clinical significance, 277–278, 277*e*
        study hypotheses, 276–277
        study limitations, 276, 276*e*
    extension of research study, 280
    implications, 279
    presentation of
        ethical issues in, 274
        figures, 275
        findings of quantitative study, 274
        narrative presentation, 274–275
        tables, 275
    recommendations, 279
    replication of research study, 279–280
    study limitations in future research, 280, 280*e*
Study limitations, 62, 139, 276, 276*e*, 280, 317, **384**
Study population, 170
Study results, in qualitative research
    communicating, 72
    utilizing, 73
Subject dropout, 141, 151, 154, 179, **384**
Subjects, availability of, 82
Survey studies, 148–149, **384**
Symmetrical distributions, 232, **384**
Synthesize, 99, **384**

Systematic random sampling, 174–175, 175*e*, **384**
Systematic review, 22, **384**

T

Table of random numbers, 171, **384**
Tables, in presentation of study findings, 275
Target population, 64, 170, 170*e*, **384**
Telenursing (TN), 305–306
Telephone interviews, 212, **384**
Testable research questions, 85, 88
Testing of hypotheses, 255
Testing threats, 141, 141*e*, **384**
Test-retest reliability, 193, 193*e*, **384**
Test statistic calculation, 258
Thematic Apperception Test (TAT), 220
Theoretical framework, 61–62, 316, **384**
Theoretical statement. *See* Propositional statement
Theory, **384**
   combining nursing/non-nursing theories, 114, 114*e*
   combining two nursing theories, 113, 113*e*
   conceptual frameworks, 115
   critiquing theoretical framework of study, 117–118, 118*b*
   from nursing, 112–113
   from other disciplines, 113–114, 114*t*
   scope of, 112*f*
   terminology, 104–106
   testing, hypotheses and, 132
   testing in nursing research, 116–117
   theoretical framework, 115
   theory generation/development, 116, 116*t*
   types of
      metaparadigm, 106–107
      middle-range theories, 110
      Neuman's systems model, 109, 109*e*
      nursing conceptual models, 107
      Orem's self-care model, 107–108, 108*e*
      paradigms, 106–107
      practice theories, 111
      Rogers's science of unitary human beings, 108
      Roy's adaptation model, 108–109
Theory of unpleasant symptoms (TOUS), 114
Theory–practice gap, 110
Time for research projects, 81
Time sampling, 215, **384**

Time-series design, 147, **384**
Title, 315, 321
Transferability, 71
Translational research, 21
Translation science, 32
Triangulation, 73, **384**
True experimental design, 143–146, **384**
   posttest-only control group design, 145
   pretest-posttest control group design, 144–145
   Solomon four-group design, 146
t test, 261–262, **384**
Two-tailed test of significance, 257–258, **385**
Two-variable studies, 84
Type I error, 260–261, 260*f*, **385**
Type II error, 260–261, 260*f*, **385**

U

Unethical research in United States, 43–44
Unimodal, 237, **385**
Univariate study, 83, **385**
Universe, 64
University Microfilms International (UMI), 98
Unstructured interview, 211, **385**
Unstructured observations, 215, **385**
U.S. Department of Health, Education and Welfare (HEW), 45
U.S. Department of Health and Human Services (DHHS), 45
U.S. Preventive Services Task Force (USPSTF), 25, 40
U.S. Public Health Services (PHS), 51
Utilization of nursing research findings
   barriers to, 293
   gap between research and practice, bridging, 294–296
   inadequate dissemination of research findings, 293–294

V

Validity of instrument, **385**
   concurrent validity, 197, 197*e*
   construct validity, 197, 198, 198*e*
   content validity, 196, 196*e*
   criterion validity, 196, 197*e*
   face validity, 195–196, 196*e*
   factor analysis, 198, 198*e*

Variability, measures of. *See* Measures of variability
Variable(s), 131, **385**
    in research question
        multiple-variable studies, 84–85
        one-variable studies, 83–84
        two-variable studies, 84
Variance, 240, 242*t*, **385**
Visual analogue scale (VAS), 221, 221*e*, **385**
Volunteers, 182, **385**

W
Watson's Theory of Human Caring, 110, 110*e*
Weighting, 172
Western Council on Higher Education for Nursing (WCHEN) project, 294
World Medical Association (WMA), 44

Z
Z-score, 240, **385**

Barrett Library
Allen College Campus
Waterloo, Iowa 50703